Nursing Studies - A Path to Success

Edited by Liliana David

Published in London, United Kingdom

Nursing Studies - A Path to Success
http://dx.doi.org/10.5772/intechopen.1001684
Edited by Liliana David

Contributors
Corné Coetzee, Cristina Maria Sabo, Dinu Iuliu Dumitrascu, Dorin Farcau, Dumisani Benedict Vilakati, Fhumulani Mulaudzi, Frøydis Vasset, Hildegunn Sundal, Hiroyuki Ogihara, Ingeborg Ulvund, Liliana David, Lynette Harland Shotton, Manaporn Chatchumni, Melita Peršolja, Miriam Chickering, Miroljub Jakovljević, Princess Busisiwe Siphiwe Mbatha, Rodwell Gundo, Rosanda Drufovka, Simangele Shakwane, Stefka Stoilova, Susan Boyer, Ulrica Lovén Wickman

First published in London, United Kingdom, 2024 by IntechOpen
IntechOpen is the global imprint of INTECHOPEN LIMITED, registered in England and Wales, registration number: 11086078, 167-169 Great Portland Street, London, W1W 5PF, United Kingdom

British Library Cataloguing-in-Publication Data
A catalogue record for this book is available from the British Library

Additional hard and PDF copies can be obtained from orders@intechopen.com

Nursing Studies - A Path to Success
Edited by Liliana David
p. cm.
Print ISBN 978-0-85466-245-6
Online ISBN 978-0-85466-244-9
eBook (PDF) ISBN 978-0-85466-246-3

For EU product safety concerns:
IN TECH d.o.o., Prolaz Marije Krucifikse Kozulić 3, 51000 Rijeka, Croatia,
info@intechopen.com or visit our website at intechopen.com.

Meet the editor

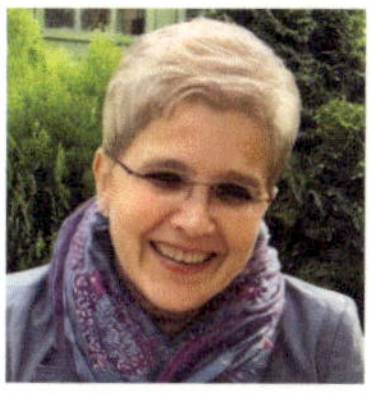

Liliana David was born in Cluj-Napoca, Romania. She inherited from her mother, a pharmacist, the passion to help sick people, and from her father, an engineer, rigorousness. She graduated from the prestigious Highschool for Nurses Cluj-Napoca and started working in emergency rooms and surgery clinics. To accomplish her training, she graduated from the Faculty of Chemistry at Cluj University and obtained a bachelor's degree in nursing. She further obtained a master's degree in clinical pharmacology and a Ph. D. in medical sciences. She is now director of the nursing program at Iuliu Hatieganu University of Medicine and Pharmacy Cluj-Napoca, head assistant and head of the lab for functional gastrointestinal investigation at Cluj County Clinical Emergency Hospital, and a representative of Romania at the European Society of Nurses in Gastroenterology (ESGENA).

Contents

Preface

It is my pleasure to introduce this book to our readers. This is one of the few books written by nurses (of different specializations) about the many issues of their vocational job. Even more, this is one of the few books dedicated to nursing including a global perspective. Indeed, we have in this book contributions coming from several continents and emerging from different cultures. But the common and strong point is the tremendous wish to offer the best-quality healthcare, providing also recommendations to train nurses in the highest quality manner. Our subtitle "A Path to Success" reflects our optimism that the present volume is really paving the road to success in the noble profession of nursing.

You will find here two sections: One is dedicated to the challenges of our profession; the second one is dedicated to various aspects of the education and training of nurses.

What are the challenges of nursing? They are numerous, and you will find in the pages of our book well-written chapters: a perspective chapter on emotional labor and the emotional overload of nurses linked to professional responsibilities; a very interesting African perspective on intimate care and body touching according to Christian African sensitivities; a useful approach to pain, displaying pathophysiology and management, pain being a symptom challenging us every day in our profession; a sensitive chapter on psychiatric illness among young adults where the Scandinavian experience is shared; a comprehensive, important overview of professional diseases of nurses, emphasizing the fragility of the nursing profession and also the need of work safety; and another chapter dedicated especially to work-related musculoskeletal disorders of nurses.

One can see from this simple enumeration how many and how important the challenges of our profession are. Understanding them and responding well to them ensures the "path to success" mentioned in our subtitle.

The second section of our book is larger, comprising a few more studies dedicated to many issues in the training and education of nurses. We have rigorously selected and included papers dedicated to the following topics. We have included a few perspective chapters. The first one is dedicated to the development of clinical competencies in nurses, proposing a standardized, well-working model. This is juxtaposed to another interesting African study on the Ubuntu model of healthcare and how it works nowadays.

The next two chapters focus on pediatric nursing training: One is from northern Europe and is dedicated to methods on how to learn clinical pediatric nursing, while the second one is coming from Japan and presents an original contribution to pediatric nursing for appropriate healthcare environment according to the United Nations Convention on the Rights of the Child.

Other chapters cover more specialized issues, like specific pathologies. Thus, another perspective chapter is dedicated to the education of patients with chronic inflammatory arthritis performed by nurses. This is continued by a contribution from the African continent to nurse education in orthopedics.

Related chapters are those dedicated to the training of nurses for caring for patients with pressure ulcers, an important problem in healthcare. The last chapter of this second section describes how to proceed with intimate care during nursing education, a topic that very few approach. I hope that you observe how complex and interesting the content of our book is.

Last but not least, I want to pay tribute to our profession. Indeed, nursing is one of the oldest professions in the world and can be defined as the job or skill of caring for people who are sick or injured (Oxford Dictionary). Nurse means "a person who cares for the sick or infirm" (Merriam-Webster Dictionary). More recently, the word "nurse" also acquired a professional meaning: "a licensed health-care professional who practices independently or is supervised by a physician, surgeon, or dentist and who is skilled in promoting and maintaining health" (Merriam-Webster Dictionary).

The etymology of the word derives from the Latin word nutricia, meaning "nourishing", and was initially used for "feeding an offspring from the breast" (Merriam-Webster Dictionary). From this original use, this noun developed its meaning to today's significance.

What can be more beautiful than our profession?

The book is dedicated not only to nurses but to any healthcare provider interested in the various aspects of medical sciences.

Special thanks are owed to the staff of our publisher who took care of the high-quality publication of this book.

Liliana David, RN, BSc, MSc, Ph.D.
Department of Nursing,
Iuliu Hatieganu University of Medicine and Pharmacy,
Cluj-Napoca, Romania

Head Assistant,
2nd Department of Medicine,
Cluj County Clinical Emergency Hospital,
Cluj-Napoca, Romania

Section 1

Challenges of Nursing

Chapter 1

Perspective Chapter: Emotional Labour – Understanding and Responding to the Emotional Challenges of Nursing

Lynette Harland Shotton

Abstract

The purpose of this chapter is to consider the emotional labour of nursing. The chapter explores the context of caring in nursing and the resulting need for nurses to engage in emotional labour. There is an overview of the origins of the term, emotional labour, before consideration of emotional labour in the context of nursing. The sources of emotional labour in nursing are covered alongside the impact of engaging in emotional labour on individual nurses, the service users they deliver care to, as well as the organisation and wider social impact. Strategies designed to support nurses and to respond to the emotional challenges of nursing are also explored.

Keywords: emotional labour, burnout, compassion fatigue, post-traumatic stress disorder, vicarious trauma

1. Introduction

It is suggested that caring is an innately human quality and one that people demonstrate toward each other through altruistic acts or feelings of concern for another person [1]. Nursing is a profession which is characterised by care and care giving is an essential feature of the nursing role. Despite the increasing complexity of modern healthcare with changes in technology, medicine and expansion of nursing roles, this has not eroded the over-riding concern of providing care.

In nursing caring occurs through two domains. Firstly, it is a noun that refers to the act of caring for people when they are unable to care for themselves. Secondly is through the adjective of being a caring nurse, which is displayed through certain actions, namely those that show compassion kindness and concern. Whilst caring is not unique to nursing it has often been considered a key quality and feature of the role and there is both an onus on the nurse to perform their nursing duties in a caring manner but also on the discipline in its wider sense to foster this, This places emphasis on employing and regulatory bodies to develop the evidence base of the caring profession and to provide the requisite mechanisms through education, training and organisational practices to achieve it [1].

IntechOpen

In nursing, caring involves being there for the patient and/or their family in what ever way is needed at the time and in the particular context. Thus, the context of providing care is complex and presents the nurse with a wide range of situations and diverse people to provide care for. This can include caring for people at different stages of the life course; those who have specific vulnerabilities and in birth and death, meaning nurses can provide care at some of the happiest and most difficult times. To do this, the nurse must draw on a wide range of skills to be able to adapt to the needs of individual patients and situations with the aim of caring and showing a caring attitude at the centre of this work [1].

Whilst many nurses join the profession to provide high quality care, the demands and complexity of the nursing role can provide a barrier to this and can have impacts both on the quality of the care delivered but also on the nurses delivering it. The increasing demands on nurses have become a key global concern and in recent years there has been recognition that countries across the globe need to do more to retain staff and to attract nurses to the profession. It is known that nurse retention is a key concern globally and many newly qualified and experienced staff are leaving the profession citing lower levels of job satisfaction, working conditions such as workload, stress and burnout, as key factors [2]. This context is known to influence recruitment and impact on the extent to which nursing is considered a desirable profession. On this basis some of the approaches recommended globally are to focus on improving the context in which nurses work and placing emphasis on support for their physical and emotional well-being, which is the focus of this chapter.

2. Emotional labour

In 1983 Hochschild [3] introduced the term emotional labour and this then generated both interest and research into this subject which focused on the impact of work on individuals at an emotional level and also the organisational structure and social relations of service jobs [4].

Hochschild [3] drew on Marxist theory that considered not only the fairness of using and paying human beings as instruments in the context of the profits made by factory owners but also focused on the human cost to the individual. Drawing a parallel between the Marxist and modern context Hochshild [3] explored the relationship between emotions that are really felt and those that are acted out for the benefit of others, using the example of commercial airlines where flight attendants were actively recruited based on their potential to project a desired company image and were then further trained to treat passengers in a certain way and to act out the idealised notion of Southern American charm and hospitality. They were expected to always smile and the connection between their smiles and the travel experience were a key focus of marketing strategies. Thus, the smile is considered an asset which reflects the company's disposition and sells a product and experience to consumers. The impact of this on the flight attends was significant and Hochschild's work revealed that the commercialisation and professionalisation of flight attendants work where they were trained to adopt a set of behaviours and working practices, which included the performance of smiling and creating a calm and warm atmosphere for passengers produced an emotional impact on them [3]. This resulted in feelings of insincerity, feeling their behaviour was contrived, with a need to suppress or what Hochschild called transmutation of their own feelings in order to sustain a particular outward image in the context of their working life, producing tensions between real and performed behaviours where seeming to love the job becomes part of the job [3].

Essentially, Hochschild's work suggests flight attendants sell their personal emotions in the labour market, as if they were a product [3]. Some flight attendants reported a deep tensions, where the process of deep acting was so stressful, they overidentified with their work and found it difficult to relax and switch off from the artificially created elation at the end of a shift but also experienced a blurring of the boundaries between their personal and professionals selves, thus becoming more at risk of stress and burnout.

In exploring the work of the flight attendant Hochschild noted that the role involved physical labour in terms of the activities associated with providing catering to passengers but also an emotional aspect relating to the mental challenges associated with caring for the passengers, looking after their safety, their comfort and providing them with a cheery and calm atmosphere. This combination of the physical and the mental is what Hochschild combined to define as emotional labour [3].

Hochschild made an important link between emotional labour and gender and suggested that emotional work and emotional labour were expressly tied to women's work and were illustrative of wider social structures that reflect social status and power [5]. Historically this connected to the role of women being homemakers and responsible for caring for children, and the resulting financial dependence on men, as well as enduring social norms relating to the belief that women are naturally more caring than men. Such social norms are manifest in the role of women in the workforce where historically they have predominantly occupied professions considered to be caring, such as nursing.

2.1 Emotional labour in nursing

Hochschild never applied the concept of emotional labour to nursing but acknowledged the application of it to professions other than flight attendants should three features of their work be met:

1. the role requires face to face or voice to voice interaction with the public.

2. there is a need for the worker to produce an emotional state.

3. there is a role of the employer through the provision of training and supervision to exercise a degree of control over the emotional activities of employees [3]. On this basis it is not surprising that her work has been applied to healthcare and in particular, nursing.

There is a clear parallel between Hochschild's assertion that emotional labour is connected to women's work and the historical development of the nursing profession, particularly the prototype for more contemporary nursing, Florence Nightingale, who is the archetypal caring female [6]. Despite the contemporary overarching narrative and reality that globally more nurses are female, men do actually have a long history in nursing that is somewhat lost to the last 200 years [7]. Indeed, Kearns and Mahon highlight many historical examples of men providing nursing care dating back to 250 BC when the first nursing school started in India where only men were considered pure enough to become nurses. By the mid-1800s as men fought and died in wars including the Crimean and American Civil wars among others, more women became nurses. Alongside this, there was an increasingly gender based division of labour which produced a context where the social concept of care became increasingly feminised and men in caring professions were considered deviant or unable to get a man's job and accompanied by the devaluing of caring and the ensuant low pay, more men were forced to seek work in occupations with higher status and better pay to provide for their families [7]. Despite this there are global efforts now to encourage men to join nursing, particularly to address the global shortfall in the nursing workforce and importantly it is recognised that men who do enter nursing, do so for the same reasons as women – to provide care. As such, it is important to understand the impact of providing care on all nurses regardless of gender to recruit and retain staff and support them to deliver high quality care to patients.

Smith 1992 was arguably one of the first to specifically identify the relevance of emotional labour to nursing and in particular to nursing students and the way they were trained [8]. In 1991 and 1992 she travelled to California to study under Hochschild in order to apply the concept to nursing. Smith wanted to explore the perception of nurses as being intrinsically caring and apply this to the context of nurse training. She asserted that in a similar way to how Hochschild uncovered that flight attendants were recruited for their personal characteristics, this also occurs in nursing where candidates who display a friendly and caring attitude are actively selected [8]. This is reflected in the approach adopted in some countries, such as England, where a values-based recruitment framework has been introduced in the National Health Service which aims to recruit the best people with personal values that align with that of the organisation [9]. Whilst recruiting those with caring qualities is important, Smith notes that the process of nurse training is designed to shape these qualities and the nursing students' identity to develop them into that of the professional and dedicated nurse who portrays the nursing image through their physical appearance and the emotional labour invested in their role [8]. Part of nurse training embeds in staff a sense of professional duty to follow organisational emotion-display rules and develop strategies to manage their emotions.

Nursing is a complex profession and the day-to-day activities involved in nursing are often both physically and emotionally demanding. These include but are not limited to the increasing organisational and professional regulatory demands placed on nurses, the exposure to the chronic and acute conditions of patients, as well as births, deaths and traumatic events experienced by their patients. It is also recognised that nurses experience physical and verbal abuse within the context of their working life given the complex nature of patients they provide care to but also some nurses experience negative interactions with peers and reported bullying from superiors [10]. These all require some form of cognitive and emotional response by the nurse, essentially, emotional labour.

It is asserted that there are two broad strategies employed by service workers, including nurses, in engaging with emotional labour. These are surface acting and deep acting [3]. Surface acting is the suppression of internally felt emotions driven by the need to adhere to organisational or occupationally desired emotions. So here, this results in hiding or faking emotions and displaying outward behaviours such as smiling, which are not consistent with the emotions they are truly feeling [11]. Deep acting is where the individual engages in or tries to experience emotional expressions which are consistent with the emotions they feel or the desired emotions. So here, this involves work on inner feelings and effort to try and regulate emotions, for example, trying to stir up a feeling we wish we had or trying to block a feeling we wish we did not. The drivers of this emotional labour are produced by organisational and professional regulatory guidelines but are also influenced by social norms, personality traits and situational factors such as the intensity of work and the interaction with service users [11].

2.2 Consequences of emotional labour

The negative consequences of emotional labour in nursing are wide ranging but can produce both a physical and emotional impact. These include emotional dissonance, burnout, compassion fatigue, secondary and post-traumatic stress and vicarious trauma [12].

2.2.1 Emotional dissonance

It is thought that because surface acting requires the suppression of internal feelings, this results in an emotional dissonance which can impact on the emotional well-being of the individual as well as job satisfaction and commitment [10]. Emotional dissonance, which has been mentioned previously in this chapter, is perhaps one of the most common negative consequences of emotional labour and is produced by the tension associated with feeling emotions but because of professional constraints being unable to express them and consequently being required to act in a way that makes the individual feel they are unauthentic, thus posing a challenge to the person's sense of self [13].

2.2.2 Burnout

The term burnout was introduced by Freudenenberger in 1974 [14] when he observed a loss of motivation and reduced commitment among volunteers who were working at a mental health clinic. Burnout is a response to excessive stress at work and is characterised by feelings of emotional and physical exhaustion. Burnout develops over time through exposure to prolonged, excessive chronic stress which has either not been successfully identified and/or managed [15]. Maslach [16] suggests that burnout is connected to a number of risk factors or dimensions and in cases where burnout presents, it is usually connected to at least one of the six dimensions of working life, shown in **Table 1**.

Whilst Maslach views burnout as being work related [16] others such as Shirom [17] refer to it as a process which may include both work and personal related circumstances that place excessive and cumulative demands on the individual. Burnout is known to impact on mental health and may lead to depression and anxiety and feelings of physical exhaustion, as well as increasing the risk of substance misuse and suicide [18]. Burnout often impacts on job satisfaction and has been cited as a key reason for staff in health and social care leaving their jobs. Equally, it is important to note that for staff experiencing burnout there are likely to be consequences for care delivery in terms of reduced quality of care and errors [19].

Burnout is often considered an occupational hazard for nurses, and it is known that the number of staff working in health and social care, particularly nurses are reporting burnout more frequently [15, 20]. Reflecting the dimensions highlighted in **Table 1**, workload is often a key factor, and this is connected to and a driver of vacancies in the sector. Alongside this, the intensity of workload is a factor where chronic and sustained workload pressures increase risk brought about by staffing levels as well as the increased demands on nurses in terms of providing care to increasingly complex patients, for example, during the global pandemic [20].

Dimension	Reason for increased risk of burnout
Workload	If workloads and the demands of work are excessive and recovery from these demands cannot be achieved.
Control	If employees have or do not believe they have sufficient control over the resources needed to complete their job.
Reward	Where employees receive or perceive they receive too little reward for their work. These rewards may be monetary but also include other rewards such as social rewards and a sense of pride in their work.
Community	Where employees doe nor feel they have positive connections with peers, senior colleagues and that there is an absence of social support.
Fairness	Where there is actual or perceived unfairness, which may include inequity of workload or financial remuneration for work.
Values	Where employees feel their job forces them to act against their own values or when they experience conflict between the organisation's values.

Table 1.
Dimensions of burnout (based on the work of Maslach) [16].

When nurses experience burnout there can be variation in how this manifests, but it is thought that for many there is an impact on physical and emotional well-being, and that this can include feelings of physical and emotional exhaustion, a sense of cynicism about one's work and feelings of moral distress brought about by a sense that they are not delivering the quality of care they would like to [15].

2.2.3 Compassion fatigue

Compassion is often considered an essential aspect of nursing care and refers to the sense of connection to another person's suffering. It is positioned as being a hallmark of good nursing and is thought to enhance care delivery and ensure that patients are treated with comfort, dignity and respect [21].

Initially described by Johnson [22] compassion fatigue is viewed as emotional, physical and psychological exhaustion induced by work-related stress. It is often associated with burnout and is thought to be a process which originates as compassion discomfort before progressing to compassion stress and ultimately culminates in compassion fatigue [23]. Whilst this implies that compassion fatigue is the result of experiencing many traumatic events over a prolonged period of time, there is also evidence that it can arise from the experience of caring for one individual or from a single event [24]. It is thought that when nurses reach the point of compassion fatigue it is extremely unlikely that compassion will be fully recovered and as such, it is not surprising that this is one of the most commonly cited reasons globally for nurses leaving the profession, which has partly contributed to an expected global shortage of 7.6 million nurses by 2030 [25].

In recent years compassion fatigue has been a key concern in nursing given the impact it has on the individual as well as employers and the wider discipline, At the individual level some of the impact is similar to the symptoms of burnout in terms of the negative effect on physical and emotional well-being where those affected may suffer from insomnia, exhaustion, depression as well as poor judgement, and failure to nurture. Research [26] also highlights the impact on patient care where compassion fatigue can lead to poor nurse–patient relationships, reduced quality of care and increased likelihood of complaints. This is felt at the organisational level and is compounded by the cost of reduced productivity, high staff turnover and difficulties in attracting new staff into nursing. Whilst employees in many sectors report experiencing burnout, it is thought that compassion fatigue is unique to those involved in caring or providing emotional support to others and is triggered by the need to use empathy and emotional energy; in other words, emotional labour.

2.2.4 Post-traumatic and secondary traumatic stress

Post-traumatic stress or Complex Post Traumatic Stress Disorder (PTSD; C-PTSD) is a mental health condition which is the result of the individual experience an event that they find highly traumatic. These traumatic events can include terrorist attacks, street violence and sexual assault. The severity of the condition varies from person to person but for some the condition can be crippling and can mean they are unable to return to their previous state of mind.

Whilst PTSD is a relatively well-known condition, there is increasing awareness of the impact of secondary trauma on individuals. This describes the impact of indirect exposure or experience of a traumatic event. As mentioned earlier in this chapter, the daily working lives of nurses often involve caring for patients during difficult times and it is known that providing this care and listening to the firsthand accounts of patients who have encountered trauma can be a traumatic and emotionally challenging experience for nurses [27]. Equally, as outlined earlier, emotional labour and both surface and deep acting are often required as nurses provide care and support and try to understand what the patient has experienced. One of the factors that compounds both identification and intervention for staff experiencing secondary trauma is the wider social narrative that assumes nurses should expect and be equipped to deal with working in this context. This can impact on ability to seek and receive support.

2.2.5 Vicarious trauma

Burnout, compassion fatigue and vicarious trauma are often referred to collectively, they are theoretically distinct. Burnout, described previously in this chapter, is a psychological strain resulting from difficult conditions and can result in emotional exhaustion, decreased motivation, low mood and delivery of poor care but it is unlikely to alter core internal belief systems. Compassion fatigue is also a reaction to the work environment and like burnout can produce similar consequences. However, vicarious trauma is thought to more closely resemble a primary traumatic response, as experienced in PTSD and C-PTSD. This can have sustained impacts on self, trust, safety and regulation [28], and therefore, this should be prioritised as a concern for nurses.

Vicarious trauma is considered with the impact on professionals who support those who have experienced trauma. It refers to the undesirable outcomes associated with this work, resulting from listing to and observing the effects of trauma from those who have received, as well as reviewing case files and evidence and being involved in providing a response, in relation to providing care and nursing intervention (Office for Victims of Crime). It is also known that clinicians may experience moral distress which can result from ethical conflicts, sometimes resulting from their own beliefs, values, and attitudes, and also from institutional limitations on the extent of care they can provide [28].

Vicarious trauma is a product of the therapeutic relationship, whereby the ability to provide empathic care to the patient produces harm to the nurse. Whilst there is a risk of experiencing vicarious trauma generally in nursing, it is thought that some settings are more likely to increase the risk. These include, but are not limited to, settings such as emergency departments, mental health services, substance misuse services, hospices, veteran services and sexual assault services. Here, the increased risk is related to levels of exposure to people who have experience trauma.

2.2.6 Additional risk factors for the individual

Alongside the consequences of emotional labour already described, there are also some individual risk factors which are thought to contribute to poor mental health and well-being. These include some of the six dimensions Maslach [16] refers to, particularly perceived and actual workload and levels of autonomy staff hold to carry out their duties. Other risks include working patterns, which is a key concern in nursing, particularly in view of the need for shift rotation in many nursing roles. There is some evidence to suggest that working shifts in itself is a potential risk, but this can be compounded by shift length, the pattern of shifts and also how the individual has control over their shift pattern and the fit with their personal circumstances [29]. Frequency and length of breaks are also a factor as well as organisational issues such as staffing levels, the quality of relationships with peers and leaders and the wider culture within the organisation.

Staff who have pre-existing mental health problems are at increased risk of negative effects associated with emotional labour as well as those with lower levels of resilience and personal support [19]. There is also evidence that staff from minority ethnic backgrounds are generally at greater risk of poor mental health [19].

2.2.7 Positive consequences of emotional labour

It must be noted that whilst emotional labour is a central feature of nursing, there are wide ranging benefits to the individual nurse of providing high quality, compassionate care. Indeed, empathic interactions with service users can bring about a feeling of pride and personal accomplishment, as well as having a motivational and energising impact on the individual's work [19]. Equally, it is suggested that nurses who work with those who have experienced trauma are sometimes protected from negative outcomes on their emotional well-being. This can be accounted for by the sense of care they provide, but also by the policies and protocols which govern practice in these complex areas and wider organisational support, which will be explored later in this chapter.

As mentioned previously, nurses are often drawn to the profession due to a desire to make a difference in the lives of their patients and are recruited on the basis of showing caring and compassionate qualities. This may explain why many nurses actually flourish when they know they are providing support to patients during their time of need. Sacco and Copel [28] refer to this as compassion satisfaction and this allows the care giver to cope with the negative aspects of their work.

2.2.8 Consequences for the organisation and profession

The negative consequences of emotional labour can have significant implications for employers in terms of staff absences, staff attrition and the delivery of poorer care, which can lead to litigation, as outlined previously. Also of great concern is the global nursing workforce shortage which produces difficult working conditions and therefore, is a key contributory factor to the mental well-being of staff.

A recent report suggests that prior to the global Covid-19 pandemic there was an international shortfall of 5.9 million nurses and many of these shortages are concentrated in low and lower-middle income countries [20]. To address this shortfall and the expected future workforce changes, it is suggested that in the next ten years 13 million additional nurses will be needed. It is accepted that the global Covid-19 pandemic has worsened the global shortage of nurses and that this has increased some of the issues outlined already in this chapter, particularly burnout, compassion fatigue and moral injury. In view of this there is a need for all countries globally to review their workforce needs and put in place measures to try to address not only retention but also desire to join the profession.

It is suggested that poor workforce planning in many countries has not only produced the significant staff shortages outlined in this chapter but has also impacted on skill mix and created a context where working conditions are not attractive to potential or existing staff [2]. Poor salary is also reported as a key factor and in recent years this has been compounded by the cost-of-living crisis facing many countries. This means that some nurses seek employment outside of the health sector in jobs with comparable salaries but less stress and better work-life balance [30].

Clearly, addressing workforce shortages and skill-mix are not straightforward and the solutions are not instant given the time it takes to train nurses, but what is key, is to retain the current workforce and support existing nurses to thrive.

2.3 Responding to emotional labour

Understanding the impact on those who experience emotional labour as part of their work is vital and this can help inform strategies to address any negative consequences. These strategies include activities at organisational and individual level.

2.3.1 Supporting staff wellbeing

It is known that in high stress environments supportive work environments can positively impact on physical mental health and well-being and also improve individual and team performance. Some of the key ways to support staff well-being include making time for team-based activities which can be in the form of formal meetings as well as more informal events. Given the changes to working conditions for many staff, particularly since the global Covid-19 pandemic it is important that staff who work from home in a hybrid way, as well as those who work alone are included in these. It is thought that good peer relationships improve morale but also create an environment where colleagues can identify any changes in behaviour and provide peer support when needed. It also provides an opportunity for colleagues to talk and share coping strategies or identify sources of support if needed.

Organisations need to provide mechanisms to support staff to look after their general health and well-being and this includes the provision of preventative services, including immunisation, as well as access to occupational health services [22]. It is also necessary to try to improve safe staffing levels and create working patterns and cultures that support staff and help them to thrive; this includes access to continuing professional development and supportive leadership. Where senior leaders are shown to care about their staff, this has a positive impact on staff morale but also helps leaders to identify and address actual and potential issues.

In some countries, England, for example, safe spaces have been created in some clinical areas, referred to as wobble rooms [31]. These spaces provide somewhere staff can go for a short break to have time out from the clinical area or to have a few moments with a colleague to share worries, experiences or just sit quietly. The idea behind the introduction of these spaces is to create a culture where it is acceptable for staff to express their emotions and feelings and also to receive support.

Clinical supervision has been used widely in nursing and provides a safe space where staff can talk about critical incidents or their experiences. However, given some of the challenges nurses face in relation to shift work and short staffing, this can be difficult to access. Similarly, education and training are thought to help in terms of raising awareness about physical and emotional well-being and ways to engage in self-care and access support. However, the pressures nurses face in terms of busy and demanding roles can impact on ability to access these resources.

Whilst there is a clear organisational role in creating a positive working environment, it is important for staff to look after themselves. This can include taking care of physical health by eating well and exercising, as well as having regular time off. This will also have an effect on emotional well-being. This chapter has outlined the role of nurses in providing compassionate care, and this should also apply to caring for themselves. Neff [32] refers to the concept of self-compassion, which refers to the way in which we treat ourselves. Neff suggests we should recognise that we are human and not be too hard on ourselves [32]. In doing this, nurses can become less critical and judgmental but also more resilient.

3. Conclusion

This chapter has introduced the context of caring in nursing and the need to engage in emotional labour within everyday nursing practice. Emotional labour requires surface and deep acting and can bring about positive and negative consequences for the individual. The negative consequences are of key concern in terms of the impact on the individual nurse, where a range of issues including burnout and compassion fatigue may manifest. These can bring about situations that compromise the delivery of high-quality care and are a key contributor to the current global nursing workforce, which compounds the situation further. Whilst addressing nursing workforce issues cannot be achieved quickly, this chapter has highlighted some of the strategies that may help to support nurses and address some of the negative consequences of engaging in emotional labour in order to not only retain them in the profession but to support them to enjoy their work and to deliver high quality nursing care.

Conflict of interest

The author declares no conflict of interest.

Author details

Lynette Harland Shotton
Northumbria University, Newcastle Upon Tyne, United Kingdom

*Address all correspondence to: lynette.shotton@northumbria.ac.uk

References

[1] Adams LY. The conundrum of caring in nursing. International Journal of Caring Sciences. 2016;**9**(1):1-12. Available from: https://www.internationaljournalofcaringsciences.org/docs/1_1-Adams_special_9_1.pdf [Accessed: December 8, 2023]

[2] Tamata AA, Mohammadnezhad M. A systematic review study on the factors affecting shortage of nursing workforce in the hospitals. Nursing Open. 2023;**10**(3):1247-1257. DOI: 10.1002/nop2.1434. Epub 2022 Oct 27

[3] Hochschild AR. The Managed Heart: Commercialization of Human Feeling. Berkely: University of California Press; 1983

[4] Wharton AS. The sociology of emotional labour. Annual Review of Sociology. 2009;**35**(2009):147-165. Available from: https://www.jstor.org/stable/27800073

[5] Theodosius C. Emotional Labour in Health Care: The Unmanaged Heart of Nursing. London: Routledge; 2008

[6] Gray B, Smith P. Emotional labour and the clinical settings of nursing care: The perspectives of nurses in East London. Nurse Education in Practice. 2009;**9**:253-261. DOI: 10.1016/j.nepr.2008.08.009

[7] Kearns K, Mahon P. How to attain gender equality in nursing—An essay. British Medical Journal. 2021;**373**:1-14. DOI: 10.1136/bmj.n1232

[8] Smith P. The Emotional Labour of Nursing. Its Impact on Interpersonal Relations, Management and Educational Environment. London: Red Globe Press; 1992

[9] Health Education England. Values Based Recruitment Framework. UK: Health Education England; 2016. Available from: https://www.hee.nhs.uk/sites/default/files/documents/VBR_Framework%20March%202016.pdf [Accessed: December 15, 2023]

[10] Lartey JKS, Osafo J, Andoh-Arthur J, Asante KO. Emotional experiences and coping strategies of nursing and midwifery practitioners in Ghana: A qualitative study. BMC Nursing. 2020;**19**(92):1-12. DOI: 10.1186/s12912-020-00484-0

[11] Badolamenti S, Sili A, Caruso R, Fida Fida R. What do we know about emotional labour in nursing? A narrative review. British Journal of Nursing. 2017;**26**(1):48-55. DOI: 10.12968/bjon.2017.26.1.48

[12] The Kings Fund. Urgent Action Is Needed to Improve Working Conditions for Nurses and Midwives. UK: The Kings Fund; 2020. Available from: https://www.kingsfund.org.uk/press/press-releases/urgent-action-needed-improve-working-conditions-nurses-and-midwives [Accessed: January 5, 2023]

[13] Yozgat U, Çalişkan SC, Ürü FO. Exploring emotional dissonance: On doing what you feel and feeling what you do. Procedia – Social and Behavioural Sciences. 2012;**58**:673-682. DOI: 10.1016/j.sbspro.2012.09.1045

[14] Freudenberger HJ. Staff burn-out. Journal of Social Issues. 1974;**30**(1):159-165

[15] Health and Social Care Committee. The Scale and Impact of Workforce Burnout in the NHS and Social Care.

UK: Health and Social Care Committee; 2021. Available from: https://committees.parliament.uk/publications/6158/documents/68766/default/ [Accessed: December 5, 2023]

[16] Maslach C. A multidimensional theory of burnout. In: Cooper CL, editor. Theories of Organizational Stress. Oxford: Oxford University Press Inc.; 1999

[17] Shirom A. Job-Related Burnout: A Review. Handbook of Occupational Health Psychology. Washington, DC, US: American Psychological Association; 2003. pp. 245-264

[18] Wei H, Aucoin J, Kuntapay GR, Justice A, Jones A, Zhang C, et al. The prevalance of nurse burnout and its association with telomere length pre and during the covid-19 pandemic. PLoS One. 2022;**17**(23):e0263603. DOI: 10.1371/journal.pone.0263603

[19] Kinman G, Teoh K, Harris A. The Mental Health and Wellbeing of Nurses and Midwives in the United Kingdom. 2020. Available from: https://www.som.org.uk/sites/som.org.uk/files/The_Mental_Health_and_Wellbeing_of_Nurses_and_Midwives_in_the_United_Kingdom.pdf [Accessed: December 5, 2023]

[20] Buchan J, Catton H, Shaffer F. Sustain and Retain in 2002 and beyond. 2022. Available from: https://www.intlnursemigration.org/wp-content/uploads/2022/01/Sustain-and-Retain-in-2022-and-Beyond-The-global-nursing-workforce-and-the-COVID-19-pandemic.pdf [Accessed: December 7, 2023]

[21] Isobel S, Thomas M. Vicarious trauma and nursing: An integrative review. International Journal of Mental Health Nursing. 2022;**31**(2):247-259. DOI: 10.1111/inm.12953bs_bs_banner

[22] Johnson C. Coping with compassion fatigue. Nursing. 1992;**22**(4):116-118

[23] Coetzee SK, Klopper C. Compassion fatigue within nursing practice: A concept analysis. Nursing and Health Sciences. 2010;**12**(12):235-243. DOI: 10.1111/j.1442-2018.2010.00526.x

[24] Cavanagh N, Cockett G, Doi CJ. Compassion fatigue in healthcare providers: A systematic review and meta-analysis. Nursing Ethics. 2019;**27**(3):639-665. DOI: 10.1177/0969733019889400

[25] Peters E. Compassion fatigue in nursing: A concept analysis. Nursing Forum. 2018;**53**(4):466-480. DOI: 10.1111/nuf.12274

[26] Wanqing X, Chen L, Feng F, Chizimuzo TC, Okoli TC, Tang P, et al. The prevalence of compassion satisfaction and compassion fatigue among nurses: A systematic review and meta-analysis. International Journal of Nursing Studies. 2020;**120**(2020):1-18. DOI: 10.1016/j.ijnurstu.2021.103973

[27] Nimmo A, Huggard P. A systematic review of the measurement of compassion fatigue, vicarious trauma, and secondary traumatic stress in physicians. Australasian Journal of Disaster and Trauma Studies. 2013;**1**:37-44. Available from: http://tur-www1.massey.ac.nz/~trauma/issues/2013-1/AJDTS_2013-1_Nimmo.pdf

[28] Sacco TL, Copel LC. Compassion satisfaction: A concept analysis in nursing. Nursing Forum. 2018;**53**(1):1-11. DOI: 10.1111/nuf.12213o

[29] Ourega-Zoé E, Dall'Ora, C. and Griffiths, P. Nurses' experiences and preferences around shift patterns:

A scoping review. PLoS One. 2021;**16**(6):e0270446. DOI: 10.1371/journal.pone.0256300

[30] McGloin S. Cost-of-living crisis impacts the nursing and midwifery professions. Occupational Medicine. 2023;**73**(2023):385-387. DOI: 10.1093/occmed/kqad057

[31] Royal College of Nursing. Healthy Workplace Toolkit. UK: Royal College of Nursing; 2021. Available from: https://www.rcn.org.uk/Professional-Development/publications/healthy-workplace-toolkit-uk-pub-009-734 [Accessed: November 31, 2023]

[32] Neff K. Self-compassion. New York: Harper Collins Publishers; 2011

Chapter 2

Advocacy for Personhood: Integration of African Christian Rituals and Intimate Care on the Touched Human Body

Dumisani Benedict Vilakati and Simangele Shakwane

Abstract

Intimate care relates to essential nursing care nurses provide that requires touching the patient's body. It is noted that the human body goes through many rituals from birth through all life stages. Rituals done on one's body symbolize the need for acceptability in the family, community, and society. The purpose was to integrate African-Christian rituals into nursing care to improve the quality of care for the touched human body. Ubuntu paradigm was used to understand the rituals and nursing intimate care practices on the human body in an African context. African-Christian leaders were sampled using snowball sampling from three Southern Africa countries (Eswatini [former Swaziland], South Africa, and Zimbabwe), and nursing practitioners were purposively sampled from two selected hospitals in South Africa. Naïve sketches and semi-structured interviews were used to collect in-depth data. Rituals of the identity of the person through naming and initiation into family and community. The body is constantly touched during ritualization and provision of care. Advocating for personhood asserts that individuals needing physical or spiritual care should be treated with dignity and respect. As a human person embraces the physical and spiritual realm, integration of nursing and spiritual care is critical for healthy families and communities.

Keywords: ubuntu, personhood, African, Christian, intimate care, advocacy

1. Introduction

The human body goes through many rituals from birth through all life stages. Rituals done on one's body symbolize the need for acceptability in the family, community, and society. The African and Christian religions are among the communities that conduct rituals on the human body. A ritual is a social construction of a body by which the person is afforded a particular sense of identity. It simultaneously empowers the person by indicating their individuality within a community [1]. Wulf further describe rituals as social constellations in which individual and communal social actions and how they are interpreted produce structures and hierarchies [2].

The rituals are performed on the body of a person. A human person is a biological entity with a capacity for certain intentional states, such as believing, desiring, and intending [3]. The human body is not an isolated entity but a biological, sociological, and ecological organism [4]. The body mediates all action; it is the medium for internalizing and reproducing social values and the simultaneous constitution of self and world social relations [1]. The body is the medium through which health and illness are experienced, it gives social meaning [5]. Thus, rituals are fundamental to human transformation and personhood. The person is guarded by three premises: cultural, religious, and healthcare. Each aspect of life is critical: a child is born into a family (cultural) and presented to the religious community and healthcare sector for identity. Acquisition of culture is a result of the socialization process. Every human being growing up in a particular society is likely to be infused with the culture of that society, whether knowingly or unknowingly, during the socialization process [6].

The body is the most individual and intimate aspect of human existence. It is inseparable from individual identity, thus difficult to distinguish between having a body and being the body [7]. The body is used to make sense of one's world as it extends beyond biological and physiological boundaries; it encompasses social and cultural dimensions [5]. The body is the site of concrete, an individual experience of tension between local cultural life and its global conditions [7]. Therefore, a person comes into existence in the reciprocal relatedness of individual and community, the human person is a holistic well-being within a web of relationships and a supreme being [8]. This proposition attests that humans have a dual nature, comprising the body and the spirit which exists beyond physical disappearance from the human world [9]. The mind finds its expression in the physical body as the body interprets what goes unseen. Clothing reveals the human essence to the world. It tells the world one story, inner thoughts, who the person is, and who they want to be. Therefore, dressing reveals personality, and cultural and religious affiliations [10]. Physical, emotional, and even spiritual closeness is established when rituals are conducted on the human body. One's body is exposed to people outside the family circle. Understanding the importance of rituals that promote healing and wholeness is vital in caring for an African human body. The culture of respect and dignity of the body can be extended to other cultural spaces, as what matters and upholding the integrity of the person.

1.1 The nakedness of the body

During the performance of rituals on the human body, the person is exposed to other people viewing and touching their naked bodies. The perspective of nakedness can be viewed within the biblical, cultural, and nursing care premises with the view of giving a voice to the body that is touched.

The book of Genesis gives credence to the story of Noah, who appeared naked and in a shameful situation (Gen 9:21–23). The act of the two sons covering the body is seen as an act of care for their drunk and naked father. Even passages that speak of the treatment of lepers are safeguards against the disease that could ravage society. Not touching the body in that context was seen as practicing care for one's body (Lev 13–14). Nevertheless, nakedness as such should not always be viewed in the negative, at least biblically. When the character Job was faced with challenges as he lost property, children and good health, he found comfort in the fact of his own body. "Naked I came from my mother's womb, and naked I shall return there. The LORD gave, and the LORD has taken away. Blessed be the name of the LORD" (Job 1:21). This is a sign of the sacredness and special nature of the body, notwithstanding the challenges one is going through. It is probably an understated fact that Jesus would have been naked when he was crucified. Jesus's torturers cast lots to determine ownership of the special garment. "And they crucified Him, and divided up His garments among themselves, casting lots for them to decide what each man would take" (Mark 15:24). Of course, the aim of Jesus' tortures was not to uplift and honor Him but rather to humiliate him even further. Yet in the story of Adam and Eve, their state of nakedness was the result of their sinning against God, nakedness was not in the world but came because of sin. In Gen 3:3 "then the eyes of both of them were opened and they knew they were naked and they sew fig leaves together and made themselves covering," thus nakedness is equated to sinfulness.

The African meaning of nakedness of the body is not far from the biblical context. As it is seen body image refers to personal construction and public projections of one's body, thus, body image involves one's perception, imagination, and emotional and physical sensation [11]. African cultures are conservative, a person is not just a product of nature, but a product of his/her culture. Culture informs the person how to relate with others, roles, norms, and expectations that shape how people relate to each other [10].

In African societies, women are often expected to cover their bodies, especially breasts, hips, and buttocks [12]. Unfortunately, the African body has been subjected to protracted racial slurs and symbolic objects of sexuality [11]. The body in its physical form, informs how it is read or perceived and what values are attached to it that inform social order. The sexual gaze on women alludes to women as objects of the male gaze, problematic ideas of what the female body should look like and defining when and how this body should be seen [13]. In some cases, women use naked body protests to illustrate their vulnerability and at the same time, naked bodies can disrupt, turning vulnerability into empowerment [14]. The unclothed body was previously read in a nonsexual manner, but now it is sexualized. Thus, the naked body is seen as irrational, uncontainable, and outside of normative constructive reason and African modernity [15]. In some instances, nakedness may be used to express vulnerability as a method of confrontation resistance and as a conflict resolution [14].

1.2 Objectives

The chapter aligns with the understanding that the human body is sacred and that each person goes through various bodily rituals for a sense of belonging. Therefore, the objectives were to:

- Explore and describe the rituals on the human body used in the African Christian religion for inclusive quality care.

- Integrate African-Christian rituals in nursing intimate care of the human body.

2. Methods

2.1 Theoretical framework

2.1.1 Ubuntu

Ubuntu can be generally defined as a worldview of African societies and a determining factor in the information of perceptions that influence social conduct [16]. Ubuntu is an African ethics that is based on ethical beliefs, and moral judgments associated with communal relationships. Ubuntu has its roots in the South African Nguni oral traditions which are made up of the prefix "ubu-" meaning being in potency or an enfolded being and stem "ntu" meaning being in actuality or unfolded being. The general impression of personhood and humanness is expressed. Therefore, ubuntu has emphasized the true meaning of being human, and what it means to be a person [17].

The notion of ubuntu places one as a person (human) bound into a community through relationships of care. Therefore, every person should be valued and respected, care and personhood cannot be separated as it gives one a sense of identity and humanness. Ubuntu refers to the critical values of group solidarity encompassing compassion, respect, human dignity, conformity to basic norms, and collective unity [18]. It advocates for communitarianism, where relations are forged and emphasizes reciprocal relationships that place an obligation on one another. Thus, a person cannot exist of themselves, as they come from a specific community that serves to nurture the realities of being human [19]. Its values represent personhood, humanity, humaneness, and morality. Many African philosophers, such as Mbiti and Ramose focus on ubuntu as a philosophy rather than practice, an ethical framework of relational justice. Ubuntu in a profound sense, implies an interactive ethic or an ontic orientation in which who and what a person can be as a human being is always shaped in interaction with others [20]. Ubuntu advocates for human connectedness with others, it assists in the facilitation of social connections. Ubuntu as a philosophy is grounded on the generic life values of justice, responsibility, equality, collectiveness, relatedness, reciprocity, love, respect, helpfulness, caring, dependability, sharing, trust, integrity, unselfishness, and social change [21]. *"Ubuntu brings the human face to every aspect of life."* In this study, Ubuntu was used as a framework to understand the human body's interconnectedness through rituals. The importance of personhood and humanness during initiation and caring for the person. It posits that every person should have a sense of belonging through identity in the family and community.

2.2 Research design

A qualitative exploratory-descriptive design was used. Qualitative research technique is a process where the research problem is studied in its natural setting, it gives room to a deeper understanding of the subject matters as they exist in their unique environment [22]. It intends to generate knowledge grounded in human experience [23]. Exploratory-descriptive design seeks to explore and describe the experiences of people. Exploratory research is a broad-ranging, purposive, systematic, prearranged undertaking designed to maximize the discovery of generalizations leading to the description and understanding of social or psychological life [24]. For this chapter, the rituals on the human body from Christian, African, and nursing perspectives were explored and described. Their descriptions gave meaning and a voice to the touched body with an in-depth understanding of the interconnectedness of human life.

2.2.1 Population and sampling

The population was divided into two groups:

2.2.1.1 Group 1: African-Christian leaders

The population were African-Christian leaders from the three countries in Southern Africa, which were Eswatini (former Swaziland), South Africa, and

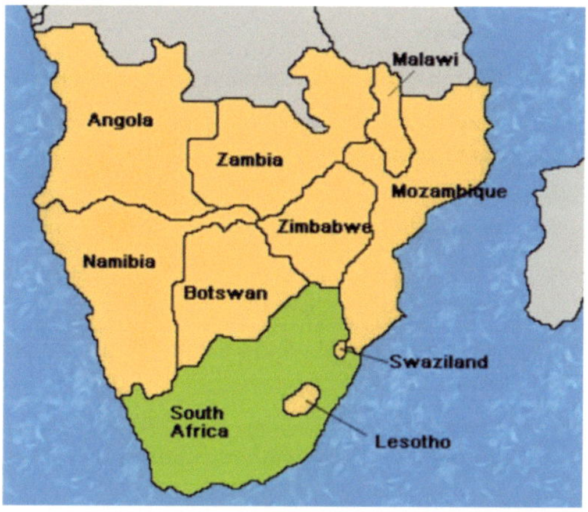

Figure 1.
Southern Africa map (from Google Maps).

Zimbabwe (**Figure 1** shows the geographic map of these countries). The individuals were involved in leadership in their churches and communities. For this group, snowball sampling was used to recruit the participants. Snowballing is a sampling method in which the participant is requested to refer individuals who meet the prescribed criteria. The first participants in the three countries were purposively selected. From there, other participants were recruited from the reference of the initial participants. Nineteen individuals participated in this group: eight African-Christian leaders from mainline churches (with a European history) such as Catholic and Lutheran, Pentecostal churches; seven African indigenous churches, such as Zionist church and three African indigenous practitioners.

2.2.1.2 Group 2: registered nurses

This group comprised of registered nurses working in two selected hospitals in midwifery, medical and surgical units. The participants were purposively recruited based on their experiences in nursing practice: three years or more experience in nursing practice and an understanding of providing intimate care to diverse patients. They were from 35 to 50 years of age. Eight registered nurses participated in the study.

2.2.2 Data collection

2.2.2.1 Naïve sketches

Naïve sketches are defined as brief essays by participants on the formulated questions, it is used to obtain descriptions of personal experiences concerning the research phenomenon, considering the social and cultural context of the study [25]. Naïve sketches were used for the African-Christian leaders. The questions were divided into four sections: Section A focused on demographic data linked to inclusion criteria, which were age, gender, and experiences as a leader in a specific group. Section B led to the discussion on the rituals for the birth of a child, and Section C care of the sick person. The participants were invited to respond to the questions in **Table 1**.

Sections	Questions
1. Birth of a child	• What happens when a child is born in your respective Christian community? • How does your religious group relate to children born of parents who are not members of the religious group? Or even children born outside what is contemplated in number 1 above? • Who is allowed to touch a newly born baby and how?
2. Life of a person	• As a child grows up, are there any practices that reinforce initiation in the group? What are these and how are they celebrated?
3. Sickness of the person	• When a person gets sick, what practices or rituals are performed on the sick person? • In your religious grouping who is allowed to touch the sick person? Where in the body can the person be touched? Is the sick person in a position to accept being touched or not?

Table 1.
Naïve sketches and semi-structured interview guide for group 1.

Author 1 emailed the information sheet, informed consent, and naïve sketches to the participants, they were requested to answer the questions as honestly as possible. After the completion of informed consent and naïve sketches, they were emailed back to author 1. The two researchers independently read the answers for completeness. Follow-up interviews were conducted to probe participants to explain the provided information for better understanding. The three Indigenous African practitioners requested to be interviewed and author 2 conducted the interviews using the questions in **Table 1** after signing the informed consent.

2.2.2.2 Semi-structured interviews

Semi-structured interviews entail having an interview guided by questions aimed at addressing the research objectives. The interview guide includes open-ended questions with follow-up probe questions with the interviewer to refer to throughout the interview [26]. The interview guide was developed to understand the caring rituals that are done on the person in healthcare institutions. Semi-structured interviews were conducted with group 2–registered nurses. Three main questions were used as a guide:

- What nursing practices are performed at the birth of a child?
- How is the healthy well-being of a person maintained during the life span?
- When a patient is admitted to the hospital, how is the body of a person cared for?
- Discuss intimate care and touch practices on the human body during hospitalization.

The interviews were conducted between June and September 2022. During the interview, a digital audio recorder was used to capture the narrative data. The participants were informed about the recording of interviews and consented. The duration of interviews was 20–30 minutes.

2.2.3 Data analysis

Narrative analysis refers to procedures used to interpret the narrative generated during data collection. The narrative meaning of data is transferred at different levels and gives greater meaning to the phenomenon experienced by the participants. Narrative analysis aims to unfold the ways individuals make sense of their lived experiences and how their telling enables them to interpret the social world and their agency within it [27].

The narrative analysis steps discussed by [27] were used to analyze data. Authors 1 and 2 independently analyze the naïve sketches and semi-structured interviews. Firstly, the authors familiarized themselves with the content and structure of the narratives by transcribing audio-recorded interviews and reading and rereading the transcripts in search of the rituals performed on the human body to understand the events, experiences, and explanations of the events. Secondly, a summary of the key elements and recording thematic ideas from the transcribed data. Thirdly, identify emotive language, imagery, or symbols used for the rituals and passages that may indicate the feelings expressed by the participant. The thematic ideas were linked to literature and theoretical framework.

2.2.4 Trustworthiness

Rigor/trustworthiness refers to the quality of qualitative enquiry and is used as a way of evaluating qualitative research [27]. Credibility addresses the rift between the participant's views and the researcher's representation of them [23]. Prolonged engagement and observations were conducted to gain an in-depth understanding of the rituals of the body. Triangulation was applied for credibility. Two multidisciplinary fields embarked on the study (Author 1—scripture scholar and theologian, and Author 2—nursing practitioner with experience in indigenous knowledge systems). Three population groups were purposively sampled which were Christian leaders, African indigenous practitioners, and nursing practitioners. Thick descriptions were provided for the reader to make a judgment about the transferability of the study to their site. Confirmability is concerned with establishing that the researchers' interpretations and findings are derived from data to demonstrate how the conclusion and interpretations were reached [23]. The audit trail was used to ensure the logical process of the research which is traceable and recorded for the reader to understand how the study was conducted. After the naïve sketches analysis, the participants were contacted to explain ambiguous statements through probing to represent the participants' views correctly.

2.2.5 Ethical considerations

The study received ethical clearance from the University of South Africa with reference number 90414357_CREC_CHS_2021. All participants were informed about the purpose and objectives of the study. The information leaflet and informed consent were given to all participants. They were informed about voluntary participation in the study, and they were free to withdraw at any time of the study. All participants signed informed consent before participating in the naïve sketches and semi-structured interviews. Participants' personal information was kept confidential by using codes and saved in password-protected files on the authors' computers. The researchers signed a confidentiality agreement to protect the identity of study participants. Permission was obtained for the photos used under the findings section.

3. Results

3.1 Participants characteristics

3.1.1 Group 1: African-Christian leaders

Seventeen (n = 17) individuals participated in this group with seven females and ten females. Seven (n = 7) Church Leaders (CL), seven (n = 7) African Church Leaders (ACL), and three (n = 3) African indigenous practitioners (AIP). The age ranges were from 36 to 60 with experiences from 3 to 35 years in leadership (**Table 2**).

No.	Participants code	Age	Gender	African-Christian affiliation	Years in leadership	Country
1.	CL-01	48	M	Lutheran	16	S Africa
2.	CL-02	36	M	Catholic	6	Eswatini
3.	ACL-01	59	F	Africa Indigenous Church	20	Eswatini
4.	ACL-02	56	M	Africa Indigenous Church	26	Eswatini
5.	CL-03	41	M	Catholic	8	Eswatini
6.	CL-04	41	M	Catholic	8	Eswatini
7.	CL-05	55	M	Catholic	27	Eswatini
8.	ACL-03	39	F	Africa Indigenous Church	3	Zimbabwe
9.	ACL-04	45	M	Africa Indigenous Church	4	Zimbabwe
10.	ACL-05	59	F	Africa Indigenous Church	20	Eswatini
11.	ACL-06	40	M	Africa Indigenous Church	6	Eswatini
12.	CL-06	27	M	Pentecostal	4	Eswatini
13.	ACL-07	45	M	African indigenous church	15	S Africa
14.	CL-07	58	F	Pentecostal	15	S Africa
15.	AIP-01	60	F	African indigenous practitioner	35	S Africa
16.	AIP-02	48	F	African indigenous practitioner	15	S Africa
17.	AIP-03	50	F	African indigenous practitioner	25	S Africa

Table 2.
Summary of African-Christian leaders' characteristics.

Participants code	Age	Gender	Unit/ward	Position	Years of experience
PRN-01	35	M	Surgical	RN	7
PRN-02	45	F	Maternity	Midwifery practitioner	8
PRN-03	40	F	Maternity	Midwifery practitioner	5
PRN-04	43	F	Maternity	Midwifery practitioner	6
PRN-05	42	F	Medical	RN	8
PRN-06	39	M	Medical	RN	7
PRN-07	49	M	Surgical	RN	10
PRN-08	50	F	Medical	RN	20

Table 3.
Summary of registered nurses' characteristics.

3.1.2 Group 2: registered nurses

Eight registered nurses were interviewed, five (n = 5) females and three (n = 3) males. They were between 35 and 50 of age. They had working experience of five years and more. Three (n = 3) from the maternity ward, three (n = 3) medical, and two (n = 2) from the surgical wards (**Table 3**).

3.2 Presentation of findings

This section presents major findings from the two population groups.

3.2.1 Theme 1: identity of a person

The identity of the person starts from conception. Pregnancy is celebrated by the expecting parents and family as the new life is to be welcomed. Once the child is born, he/she is given a name and welcomed into the family. Three sub-themes are discussed which are the *protection of an infant, naming ritual, and initiation into the family and community*.

3.2.1.1 Sub-theme 1: protection of an infant

The protection of the unborn child begins in the womb. Rituals in the birth of a child start from conception the child and parents perform the necessary rituals that will assure the safety of both the mother and the child [28]. African Traditional medicines are used for protection.

> *"During pregnancy, the woman is given isihlambelo and imbiza to assist with progress of labour and pains during childbirth" (AIP-03)*

Isihlambelo is an oral African Medicine taken in the third trimester for quick labor, fetal growth, and well-being [29]. Whereas *imbiza* herbs are said to facilitate pregnancy by preparing the uterus to accept the fetus and are mostly used in the cleansing process during pregnancy [30]. When birth occurs at home, men and people in a state of impurity are forbidden to be present in the house where the delivery place as the child will be ashamed to be born [31] leading to prolonged labor.

The midwifery practitioners emphasized the protection of the fetus using antenatal healthcare services.

> *"As midwives, we provide care to the mother and the child during pregnancy. The women are always encouraged to start antenatal clinic once they notice that they are pregnant so that we can identify pregnancy problems for the mother and foetus" (PRN-02)*

Antenatal care is a unique preventative public health initiative and intervention offered routinely to pregnant women, with the overall objective of improving the outcomes for the mother and child through early detection of complications [32]. The Department of Health advocates for eight visits to receive significant care in which pregnancy is monitored through health promotion screening, diagnosis, and disease prevention [33].

Within South Africa, midwifery practitioners expect pregnant women to use traditional medicines.

> *"Sometimes pregnant women come to the clinic late or they do not attend at all as they believe in traditional medicines. We normally educate women to use it carefully to avoid complications and even when following their practices, they must come to the clinic so that we can test to see if they are fine, including the baby. At times they overdose the traditional medicines, and we have to deal with maternal and neonatal emergencies" (PRN-04)*

Understanding African traditions is important in midwifery care, to support women in their pregnancy journey, which can be stressful. Traditional medicines must be administered safely to prevent complications such as premature labor, fetal distress, and uterine rupture due to excessive uterine contractions [29].

After birth, the child is protected from the outside world by keeping him/her in a safe space. The mother and child remain in a room for three months or until "ukuwa kwenkaba" (the fall or drying up of the umbilical cord) as it symbolizes the growth of the child.

> *"the child goes out after three months when the umbilical cord has dried up (inkaba iwile) and ukhakhayi luvalekile "closure of fontanelle". Even when you go out with the child, you must cover the child so that he/she cannot get evil spirits." (AIP-01)*

It is also believed that a small child can easily get various spirits that may affect the child negatively.

> *"There are people who carry strong medicines which are not good for the child. the child senses it and responds with their bodies by getting sick. Sometimes the fontanelle is affected "ukwehla kokhakhayi" [sunken fontanelle]," (AIP-02)*

Sometimes traditional medicines are given to the child, especially through small cuts through the skin (ukugcaba).

> *"to protect the child, we make small cuts on the body and put powdered medicine which will be absorbed into the body. The specific areas of the body are culturally specified, but the important part is the head" (AIP-01).*

During the period when the mother and child are excluded from public life, the woman is treated specially for three months, this time enables the nursing mother to recover and take proper care of the baby [31]. Interestingly, one Christian leader acknowledges the duties of family and midwifery practitioners during the birth of the child:

> *"The first person to touch a newborn baby is the midwife who helps in the delivery of the child. Then mother of the baby to receive him or her after delivery. At home family members who can handle the baby with care would hold the baby to welcome him or her into the family" (CL-02)*

In nursing practice, immunization is administered to protect and strengthen the immune system of the child.

> *"When the child is born, his/her immunity is weak, therefore at birth or before discharge, the child is immunised. We follow the Expanded Immunisation Programme which starts at birth to 12 years of age. When the child is immunised three drops for polio prevention are given and an injection on the left arm is given in such a way that it will make a mark as a sign that the child was successfully immunised for Tuberculosis. The child is then registered in the institution birth register and the Road to Health card is given and is used to record all consecutive immunisations" (PRN-02)*

Immunization is used to improve the children's immune system. It assists in preventing dangerous preventable diseases that, if not administered may result in malnutrition and child development delays [34]. In South Africa, the expanded program on immunization was introduced in 1994 as a powerful and cost-effective public health program to improve child survival [35]. Through an immunization program, the children's right to health, safety, development, and survival is promoted.

3.2.1.2 Sub-theme 2: naming ritual

Naming is a ritual used to give identity to a child. The parents or family does the naming of the child. The name gives meaning and direction to the life of the child.

> *"[...] the name has meaning which the child will follow in life [...]. Sometimes the name is more of the circumstances of the pregnancy, the relationship of the family especially the parents [...]". (AIP-02)*

> *"[...] giving a good name to a child is important as it becomes the way of life, if given the name of a family member who was not a good person, the child will follow it and cause chaos in the family and community" (AIP-01)*

> *"In the Christian community, the parents or family who offer the child to the church give the name to the child. As Christian leaders, we only advise parents on the importance of their children's names. Giving a positive name to a child is always encouraged. Because when we bless the child, he/she is called by the given name and it reveals the future path of the child". (CL-07)*

The participants believed that the infant comes from the spirit world with important information and is bringing unique talents and gifts to the family and community. On this basis, the naming of the child is an important occasion marked by rituals. The naming ritual takes place a few days after the birth of the child, he/she receives a personal name which marks entry into the family, prayers are offered, and ancestors are invoked [31].

The child has to be treated with love and dignity, a sacred being that needs to be respected:

> *"Each human person is made in the image and likeness of God, irrespective of their social background. All children deserve to be treated with dignity for human life is sacred" (CL-03)*

In nursing care, when a child is born, the surname of the mother is used to identify the child "Baby [surname of the mother]". This practice is within the South African Family law which advocates for the child's right to a name.

> *"As midwives, we do not interfere with the naming of the child. We have social workers from Home Affairs who come to the unit to assist mothers in registering their children before they are registered. This works well if the mother has the name of the child. But if that is not the case, the birth confirmation documents are given to the mother on discharge to go to Home Affairs to register the birth of the named child" [PRN-02]*

Section 28 of the South African Constitution states that "every child has the right to a name and nationality from birth." Therefore, the birth of the child must be registered within 30 days after delivery and be in the possession of a birth certificate. The birth certificate provides the person's identity and thus gives the child the human right to equality, freedom of movement, and dignity.

3.2.1.3 Sub-theme 2: initiation into family and community

When a child is born, he/she must be welcomed into the family and community. This act is linked to the Ubuntu practice, which advocates for solidarity and communal living. Within the Christian community, a child is baptized, in African practice, a child is blessed and in nursing care, immunization is used to strengthen the immune system.

3.2.1.3.1 Initiation through Baptism

The baptism of a child and an adult are distinct. For mainline churches (Catholic and Lutheran), baptism can be performed to infants. This is done to welcome the child to the church family and protect him/her from evil spirits.

> *"The religious group mainly in charge of baptism of the child, whereby the Godparents and priest touches the baby during baptizing" (CL-01)*

> *"A newborn child is a gift from God. Christians celebrate birth by welcoming the child into the church through the sacrament of baptism of which the sponsor and parents pledge to walk them (children) in the way of Christ" (CL-05)*

Baptism is a ritual through which new members are engrafted into the body of Christ and it is a symbolic guarantee that a person has become a member of the

DOI: http://dx.doi.org/10.5772/intechopen.1004213

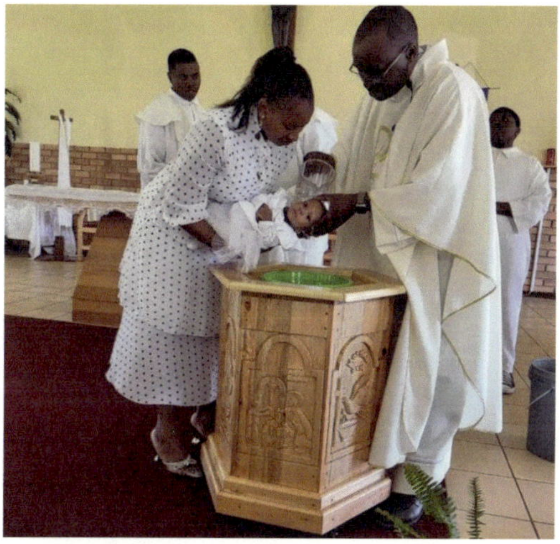

Figure 2.
Baptism of an infant.

Christian church [36]. Baptism is a sacrament by which people are incorporated into the Church, built into a house where God lives in spirit, thus, the sacrament creates a bond with all who abide by it [37]. **Figure 2** shows a child being baptized. The priest pours holy water on the forehead for the cleansing and purification of the child.

When a child is baptized, the priest touches the chest of the child as he makes the sign of the cross. After this, he will pour water on his/her forehead and thereafter anoint the forehead with oil. The symbols of the sign of the cross, water, and oil are used to purify any sin, which is considered an evil spirit [37].

In some Christian churches, the dedication ceremony is conducted for the young children. The parents dedicate the child to God:

> *"Dedication is a ceremony whereby the child might even wear beautiful white clothes. Parents can even invite relatives to come and witness the dedication. At church, the child will be dedicated to God and prayed for" (CL-16)*

3.2.1.3.2 Initiation through blessing

In African churches, baptism is only conducted when a person is an adult and can make an informed decision. When the child is young, she/he is blessed using water and incense. Therefore, a young child is welcomed into the family by introducing him or her to the ancestors and blessing.

> *"The parents present their child to church through the senior member (pastor). The pastor blows incense in his/her direction for blessing. The child is brought for blessing after three months from birth" (ACL-05)*

The initiation rituals such as baptism, blessing, and dedication welcome the child into the family and community. It symbolizes a sense of belonging and personhood. These practices are linked to the ubuntu principles that perceive the sense of self to the family and part of the community. In the photo below children are presented by parents and Godparents to the priest for blessing (see **Figure 3**).

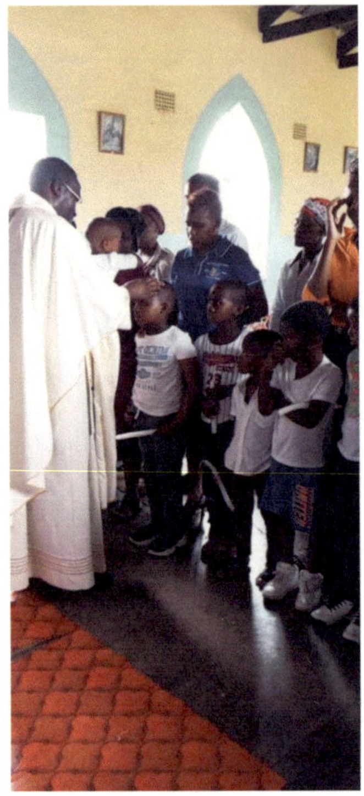

Figure 3.
Children receiving a blessing from a priest.

3.2.2 Theme 2: preservation of the person's life within the community

3.2.2.1 Sub-theme 2.1: meaning of the body

In the African context, the body is the vessel for the ancestors, which needs to be respected and honored.

> *"we respect the body, as people who have the spirit of the elders. We do not perform rituals when we are not well [during menstrual periods]. When my body is not well, I will burden the person I am praying for, for example when I am on my monthly periods as a woman, I do not pray for the person because we respect his/her body."* *(AIP-03).*

The body is the subject of practice and the object towards which much of that action is directed, it gives cultural identity and visibility to the ancestors both in family, society and moral life [38].

For Christians, the body is considered the Temple of God. In the Gospel of John 2:19, Jesus referred to His body as a temple and Apostle Paul in the letter to the Corinthians 6:19–20, explains. "Do you know that your bodies are temples of the Holy Spirit, who is in you, whom you have received from God? You are not your own, you were brought at a price. Therefore, honour God with your bodies"

In nursing, the body is a physical, mental, and spiritual being that is controlled by the patient's cultural and religious systems.

> *"As a nurse I respect the person according to the patient's belief system, first treating the body with dignity, respecting their ancestors or God in them. I ask the patient what their family practice is so that I can treat them accordingly" (PRN-01)*

3.2.2.2 Sub-theme 2.2: caring for the sick body: the healing ritual

Illness may be inevitable; therefore, the body may go through physical, mental, and spiritual difficulties that require interventions.

Before African indigenous practitioners intervene in the illness of an individual, they need to consult the ancestors through prayer or throwing of bones to get the message relating to the illness.

> *"The sick person needing help comes to eNdumbeni "consultation room" and I consult with his/her ancestors to understand the illness and how it can be solved. I listen to the message and deliver it to the person." (AIP-03)*

> *"During ukuhlola "consultation" with the ancestors, they will give directions on how to treat the illness and we give the information to a sick person. He/she is free to make a decision to be treated or not." (AIP-01)*

Figure 4 shows an African indigenous practitioner during a consultation session in the eNdumbeni.

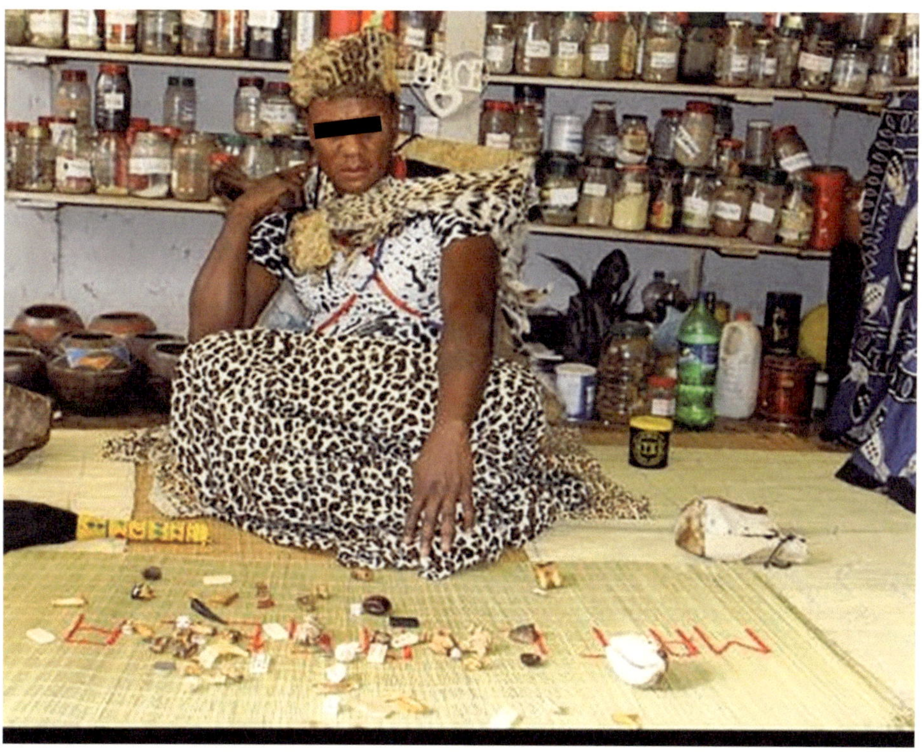

Figure 4.
African Indigenous Practitioner consulting in eNdumbeni.

The Catholic church prescribes the sacrament of healing which is spiritual and physical and can be done in the church, home, or hospital.

> *"We have the sacraments of healing. Spiritual healing is related to the sacrament of confession sins and physical healing which is the sacrament of anointing of the sick. The priest touches the sick person by laying of hands on the head. The oil is also used to anoint the forehead and hands. The sick person always must request the sacrament or a relative consent if the patient can no longer do it himself or herself"* (CL-04)

Patients come to the hospital when they have exhausted all the care available in the safe home environment. When providing basic nursing care, physical exposure of the body is experienced.

> *"We conduct a physical examination, bathing the patient and elimination- inserting a urinary catheter or serving a bedpan. During this procedure, we see the naked body of the patient and touch their bodies. These are very sensitive procedures, at times embarrassing for me as a nurse and a patient receiving care"* (PRN-08)

Being naked or nearly naked can be a major constraint in quality nursing care as the patient and nurse must negotiate a safe space for this care with mutual respect [39]. It is in the hospital space where the human body is exposed to diverse healthcare practitioners, therefore, the promotion of privacy and careful exposure of the patient's body should be well-planned to improve the quality of life for the patients.

Gender issues are critical in nursing and African indigenous practices as proximate physical contact occurs in a private space. The female African indigenous practitioners and church leaders expressed the limitations in providing interventions to male clients:

> *"When performing healing rituals on the person, when he is a man, we give them instructions on what to do, like "ukufutha" [steaming], I don't put him on it as I cannot see him naked. I give him instructions such as going to the room and undressing and then using the steam etc. If it is a woman, I go in with her and help her in the process. Ukugcaba (small cuts on the skin to put powder medicine] is done [...]."* (AIP-02)

> *"The prophet(s) and leaders depending on gender can touch the person. Touching can be done in any part of the body with dignity being observed. The decision of the sick person whether to be touched or not is respected. In case of severe illness, their relatives are asked for consent"* (ACL-03)

The importance of giving information to a participant in a ritual and allowing them to make an informed decision gives them the form of dignity and reclaiming their personhood during illness.

4. Discussions

The chapter attempted to explore and describe the rituals on the human body used in the African Christian religion for inclusive quality care. Also, to integrate African-Christian rituals in nursing intimate care of the human body. Two major themes emerged from the findings: *Identity of a person and the preservation of the person's life in the community.*

The African and Christian religions are among the communities that conduct rituals on the human body. A ritual is a social construction of a body by which the person is afforded a particular sense of identity. The body mediates all action; it is the medium for internalizing and reproducing social values and the simultaneous constitution of self and social relations. As the body is constantly touched, the rituals on the human body must be integrated to enhance one's identity as a person worthy of being respected and cared for. This section looks at rituals in three contexts: Christianity, Africanity, and nursing practice.

4.1 Identity of a person

When the child is born, he/she needs to be protected from the impurities of the world's spirit and environment. The participants expressed the meaning of an infant's weak immune system and evil spirits.

The naming of the child is important as it gives meaning to the future of the child. When a child is born in the hospital, the midwifery practitioners deliver the infant and keep warm to prevent hypothermia (kept dry, warm, and safe). The child is not washed until 24 hours after delivery. The first bath is important as it assists in the observation of the baby and the mother is welcome to participate in this activity. Before the infant is released from the hospital, he/she is immunized in the presence of the mother. The first immunization for TB and polio protects the child from contracting the communicable disease at a young age. The mothers are taught on how to take care of the umbilical cord: keep it dry to avoid infection.

The child is initiated into the family and community through baptism and blessings. In Christian churches, baptism symbolizes cleansing and purification from any sin and unites one with God. Through blessing, the child is welcomed into the family and community.

The practice of the Christian church is in such a way that the rituals contain an element of touching the person. This is true for baptism and other rituals that accompany the initiation of the human person into the Christian Church. The New Testament presents a more liberal approach to the body, especially regarding touching it: John the Baptist baptized people in the river Jordan (Mk. 1:4–5). Baptizing a person requires pouring water over the other person as the baptizer stands close to them. Jesus would even go so far as to touch people with various diseases, which was seen to be taboo. He touched a sick mother-in-law of Peter (Mk. 1:31), he touched the leper (Mk. 1:40–42), the woman who suffered a hemorrhage touched him, and he touched the dead daughter of Jairus (Mk 5:21–43). With the example of Jesus touching the other, in the Christian religion, touching a diseased body becomes standard as James exhorts thus: *"Is anyone among you sick? Let him call for the elders of the church, and let them pray over him, anointing him with oil in the name of the Lord. And the prayer of faith will save the sick, and the Lord will raise him up. And if he has committed sins, he will be forgiven"* (James. 5:14–15). Through the scriptures, the sacraments find a way into human life.

4.2 Preservation of the person's life within the community

The participants perceived the human body as a sacred vessel for the ancestors and a temple for God. This places value on the importance of a human person. The bodies distinctively bear emblems of cultural identity and visible ideologies that organize both society and individual life [38].

The body is so valued in the Christian religion that Paul would call it the Temple of the Holy Spirit (Cf. 1 Cor. 6:19–20). He also used the metaphor of the body to teach about the unity that is supposed to exist within the Christian community (Cf. 1 Cor. 12:12–27). As a result, the body is good to be cared for and protected. Caring for the body is foreseen even before the person is born, as she/he is viewed as desired by God. For this reason, the prophet Jeremiah says, *"Before I formed you in the womb, I knew you, before you came out of your mother's womb, I consecrated you and constituted you a prophet for the nations"* (Jer. 1:5). Therefore, speaking of being known in the womb brings out the utmost respect for the human body. The person should still be valued notwithstanding how he was conceived, where he was born what race or religion he belongs to and even his orientation.

The body plays a crucial role in assigning meaning to the experiences of illness and provides guidance on what actions are required for social experiences [5]. Therefore, humans have a dual nature comprising of the body and spirit which continue to exist beyond physical disappearance [9]. Elders in the family (immediate or extended) are responsible for caring for their loved ones. Same gender is used; therefore, cross-gender is not accepted. The children cannot see or touch the naked body of their parents. Before outsourcing this care, the indigenous healer is consulted to "throw bones"—consult the ancestors to see what needs to be done for healing. The incense, water, and indigenous plants are used for cleansing and as a form of medication. During these rituals, a body is repaired and refashioned through rites of healing [1]. The healing ritual enables the participants to communicate with the spirit world and is possible through the intermediary of priests or ritual leaders who will consult divinity on behalf of the participants and relate the message from the spiritual realm to them [28].

When the attempts fail, the individual will seek further management in the hospital. This is done as the last resort and, at times may seem a failure for the family. Thus, becomes critical for healthcare practitioners to understand the diverse backgrounds of their patients for professional autonomy and empathetic care. During the patient's admission to the hospital, basic nursing care requiring touch is provided to maintain the patient's well-being. Procedures such as bed baths, and insertion of urinary catheters are implemented. These procedures are considered intimate as the patient and nurse share a confined private space. Intimate care can be defined as task-oriented care that requires proximity between the patient and nurse [40]. The patient is given an identity belt to identify them while in the hospital using their names and allocated hospital numbers. Hygiene, elimination, and nutrition including medication are provided to enhance the patient's healing. The identity of the person is validated through rituals of naming, and initiation (baptism, blessings, and dedication) into the family and community. Symbols such as water, oil, incense, etc. are used to transform the body. A sense of belonging assists in maintaining the multifaceted human person: body, mind, and spirit.

5. Conclusion

This chapter sought to advocate for integrated personhood. To arrive at this, an exercise was made to integrate African Christian rituals and intimate care on the touched human body. The chapter concentrated on three countries in Southern Africa, namely Eswatini (former Swaziland), South Africa, and Zimbabwe. Some direct interviews were conducted with people who subscribe to different belief systems. This included adherents of African indigenous churches, mainline churches (those with a European background), Pentecostal churches and African indigenous practitioners. Semi-structured interviews were also conducted with registered nurses in selected hospitals. The important matter, or area of convergence, is that all the groups are for the advancement of the human person, that is for integrated personhood. This includes rituals that require the priest, leader, or elder to touch the human body. It is thus urgent that among these groups there must be constant sharing of experiences and advancements in practice. When confronted with a sick body, it is required that this body benefits from the experiences of the rituals on the human body so that healing may take place. When this is done there is an assurance that the body is treated with respect and dignity.

Acknowledgements

We acknowledge all participants who shared their valuable knowledge on the subject. This study is funded by the South African National Research Foundation Thuthuka Grant Reference: TTK210318590345.

Conflict of interest

The authors declare no conflict of interest.

Author details

Dumisani Benedict Vilakati[1] and Simangele Shakwane[2*]

1 Diocese of Manzini, Eswatini and University of South Africa, South Africa

2 University of South Africa, Pretoria, South Africa

*Address all correspondence to: shakws@unisa.ac.za

References

[1] Bell CM. The ritual body and the dynamics of ritual power. Journal of Ritual Studies. 2005;**4**(2):299-313. Available from: https://scholarcommons.scu.edu/rel_stud

[2] Wulf C. Education as transcultural education: A global challenge. Educational Studies in Japan International Yearbook. 2010;**5**:33-47

[3] Baker LA. The biology of relationships: What behavioral genetics tells us about interactions among family members. De Paul Law Review. 2007;**56**(3):837-846

[4] Yun JY. The nonhuman turn and the body in the Anthropocene in Thomas Day's Seven Seconds to Become an Eagle. Neohelicon. 2020;**47**(1):17-25. DOI: 10.1007/s11059-020-00521-6

[5] Moorley CR. Experiences of African-Caribbean women of their body after stroke. Nursing Times. 2018;**114**(5):52-55

[6] Idang GE. African culture and values. Phronimon. 2015;**16**(2):97-111

[7] Larsen SE. The body between intimacy and globalization. Journal of Aesthetics & Culture. 2013;**5**(1):22673

[8] Dolamo RTH. A trinitarian theology of creation: An ethical perspective. HTS Teologiese Studies/Theological Studies. 2019;**75**(1):1-8

[9] Iheanacho NN. Religio-cultural foundation and resources of human relations in Africa. Sociology Mind. 2016;**06**(02):65-74

[10] Okpokwasili O. Nudity, women and morality in a contemporary Nigerian society: A philosophical discourse. Nnadiebube Journal of Philosophy. 2021;**5**(1):152-165

[11] Oloruntoba-Oju T. Understanding Human Sexuality Seminar Series Body Images, Beauty Culture and Language in the Nigeria, African Context. Nigeria: African Regional Sexuality Resource Centre; 2007

[12] Mathebula M. Nakedness as decolonial praxis. Body & Society. 2022;**28**(3):3-29. DOI: 101177/1357034X221105353

[13] Jimlongo G. When women have reached the end of their politics: Nakedness as resistance. In: National Award: Best Honours Essay. South Africa: Rhodes University; 2018

[14] Tamale S. Nudity, protest and the law in Uganda. Feminist Africa. 2022;**22**:52-86

[15] Mathebula M, Canham H. The affective afterlife of naked body protests. Feminism & Psychology. 2022:1-18. DOI: 10.1177/09593535221120482

[16] Mokgobi MG. Understanding traditional African healing. African Journal for Physical Health Education, Recreation and Dance. 2014;**20**(Suppl. 2):24-34

[17] Ewuoso C, Hall S. Core aspects of ubuntu: A systematic review. South African Journal of Bioethics and Law. South African Medical Association. 2019;**12**(2):93-103

[18] Rautenbach C. Legal reform of traditional courts in South Africa: Exploring the links between ubuntu, restorative justice and therapeutic jurisprudence. Journal of International

and Comparative Law. 2015;**2**(2):275-304. DOI: 10.4314/pelj.v14i4

[19] Kroeze IJ. Once More uBuntu: A Reply to Radebe and Phooko IJ Kroeze. PER/PELJ. 2020;**23**:1-23. DOI: 10.17159/1727-3781/2020/v23i0a8048

[20] Cornell D, Van Marle K. Exploring Ubuntu: Tentative reflections. African Human Rights Law Journal. 2009;**5**(2):195-220

[21] Mayaka B, Truell R. Ubuntu and its potential impact on the international social work profession. International Social Work. 2021;**64**(5):649-662

[22] Akinyode BF, Khan TH. Step by step approach for qualitative data analysis. International Journal of Built Environment and Sustainability. 2018;**5**(3):163-174

[23] Nowell LS, Norris JM, White DE, Moules NJ. Thematic analysis: Striving to meet the trustworthiness criteria. International Journal of Qualitative Methods. **16**(1)

[24] Hunter DJ, Mccallum J, Howes D. Defining Exploratory-Descriptive Qualitative (EDQ) research and considering its application to healthcare. Journal of Nursing and Health Care. 2019;**4**:1-7. Available from: http://eprints.gla.ac.uk/180272/http://eprints.gla.ac.uk

[25] Moagi MM. Student nurses' experiences in the clinical psychiatric learning environment: The use of drawings and naïve sketches in qualitative health research. African Journal for Physical. 2014;**1**:132-141

[26] Adeoye-Olatunde OA, Olenik NL. Research and scholarly methods: Semi-structured interviews. JACCP Journal of the American College of Clinical Pharmacy. 2021;**4**(10):1358-1367

[27] Liamputtong P. Qualitative Research Methods. 4th ed. Australia: Oxford University Press; 2013

[28] Ogunleye RA. Ritual efficacy in traditional African environments. The Journal of Pan African Studies. 2014;**16**(10):209-221

[29] Mudonhi N, Nunu WN. Traditional medicine utilisation among pregnant women in Sub-saharan African countries: A systematic review of literature. The Journal of Health Care. 2022;**59**:1-10

[30] Ramulondi M, de Wet H, Ntuli NR. The use of African traditional medicines amongst Zulu women during childbearing in northern KwaZulu-Natal. African Journal of Reproductive Health. 2022;**26**(1):66-75

[31] Nwadiokwu CN, Nwadiokwu ES, Favour EN, Okwuazun ME. Rites of passage African traditional region. International Journal of Education and Research. 2016;**4**(9):41-50

[32] Hofmeyer GJ, Menrop L. Time for "basic antenatal care plus" in South Africa? SAMJ. 2015;**105**(11):902-903. DOI: 10.1016/S0140

[33] Nxiweni PZ, Oladimeji KE, Nanjoh M, Banda L, Anyiam FE, Hyera FLM, et al. Factors influencing the utilization of antenatal services among women of childbearing age in South Africa. Women. 2022;**2**(3):285-303

[34] Le Roux K, Akin-Olugbade O, Katzen LS, Laurenzi C, Mercer N, Tomlinson M, et al. Immunisation coverage in the rural Eastern Cape - Are we getting the basics of primary care right? Results from a longitudinal prospective cohort study. South African Medical Journal. 2017;**107**(1):52-55

[35] Wiysonge CS, Ngcobo NJ, Jeena PM, Madhi SA, Schoub BD, Hawkridge A, et al. Advances in childhood immunisation in South Africa: Where to now? Programme managers views and evidence from systematic reviews. BMC Public Health. 2012;**12**

[36] Ikenna E. Misconception of rituals as basis for condemnation of African traditional religion ... 43 misconception of rituals as basis for condemnation of African traditional religion among contemporary religious practitioners: A call for re-orientation. Social Sciences, Peace and Conflict Studies (IJMSSPCS). 2021;**4**:43-50

[37] Rite of Christian Initiation of Adults: Introductory Material. International Commission on English in the Liturgy: England & Wales. 1985:1-45

[38] Grillo GS. African rituals: The place of rituals in african religions. 1st ed. England: The Wiley-Blackwll Companion to African Religion; 2012

[39] Ceroni P, Martins CL, Antoniolli L, Cardozo-Gonzales RI, Dal Pai D, Echevarría-Guanilo ME. Patient's body exposure through the look of the nursing academic. Revista de Pesquisa Cuidado é Fundamental Online. 2015;7(4):3148-3162

[40] Shakwane S, Mokoboto-Zwane S. Demystifying sexual connotations: A model for facilitating the teaching of intimate care to nursing students in South Africa. African Journal of Health Professions Education. 2020;**12**(3):103

Chapter 3

Pain and Pain Management

Manaporn Chatchumni

Abstract

Nurses specialising in pain management can have a significant role in postoperative pain care. As integral members of the healthcare system, nurses should adhere to evidence-based practice guidelines to ensure optimal patient treatment. This paper focuses on the interplay between professional practice and the clinical setting, enhancing our comprehension of professional and practice-based knowledge advancement. Future studies will further expand our insights into the culture and methodologies of a specific cohort of nurses, ultimately enhancing their expertise and practice in specialised pain management. This paper will unquestionably contribute valuable knowledge to the nursing profession and its practices. From the patients' perspective post-surgery, effective pain management is closely tied to their overall health and well-being.

Keywords: pain, pain management, nursing practice, postoperative pain, patient's pain

1. Introduction

An individual's subjective experience of pain can be described as the individual's own description of the sensation and the time at which they report that it occurred. "Believe the patient" is a premise that McCaffery and Pasero state in their book Pain: Clinical Manual [1], and this idea is consistent with that approach. Both the unpleasant sensory and emotional components that are associated with actual or potential tissue damage, as well as the perception of such damage, are included in the concept of pain. The World Health Organisation's International Classification of Diseases, Eleventh Revision (ICD-11) [2] defines chronic pain as pain that lasts for more than 3 months or that happens repeatedly during that time period.

Nurses who specialise in pain management greatly enhance postoperative pain care [3, 4]. It is imperative that nurses, who are essential components of the healthcare system, adhere to evidence-based practice guidelines in order to guarantee the best possible treatment for their patients [3, 4]. Increasing our understanding of the progression of professional and practice-based knowledge is the purpose of this paper, which focuses on the interaction that occurs between clinical settings and professional practices. In subsequent research, we will be able to gain a deeper understanding of the culture and approaches utilised by a particular group of nurses, which will ultimately lead to an improvement in their level of experience and practice in the field of specialised pain treatment. This research will undoubtedly contribute valuable knowledge that will benefit the nursing profession and its practices. Effective pain management is closely related to patients' general health and well-being, as they perceive it after surgery.

2. Anatomy and physiology

One of the most common symptoms that can be seen in hospitalised patients is pain [3–7]. Acute pain usually results from damage to the tissue and lasts only a short while before going away in 3 months as the injured tissues mend. On the other hand, chronic pain persists beyond the healing phase and continues to be experienced long after the individual has recovered from the acute injury or disease. Inherently subjective in nature, pain is a phenomenon that encompasses both physiological and psychological components [8–10]. It is a multidimensional phenomenon.

An important protective mechanism that involves numerous interacting peripheral and central mechanisms is the somatosensory system's ability to identify unpleasant and potentially tissue-damaging stimuli. The term "nociception" refers to the brain processes that are responsible for the encoding and processing of noxious stimuli. Nociceptor activation and subsequent conversion into action potentials for transmission to the central nervous system are necessary for noxious stimulus detection. The nociceptive impulses are set off by chemical, thermal, or mechanical injury, which stimulates the nociceptors [8–10].

Nociceptive primary afferents contain both lightly myelinated A-delta fibres (diameter 2–5 mm) and slow-conducting unmyelinated C-fibres (diameter < 2 mm). These fibres are widely dispersed throughout the body, including the skin, muscles, joints, viscera, and meninges. The fibres go into the spinal cord's dorsal horn and connect at various locations, including Ad at Rexed laminae II and V and C at Rexed laminae II. On the contralateral side, the substantia gelatinosa, also known as lamina II, is responsible for integrating these inputs, and second-order neurons are responsible for forming the ascending spinothalamic and spinoreticular pathways (**Figure 1**).

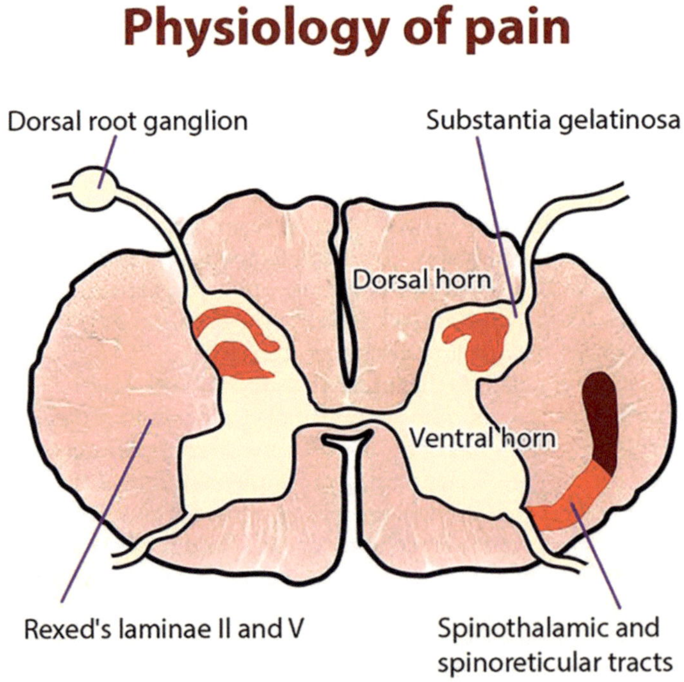

Figure 1.
Physiology of pain 1.

The inhibitory interneurons in the substantia gelatinosa are stimulated by the bigger Ab fibres leading "touch" and descending pathways, which in turn suppress the nociceptive inputs from the C fibres. The gate theory of pain is founded upon this concept. Altering the neural route that transports pain from its point of origin at the nociceptor to its interpretation within the central nervous system can be accomplished by the application of a number of different agents [8–10].

Pain can be either acute or chronic, and it may persist even after tissue repair. Managing pain effectively requires adhering to a number of core principles, including assessing and meticulously documenting pain as well as evaluating the effectiveness of interventions. Surgical pain management is seen as an ethical requirement and a basic human right. Standards for pain management were initially developed by the Joint Commission on Accreditation of Healthcare Organisations (JCAHO) in 2001 [5, 6]. One of these guidelines emphasised how important it is to consider the assessment of pain to be the "fifth vital sign."

In 1965, Professors Ronald Melzack and Patrick Wall published the seminal "Pain Mechanisms: A New Theory" [9], which laid the groundwork for the Gate Control Theory of Pain. Pain perception is like being a "passive receiver of messages," according to an expansion of this notion that came out in 2013 [9].

2.1 Types of pain

Various criteria can classify pain, including the physiological mechanisms responsible for it, the level of intensity, the temporal aspects, the specific tissues affected, and the syndromes linked with it [8, 10]. The following are the criteria that are being considered:

1. Pain Physiology: Pain can be characterised as nociceptive, neuropathic, or inflammatory based on the underlying physiological processes.

2. Intensity: Pain severity can be classified as mild, moderate, or severe and is frequently quantified using a numeric pain rating scale ranging from 0 to 10.

3. Time Course: We can classify pain as acute or chronic based on its length.

4. Type of Tissue Involved: Pain can originate in a variety of tissues, including skin, muscles, viscera, joints, tendons, and bones.

5. Syndromes: Certain illnesses, such as cancer, fibromyalgia, migraine, and others, may produce different pain patterns.

6. Psychological state, age, gender, and cultural background can all impact how pain is perceived and managed.

The clinical assessment and management of pain can be aided by the pain classification system. There are three types of pain: acute, chronic, and acute-on-chronic. Chronic pain, in contrast to acute pain, is often persistent, lasting 3–6 months or longer, and has even been characterised as an illness in and of itself rather than just a symptom of a pathological condition. While surgical procedures are the most common cause of acute pain, trauma, and medical conditions, including myocardial infarction and colic, can also contribute to this type of discomfort. Acute pain serves as a protective mechanism to alert the body to impending or existing tissue harm. This causes the action to be interrupted, it draws attention to the location of the damage, and it encourages behaviour in order to get away from the unpleasant stimuli. This syndrome is known as acute-on-chronic pain, and it occurs when a person taking analgesics for chronic pain experiences abrupt, severe flare-ups or breakthrough pain. It is present in 70 per cent of people who suffer from chronic pain.

Pain can range from low to moderate to severe, depending on the context. It is possible that a patient is experiencing more than one kind of discomfort. There may be a combination of nociceptive and neuropathic pain in a particular clinical condition. Both acute and chronic pain are crippling, and a person's mental health can have an impact on their pain levels. Patients suffering from persistent or unmanageable pain frequently experience severe affective (emotional) disturbances, which is a compelling but usually maladaptive state. More than 20% of the global population experiences chronic pain, and 20% of all physicians' visits are attributed to this condition. An increasing number of people around the world are unable to work due to chronic discomfort. Many people with chronic pain do not know what causes it. The gradual onset of this condition is accompanied by feelings of powerlessness and despair. Since chronic pain is never-ending and never-going, it increases the risk of psychological and emotional complications, including anxiety and depression, for the person experiencing it. Anxiety and depression can make the discomfort worse. There are situations when pharmacological approaches to the treatment of chronic pain are not successful.

2.2 Pain assessment

The process of assessing an individual's pain is the first stage of history-taking and physical examination. A thorough physical examination, a detailed medical history, a "pain history," and an evaluation of any functional impairment or treatment-related side effects are all necessary components of an accurate assessment of acute pain. It is crucial to do assessments at suitable intervals when managing severe pain. It is helpful to differentiate between the various types of pain, since the most likely duration of the pain and the response to analgesic techniques can vary from one type of pain to another. This assessment requires the use of appropriate measurement instruments to ensure consistent evaluation in both restful and active phases [11, 12]. As described in 2010 and 2011 [12] by Richard, Powell, Herr, Coyne, and McCaffery, the PQRST Method for Pain Assessment provides a methodical way to comprehend and treat pain. This strategy includes the following questions frequently posed by healthcare providers:

P (Provoking factors): What causes the pain to become more severe or to be triggered? What causes it to improve or make it worse? Q (Quality): How would you describe the pain's characteristics? Are there any other ways to describe it, such as tingling, scorching, stabbing, or shooting?

R (Region and Radiation): Where is the pain located, and does it spread to other parts of the body? S (symptoms and severity): How severe is the pain? Does it interfere with your daily activities? Could you please tell me how severe the discomfort is, from 1 to 10? Prior to employing this scale with a patient, it is imperative to elucidate the significance of the numerical values. The numerical values on the scale indicate the level of pain, ranging from no pain (0) to the worst possible pain (10). Healthcare workers frequently describe the 0–10 scale and ask patients to identify the corresponding number.

T (Timing and Treatment): Does the discomfort come and go, or does it occur frequently? Did the onset occur abruptly or progressively? How frequently does it occur, and how long does it last? Is there a particular time of day when the pain is more intense, such as in the morning? Does the pain worsen before or after meals?

Triage: The first foundation for triage in a hospital setting is established by employing guidelines for pain management. This strategy assures rapid service and immediate medical reaction, and it serves as a model for patient care in hospitals. Additionally, it makes communication between the physicians and nurses who are responsible for the delivery of treatment easier.

Measuring pain is complicated because it is hard to define. Assessing the level of pain that a person is experiencing can be rather challenging. To evaluate this, the individual patient's personal report is typically used to evaluate this. The effects of medication, mood, and sleep disruption on these self-reporting measures are unclear. Hyperalgesia (e.g., mechanical withdrawal threshold), the stress response (e.g., plasma cortisol concentrations), behavioural responses (e.g., facial expressions), functional impairment (e.g., coughing and ambulation), or physiological responses (e.g., changes in heart rate) may occasionally serve as supplementary indicators. One way to increase awareness and use of pain assessment is to record pain intensity as "the fifth vital sign." is one way to do that. It is important to measure pain regularly and repeatedly in order to determine if analgesic medication is effective over time.

The physiological instrument alone is insufficient for pain measurement. The most effective clinical instrument would have physical (physiological), behavioural, and self-report components. Physiological markers of pain, however, can be extremely helpful in assessing a patient's pain experience in critically ill and unconscious individuals [8, 9].

Physiological manifestations of pain include the following:

a. Tachycardia may manifest;

b. Alterations in respiratory rate and depth of respiration may occur, manifesting as oscillations, contractions, or a shift in pattern;

c. The development of hypertension may follow;

d. A decrease in oxygen saturation;

e. Sweating;

f. High blood glucose;

g. Poor organ perfusion;

h. Decreased gastric acid secretion;

i. Decreased gastrointestinal motility;

j. Pallor or flushing sensation; and

k. Pupillary dilatation.

The occurrence of neuropathic pain, surgical or other complications, or uncontrolled pain should always cause a re-evaluation of the diagnosis. Consideration

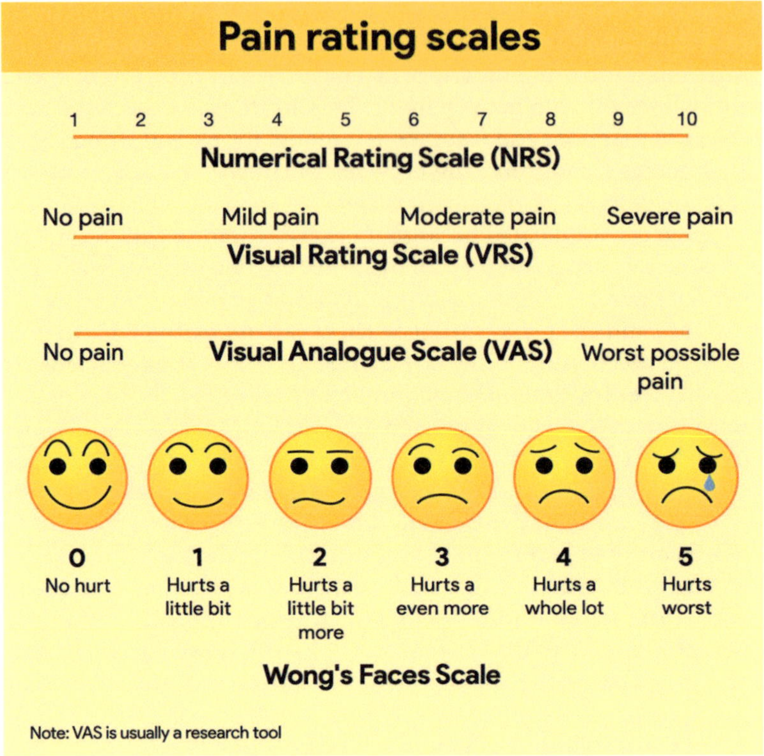

Figure 2.
Pain rating scales.

should be given to having the case reviewed by a specialist group or acute pain service. While there are multidimensional pain scales, unidimensional scales are more commonly employed for post-surgical pain evaluation due to their practicality. Departmental choice is taken into consideration when selecting from the often-described possibilities (**Figure 2**). It may be difficult to get accurate self-reports of pain from certain patients, such as those with impaired consciousness or cognitive impairment, very young children, very old patients, or in cases where communication breaks down because of language barriers, reluctance to cooperate, anxiety, or extreme nervousness. In these cases, it is necessary to use alternative pain evaluation tools, such as the FACES visual scale.

The abbreviation "FACES" is widely used in healthcare settings, especially in pediatric care and pain assessment. This acronym refers to the "Faces Pain Scale," a popular and easy-to-understand method of measuring the severity of pain, particularly in people who have trouble expressing themselves verbally. From happy or neutral features to faces showing escalating degrees of misery or pain, the Pain Scale usually has a variety of expressions to choose from. The abbreviation "FACES" can be broken down into the following:

1. F – Faces: The faces used in the pain scale are what this refers to visually. These expressions cover a wide spectrum of human emotions, from contentment and happiness to sorrow and distress.

2. A – Assessment: The Faces Pain Scale is designed to measure the intensity of pain. It gives patients a consistent way to express their pain levels by pointing to the face that best fits their emotions.

3. C – Communication: When verbal communication is difficult or nonexistent, the Faces Pain Scale can help patients and healthcare providers communicate more effectively. Instead of only describing their suffering verbally, it lets them show how much they're hurting.

4. E – Evaluation: Medical professionals can track the evolution of pain levels with the use of the Faces Pain Scale. Providers can monitor whether pain is improving or increasing and alter treatment programs appropriately by comparing the patient's selected face on the scale during several evaluations.

5. S – Standardization: The Faces Pain Scale offers a standardized way to measure pain, allowing for simpler comparisons of pain levels across various people and environments.

Pain assessment techniques are made more consistent and reliable by this standardization. The Faces Pain Scale is a useful instrument for pain assessment and management in healthcare settings, especially for people who may have trouble verbalizing their pain experiences. The expansion of "FACES" emphasizes its main components and goals.

3. Pain management

It is essential for nurses to make diagnoses in order to properly identify and treat patients who are experiencing pain. The management of pain, particularly in surgical settings, is a multidimensional process [4, 8, 12], and this suggests that postoperative patients may continue to experience difficulties in their recovery. Pain management, which is a fundamental nursing duty, is an essential component of postoperative hospital care. One must be aware of the ways in which nursing practices are influenced by cultural norms and expectations in order to learn how to properly treat pain [4, 12, 13]. It is of the utmost importance to acknowledge that pain that is not treated effectively might worsen and result in more severe acute pain, along with additional negative repercussions [12, 13].

Although medical knowledge has progressed and new ideas on pain physiology and pain management have emerged, the World Health Organisation's (WHO) analgesic ladder has served as a useful and straightforward framework for pharmaceutical pain management since 1986. Patients who suffer from chronic non-cancer pain (CNCP) should continue to use the analgesic ladder. According to the findings of Yang and colleagues [12] research, the WHO analgesic ladder for cancer pain is not suitable for the management of CNCP at the present time (**Figure 3**). The updated protocol is structured as a four-step ladder, with integrative therapies being implemented at each level to decrease or eliminate the use of opioid analgesics. Interventional therapies are evaluated at step 3, and if non-opioids and weak opioids are unsuccessful in managing CNCP, strong opioids can be upgraded. It has been suggested as a straightforward and helpful guideline by the WHO for analgesia in previous years,

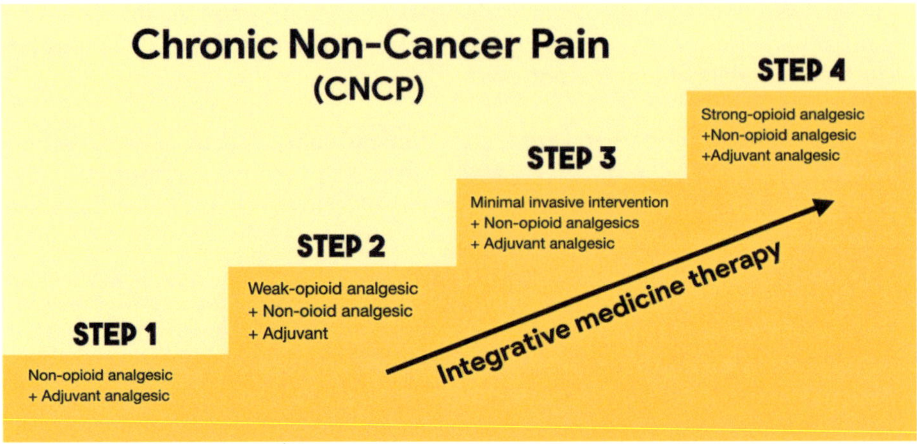

Figure 3.
Chronic non-cancer pain.

but it is not applicable to the present application of CNCP management. As a means of controlling chronic non-specific pain (CNCP), it is recommended to use a revised four-step analgesic ladder that is in line with the principles of integrative medicine and least-invasive therapies.

WHO analgesic ladder states that there are three stages that make up the progression of the level of pain that is experienced. The utilisation of non-opioid adjuncts, such as paracetamol, aspirin, or non-steroidal anti-inflammatory medications (NSAIDs), is the initial step in the process. It is possible to supplement step 1 medicine with weak opioids (such as codeine or tramadol) if the pain remains uncontrolled or is getting worse. Stronger opioids are added to the treatment plan for moderate to severe pain, or for pain that does not go away or gets worse after step 2. The term "multimodal analgesia" applies to each of these approaches. Though used in reverse order in cases of acute pain, the analgesic ladder is an essential component of individual patients' analgesic plans, along with complementary therapy. There are multiple areas of action for analgesics. There are a variety of painkillers, some of which work locally to reduce inflammation-related pain (e.g., non-steroidal anti-inflammatory drugs; NSAIDs); others modify transmission in the dorsal horn; yet others influence the central component and emotional aspects of pain (e.g., opioids and antidepressants); and still others modify nerve conduction (e.g., local anaesthetics).

There is a correlation between effective pain control and better postoperative mobility, which includes activities such as turning over in bed, sitting at the bedside, standing, and walking. Efficient management of pain results in favourable outcomes on multiple levels, including those for the patient, the care unit that the patient is assigned to, and the hospital as a whole.

Among these outcomes are the reduction of complications and suffering for the patient, the enhancement of the quality of care, the enhancement of interdisciplinary teamwork, the establishment of effective referral procedures, and the development of pain management practices within the nursing team [4, 13–17]. A decrease in readmissions, a shorter length of stay in the hospital, a reduction in medical costs, and an increase in patient satisfaction are all results experienced by hospitals [14–17]. Activities that comprise pain management include appropriate nursing interventions, administration of pain medication, and provision of information and guidance. Active listening, demonstrating empathy, and the utilisation of physical measures such as breathing exercises, turning and positioning, wound care, therapeutic temperature applications, and massages are all examples of therapies that may be utilised.

Additionally, psychological and behavioural treatments, such as cognitive-behavioural approaches, stress management, patient and family education, self-management counselling groups, and collaboration with multidisciplinary teams of experts, play an important part in the provision of pain management services. The term "quality" has long been defined by nurses as the observance of quality care standards, yet, patients frequently have an unclear understanding of what constitutes quality treatment [4, 13]. As a means of establishing a common understanding of quality care, this study highlights the significance of enhanced communication between nurses and patients. There is a direct correlation between patient happiness and the likelihood that they will seek additional treatment at a facility that is well-known for providing high-quality care. Patient intent to suggest a facility is of the utmost significance in today's healthcare environments, which are characterised by intense competition and a strong emphasis on economic factors. It has been found in previous studies that patients and healthcare personnel, such as physicians and nurses, are frequently held responsible for inadequate pain treatment. Possible patient-related obstacles may arise from apprehensions over the adverse effects of pain medicine and a refusal to take prescribed medications.

It is intriguing to consider the possibility that the prevalent patterns and rituals in nursing culture, as highlighted by an intriguing discovery by Chatchumni and colleagues [4], could impede the acceptance of innovative multimodal care models, the utilisation of research, and evidence-based practices. This may help to explain why nurses do not always give hospitalised postoperative patients proper pain management.

A crucial component of postoperative patient care is the management of pain that patients experience following surgery. There can be no moral or ethical justification for failing to alleviate pain. Relieving pain effectively is a crucial component of high-quality care. Timely and consistent pain evaluation, on par with other essential health indicators, together with appropriate intervention by all healthcare professionals, possibly utilising acute pain services, will result in enhanced patient outcomes and satisfaction. This can be achieved by providing instruction, implementing departmental protocols, conducting regular practice audits of practice, and providing feedback to the professionals involved.

According to the Nursing Diagnoses Definitions and Classification [18], nursing diagnoses can encompass, among other things, the following, depending on the evidence that is available:

1. Acute pain related to tissue trauma or injury.

2. Ineffective airway clearance related to severe chest pain, which could impair their ability to clear secretions.

3. Ineffective breathing patterns related to pain and respiratory difficulties may make patients hesitant to take deep breaths.

4. Impaired mobility related to conditions such as fractures or arthritis.

5. Knowledge deficits related to a lack of information.

6. Anxiety related to past experiences.

7. Sleep pattern disturbance related to increased pain.

3.1 Non-pharmacological pain management approaches

Both psychological and physical forms of therapy are available. Therapies address a variety of aspects of the human condition are addressed by therapies. Physiotherapy, heat and cold treatment, massage, relaxation techniques, music therapy, and self-hypnosis are the six components that make up the approach.

Psychotherapy is an effective method for improving self-management skills in the context of pain by addressing the social, emotional, cognitive, and behavioural aspects that cause and contribute to pain-related dysfunction and misery. Chronic pain has the potential to foster the formation of maladaptive thoughts and actions that impair daily functioning, exacerbate psychiatric distress, or extend the duration of pain perception [12–17, 19, 20].

Cognitive-behavioural therapy (CBT): Both personal thoughts and physical injury can have an impact on one's perception of pain. One of the cornerstones of CBT is the idea that dysfunctional ways of thinking lead to the perpetuation of distressing emotions and problematic behaviours. Cognitive-behavioural therapy (CBT) relies on the patient's ability to recognise negative beliefs about pain and substitute them with more constructive ones. Individuals suffering from chronic pain often find relief through cognitive-behavioural therapy (CBT) [12].

Relaxation techniques: These can help you calm down, get rid of stress, and feel less pain. Some strategies that people often use to relax include aromatherapy, which involves using certain scents to alleviate tension and discomfort and promote relaxation. Additionally, it makes use of oils, extracts, and smells derived from flowers, herbs, and trees. During massages, facials, and baths, the ingredients can be inhaled directly into the lungs or applied directly to the body. These techniques involve deep breathing, which is beneficial for relaxation and has the potential to reduce pain.

Guided imagery is a therapeutic technique whereby patients concentrate on mental pictures to induce positive emotions or a state of relaxation. One learns to prioritise the image over their discomfort [13–17, 19, 20].

Music therapy has the potential to lift spirits and rev up energy levels. By causing the body to release endorphins, it may be able to assist in the reduction of pain. According to Lopez and colleagues [13], music can be used in conjunction with any of the other approaches described, including relaxation and distraction.

Self-hypnosis is a technique that allows a person to focus their attention on something other than the sensation of pain. One strategy is to tell oneself encouraging things, such as how one can ignore or view the discomfort in a positive light [13].

The nursing profession commonly makes use of the following concepts: environment, health, care, humanity, adaptation, and body, soul, and spirit. The term "integrative nursing" describes a style of care that considers the whole person in their unaltered form. The goal of integrative nursing is to treat the whole person, not just their symptoms, by considering the patient in context with their physical environment. In order to research integrated nursing, which is a means of providing patients with aid in obtaining optimal health by utilising both activities and the environment [17], the purpose of this study is to investigate integrated nursing. The body, the soul,

DOI: http://dx.doi.org/10.5772/intechopen.1004731

and the spirit all benefited from the sounds that were included in the anthology. The use of five guiding principles and standards of practice is the foundation upon which holistic nursing is founded, as indicated by previous research. The objectives encompass a wide range of topics, such as: holistic theory, ethics, and philosophy; holistic care; holistic communication; holistic practice standards that respect cultural diversity and therapeutic settings; holistic education and research; and holistic self-care for nurses. The educational programme for pain management based on evidence greatly enhanced nurses' understanding of the symptoms, consequences, and treatments for uncontrolled pain. The education programme and pain management algorithm led to an increase in patient satisfaction with pain management, as evidenced by increased ratings on the Healthcare Providers and Systems Pain.

4. Conclusion

The culture among nurses in the field of pain management may impact the postoperative pain care provided. The nurses, who are essential components of the healthcare system, should adhere to the criteria for evidence-based practice in order to provide patients with the highest possible level of care. This study's concentration on the dynamic relationship between clinical settings and professional practices will improve our understanding of professional development and practice-based knowledge. The results of subsequent studies will enhance our knowledge of one group of nurses' practices and culture. Acquiring this knowledge will play a crucial role in elevating the consciousness and implementation of pain management within this specialised cohort. This research will undoubtedly generate insights into nursing and its practices. The health and well-being of patients who have just undergone surgery are inextricably tied to proper pain management from their point of view.

Conflict of interest

The authors declare no conflict of interest.

Author details

Manaporn Chatchumni
School of Nursing, Rangsit University, Pathumthani, Thailand

*Address all correspondence to: manaporn@rsu.ac.th

References

[1] McCaffery M. Nursing Practice Theories Related to Cognition, Bodily Pain, and Man-Environment Interactions. Los Angeles: University of California at LA Students Store; 1968

[2] Barke A, Korwisi B, Jakob R, Konstanjsek N, Rief W, Treede RD. Classification of chronic pain for the international classification of diseases (ICD-11): Results of the 2017 international World Health Organization field testing. Pain. 2022;**163**(2):e310-e318. DOI: 10.1097/j.pain.0000000000002287

[3] Hinkle JL, Cheever KH. Brunner & Suddarth's Textbook of Medical-Surgical Nursing. 13th ed. Philadelphia: Wolters Kluwer, Williams & Wilkins; 2014. pp. 212-236

[4] Chatchumni M, Namvongprom A, Eriksson H, Mazaheri M. Treating without seeing: Pain management practice in a Thai context. Pain Research and Management. 2016;**2016**:9580626. DOI: 10.1155/2016/9580626

[5] Frasco PE, Sprung J, Trentman TL. The impact of the joint commission for accreditation of healthcare organizations pain initiative on perioperative opiate consumption and recovery room length of stay. Anesthesia & Analgesia. 2005;**100**(1):162-168. DOI: 10.1213/01.ANE.0000139354.26208.1C

[6] Gordon DB, Dahl JL, Miaskowski C, McCarberg B, Todd KH, Paice JA, et al. American pain society recommendations for improving the quality of acute and cancer pain management: American pain society quality of care task force. Archives of Internal Medicine. 2005;**165**(14):1574-1580. DOI: 10.1001/archinte.165.14.1574

[7] The Oregon Pain Guidance Group (OPG). A Provider and Community Resource: Pain Treatment Guidelines. Oregon, United States: The Oregon Pain Guidance Group (OPG); 2016. Available from: https://professional.oregonpainguidance.org/wp-content/uploads/sites/2/2014/04/ OPG_Guidelines_2016.pdf

[8] Koneti KK, Jones M. Management of acute pain. Surgery (Oxford). 2016;**34**(2):84-90. DOI: 10.1016/j.mpsur.2015.11.008

[9] Melzack R, Wall PD. Pain mechanisms: A new theory: A gate control system modulates sensory input from the skin before it evokes pain perception and response. Science. 1965;**150**(3699):971-979

[10] Herr K, Coyne PJ, McCaffery M, Manworren R, Merkel S. Pain assessment in the patient unable to self-report: Position statement with clinical practice recommendations. Pain Management Nursing. 2011;**12**(4):230-250. DOI: 10.1016/j.pmn.2011.10.002

[11] Soenarto RF, Sukmono B, Findyartini A, Susilo AP. Improvement in medical students' knowledge on chronic pain assessment through integrative learning approaches: A randomized controlled trial. Frontiers in Pain Research. 2023;**4**:1210370. DOI: 10.3389/fpain.2023.1210370

[12] Yang J, Bauer BA, Wahner-Roedler DL, Chon TY, Xiao L. The modified WHO analgesic ladder: Is it appropriate for chronic non-cancer pain? Journal of Pain Research. 2020;**17**(13):411-417. DOI: 10.2147/JPR.S244173

[13] Powell RA, Downing J, Ddungu H, Mwangi-Powell FN. Pain history and pain assessment. In: Guide to Pain Management in Low-Resource Settings. Vol. 67. Washington, United States, Kampala, Uganda: International Association for the Study of Pain; 2010. Available from: https://www.aped-dor.org/images/diversos/documentos/iasp_guide.pdf#page=79

[14] Lewis MJ, Kohtz C, Emmerling S, Fisher M, Mcgarvey J. Pain control and nonpharmacologic interventions. Nursing. 2018;**48**(9):65-68. DOI: 10.1097/01.NURSE.0000544231.59222.ab

[15] Chatchumni M, Eriksson H, Mazaheri M. Core components of an effective pain management education programme for surgical nurses: A Delphi study. International Journal of Qualitative Studies on Health and Well-Being. 2022;**17**(1):2110672. DOI: 10.1080/17482631.2022.2110672

[16] Herdman TH, editor. Nursing Diagnoses 2012-14: Definitions and Classification. Hoboken, New Jersey, United States: John Wiley & Sons; 2011

[17] DeVore J, Clontz A, Ren D, Cairns L, Beach M. Improving patient satisfaction with better pain management in hospitalized patients. The Journal for Nurse Practitioners. 2017;**13**(1):e23-e27. DOI: 10.1016/j.nurpra.2016.07.020

[18] NANDA International. Nursing Diagnoses: Definitions and Classification 2009-2011. West Sussex, UK: Wiley-Blackwell; 2009

[19] Chatchumni M, Eriksson H, Mazaheri M. A scoping review of pain management education programs (PMEPs): Do they prepare nurses to deal with patients' postoperative pain? Pain Research and Management. 2020;**2020**:4062493. DOI: 10.1155/2020/4062493

[20] Eaton LH, Meins AR, Zeliadt SB, Doorenbos AZ. Using a mixed methods approach to explore factors associated with evidence-based cancer pain management practice among nurses. Applied Nursing Research: ANR. 2017;**37**:55-60. DOI: 10.1016/j.apnr.2017.07.008

Chapter 4

Mental Illness among Young Adults in Primary Care and Community Context

Ulrica Lovén Wickman and Corné Coetzee

Abstract

Nurses are important in primary care and community contexts to apply actions and interventions to the needs and interests of young adults. This chapter aims to explore health-promotive actions for young adults with mental illness and move nursing theories into the context. The journey of recovery from substance use disorder is a complex and multifaceted process, particularly poignant in the lives of young adults. This developmental period is marked by identity formation, exploration, and navigating societal expectations. Recognizing and understanding the dynamic nature of recovery, the pivotal role of social support, and the inherent resilience of this population provides a foundation for developing targeted interventions. Another aspect is to enrich the development of skills for nurses by the use of more knowledge of nursing theories. Primary prevention efforts should be tailored to meet the needs of both nurses and young adults. These thoughts are both challenging and create new possibilities. Furthermore, nurses need more knowledge, which will give them the opportunity to make a difference.

Keywords: community, intervention, mental health, mental illness, nursing, perspectives, primary care, young adults

1. Introduction

Mental illness is a widespread public health problem, and a large proportion of those who suffer from it are young adults. Young adults are overrepresented among people with mental illness, and the condition can cause both physical and psychological problems. It creates a huge barrier of suffering, financial loss through a dysfunctional working life, and reduced quality of life. There is a stigma around mental illness, which is often considered to be due to a lack of knowledge about mental illness. This constitutes a basis for poorer treatment [1]. This, in turn, constitutes a basis for poorer treatment [1, 2]. Adolescents and young adults hold stigmatizing beliefs about mental health treatments, health professionals, and access to care. The sources of these beliefs remain unclear, although some may be influenced by culture [2].

Mental illness encompasses a spectrum of health conditions characterized by alterations in emotion, cognition, and behavior. Despite its prevalence and impact, the absence of definition underscores the complexity of this phenomenon. Serving as an overarching term, mental illness incorporates diverse conditions that vary in duration and intensity, collectively impinging on a young adult's capacity to navigate and adapt to daily life challenges. This term encompasses a wide array of mental illness, spanning from severe psychiatric disorders to milder and moderate conditions. The array of mental illness includes well-known conditions such as depression, schizophrenia, autism spectrum disorder (ASD), anxiety disorders, obsessive-compulsive disorder, adjustment disorder, eating disorders, personality disorders, attention deficit hyperactivity disorder (ADHD), and substance use disorder (SUD). Each condition presents unique challenges, affecting young adults to varying extents [3].

Young adults' experiences from primary care are described as facing difficulties in accepting help, relational preconditions, structural and organizational hindrances, and satisfaction with youth-focused mental health interventions. They experience difficulties in accessing and receiving proper help from primary care. Further, they do not believe in recovery from mental illness, and they also express a lack of mental health literacy [4]. Primary care nurses (PCN) are advanced nurses in primary care or community context. Further, in the text, nurse or nurses will be mentioned.

On average, young students spend 3.38 ± 0.80 h on social media. Most-used social networks are shown as YouTube (98.8%), WhatsApp (98.4%), Facebook (93.2%), Instagram (88.1%), and Snapchat (48.5%) or TikTok (47.3%). The main reasons why students use these networks are shown as primarily socialization (49.0%, n = 209) and entertainment (31.1%, n = 133) [5].

Prevalence of loneliness for adolescents ranges from 9.2% in South-East Asia to 14.4% (12.2 to 17.1%) in the Eastern Mediterranean region. The lowest prevalence of loneliness is observed in northern European countries (2.9, 1.8 to 4.5% for young adults and the highest in eastern European countries (7.5, 5.9 to 9.4% for young adults [6].

About one in ten young adults has an income that is below the threshold for what is required for a reasonable standard of living, and about one in four young adults has had difficulties meeting their current expenses. The economic vulnerability of young people draws attention to the fact that there are large differences in the financial situation of young adults aged 20–25. The majority of the group has good living conditions, but there are large differences within the youth group. The higher financial income relates to higher self-esteem [5]. Data from suicide research indicates that in the age group 15–24 years, the number of suicides has increased by approximately one percent per year over the past 20 years [7].

2. Recovery perspectives among young adults with substance use disorder

Substance use disorder (SUD) is understood as a biopsychosocial disorder. Young adults who want to stop using substances or improve their well-being while using substances need to undergo a recovery process [8]. The road to recovery for young adults living with mental illness is often long and looks different depending on the condition and problem. SUD and recovery should be understood using the same coherent approach – as an interplay between biological and psychological factors and social, political, and cultural contexts [8]. Recovery is a way to achieve developmental milestones shared by other young adults and a way to return to normalcy. It is described as multifaceted, with many participants citing the integral role that mental health played in their substance use disorder (SUD), and the need to address this in their recovery. Recovery from SUD is therefore increasingly recognized as a dynamic and individualized process, encompassing various dimensions such as physical, emotional, and social well-being [9]. The interplay of physical, emotional, and social dimensions in their recovery process underscores the need for comprehensive, holistic interventions [9]. Young adults feel stressed that recovery from substance use disorder (SUD) has to be self-motivated and is a process that requires consistent work. The recovery perspectives of young adults unveil narratives of transformation marked by both vulnerability and strength.

The challenges faced by young adults in recovery are manifold, ranging from societal stigma to internal struggles with identity and purpose [10]. Despite these hurdles, many exhibit remarkable resilience, drawing on factors such as self-efficacy, motivation, and a sense of purpose to sustain their recovery efforts [11, 12]. Unfortunately, there are societal barriers that reduce the opportunities for young adults with mental health challenges to enter the job market and advance in their careers. Societal attitudes, various policies, and organizational practices are examples of such barriers [13]. In working life, young adults with mental health challenges are seen as less attractive to hire, and difficulties in meeting work demands are reported by young adults with mental illness [14]. This can lead to mental health challenges, ultimately resulting in sick leave [14, 15].

For young adults involved, recuperation served to attain the developmental goals common among their peers, aiming to regain a sense of "normalcy." They depicted recovery as a complex journey, with a significant emphasis on the pivotal role of mental health in their SUD and the necessity to address it during their recovery. Young adults emphasize that the recovery process from SUD had to be driven by their own motivation and demanded unwavering, continuous effort [12].

Furthermore, they highlighted the need for access to professional and social support during the recovery process [8]. Young adults, in particular, often rely heavily on their social networks for encouragement and validation [16]. Primary care, peers, family, and community support can serve as crucial catalysts or barriers to recovery.

3. The perspective of nurses meeting young adults with mental illness in primary care or community context

The most common way for a person with mental illness is contact with a primary care nurse (PCN) [17]. Effective treatment of young adults with mental illness provides them with the opportunity to be actively involved in their care. A reciprocal relationship marked by dedication from healthcare professionals enhances patient engagement. Nurses engaging with young adults affected by mental illness underscore the critical role of knowledge in this context. A profound understanding of mental illness enables the comprehensive collection of patient history and facilitates appropriate referrals for specialized assistance. Emphasizing the importance of accessing the right healthcare professional for mental health concerns, Nurses reveal a disconcerting reality – they perceive that young adults grappling with mental health issues often experience a lapse in the provision of adequate care. Furthermore, nurses lament the inadequacy of resources and knowledge within primary care settings, asserting that this deficit impedes the establishment of a trustworthy therapeutic relationship with young adults affected by mental illness (**Figure 1**) [18].

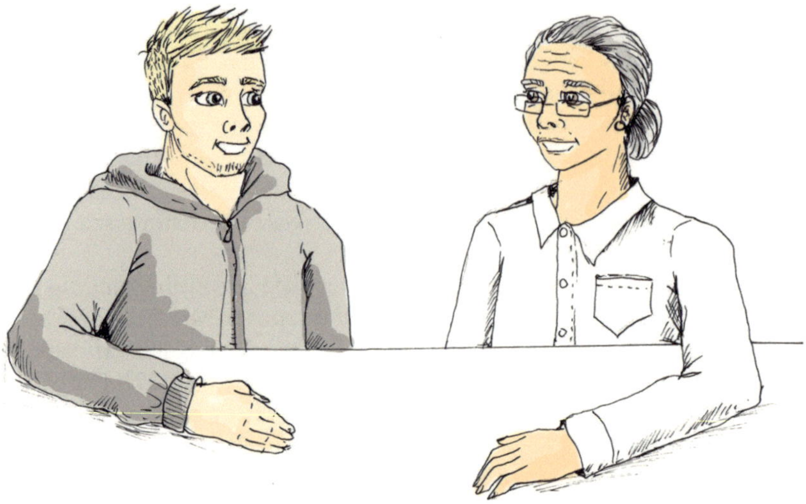

Figure 1.
The therapeutic relationship illustrated by Aline Grindatto.

The experience of nurses engaging with young adults with mental illness is characterized by a recognition of the considerable time investment required for these young adults. Furthermore, there is a discernible upward trend in the number of young adults presenting with mental illness in primary care [18]. These young adults encounter difficulties in accepting assistance, contend with relational barriers, grapple with structural and organizational impediments, and express satisfaction with mental health interventions [4]. This encounter is described as emotionally challenging by nurses, who convey a sense of frustration and helplessness in their work with mental illness [18].

The confluence of numerous demands and societal pressures exerted on young adults, emanating primarily from educational institutions and broader societal expectations, has the potential to evoke a sense of frustration among nurses. This frustration, in turn, contributes to an increased complexity in managing their interactions. The nurses articulate that the escalating demands and pressures on young adults serve as significant contributing factors to the onset of mental illness, with contemporary society being identified as a source of heightened stress.

The strategies of "Listen, confirm, and dare to ask" have demonstrated significance in comprehending the experiences of young adults when they seek assistance at health centers. The study established that young adults are frequently perceived as delicate, underscoring the importance of active listening and trust-building as pivotal tools in facilitating effective communication. The exploration of family dynamics and social networks emerges as an integral component of these conversations [18].

4. Theories in nursing for recovery

4.1 The tidal model

The Tidal model is considered a person-centered and holistic theory. The theory was created in the late 1990s. The model is based on a philosophical approach to recovery and to the identification of mental illness. The focus is on a person's stories, the person, and their experiences. The theory states that healthcare professionals need to learn about these stories and experiences to provide the right support and help young adults living with mental illness. One part of the model is described as the commitment of the healthcare professionals. The commitment determines whether a genuine relationship with the person can be created or not. With a genuine relationship, life problems can be identified. The commitment strengthens the relationship, which contributes to the development and recovery of the young adult. Through guidance to the right choice in life, the young adult is guided through difficulties in life. The greatest need for young adults with mental illness is support, and they need someone who can meet their needs without being drawn into the process themselves. The experiences need to be shared with someone. As nurses become involved in young adult's problems, they get to share stories, and they need to show that they are not afraid to meet the person where they are with their life problems. The theory points out that nurses should not be emotionally or spiritually affected in the process. The nurse is seen as a help to the young adult to regain control over life, the life conditions, the experiences, and continue the life journey. Autonomy and empowerment are at the center [19].

The theory was first created for acute psychiatric care but is seen to be relevant in other care units such as primary care and community contexts. The study of nursing theories, Phil Barker's model, brings contributions to the theoretical framework of nursing when thinking of concepts that make up the metaparadigm of science nursing, contributing to care science. Contributions to nursing practice, enabling person-centered care and experiences of the young adults, giving voice to subjects and reorienting the mental health care paradigm. The theory emphasizes a paradigm for mental health nursing, with a view to interdisciplinary work and the empowerment of nurses and subjects in mental illness [19].

Numerous studies in mental health nursing care draw upon the Tidal model. This model remains in a continuous state of development, enjoys international utilization and manifests in diverse life cycles within various services pertaining to mental and psychiatric health nursing practices. It is advisable to conduct research that delves deeper into the theoretical concepts, refining the model and tailoring it to the varied contexts within mental health [19].

4.2 Mental health continuum: flourishing

As a persistent and substantial deviation from normal functioning, mental illness impairs the execution of social roles, and it is associated with emotional suffering. The mental health continuum applies an operationalization of mental health as a syndrome of symptoms of positive feelings and positive functioning in life. It summarizes the scales and dimensions of subjective well-being, which are symptoms of mental health. The presence of mental health is described as flourishing; the absence of mental health is characterized as languishing in life. Positive functioning consists of six dimensions of psychological well-being: self-acceptance, positive relations with others, personal growth, purpose in life, environmental mastery, and autonomy. However, there is more to functioning well in life than psychological well-being. Positive functioning includes social challenges and tasks and is expressed in five dimensions of social well-being. Psychological well-being represents more private and personal criteria for evaluation of one's functioning, and social well-being epitomizes the more public and social criteria whereby people evaluate their functioning in life. These social dimensions consist of *social coherence, social actualization, social integration, social acceptance, and social contribution* [20].

4.3 The self-determination theory

The self-determination theory (SDT) is a well-researched theoretical framework that can be applied to gain a better understanding of recovery [21]. A motivational theory that posits three fundamental human needs (autonomy, competence, and relatedness to others), the self-determination theory shows striking similarity to basic ideas on recovery [22]. Social environments that contribute to the development of these three basic needs are autonomy-supportive, well-structured, warm, and responsive. Autonomy-supportive environments foster the growth of young adults' intrinsic motivation by cultivating their inner resources. Internal motivation refers to "the inherent tendency to seek out novelty and challenges, to extend and exercise one's capacities, to explore, and to learn." Such motivation reflects our human capacities, the need to explore, show curiosity, express interest, and seek mastery. The achievement of internal motivation likely occurs as young adults progress to more advanced stages of recovery. An assumption in SDT is that motivation exists on a continuum ranging from amotivation (lack of motivation to engage) to extrinsic motivation or intrinsic motivation, with intrinsic motivation being the most effective in well-being and ongoing behavior. Communication within autonomy-supportive environments relies on informal and noncontrolling language, emphasizing collaboration and understanding [21].

5. Application of theories and opportunities of nursing to promote health for young adults in communities and primary care

The young adult's story represents the start and endpoint of the helping encounter. It embraces not only an account of the young adult's distress but also the young adult's hope for its resolution. The Tidal model seeks to help young adults express their experiences in a version of "their story." The nurse needs to demonstrate a capacity to listen actively to the young adults' story and help to record their story in their own words at every stage of the caring relationship. By valuing – and using – the young adult's own language, the nurse shows the simplest, yet most powerful, respect for the young adult. The nurse helps the young adult express their understanding of personal anecdotes, similes, or metaphors [19]. The Tidal model features commitments described in fundamental values that represent the essence of the therapeutic process. Specific competencies that nurses should have and which facilitate the use of the model in primary care and community context [23, 24].

The SDT approach helps young adults grasp the purpose behind it, reinforcing their sense of autonomy and engagement in the recovery process. Moreover, autonomy-supportive environments promote respect for diverse perspectives, fostering an atmosphere of mutual understanding and open communication. By valuing and acknowledging different perspectives, these environments contribute to a more inclusive and enriching recovery experience. The SDT can also be used to examine work motivation and implementation strategies within primary care and community organizations [21]. The flouring perspective is important according to the positive functioning with dimensions of psychological well-being with self-acceptance, positive relations with others, personal growth, purpose in life, environmental mastery, and autonomy. Positive functioning also includes social challenges and represents private areas of functioning. The social dimensions are also an important aspect of the flourishing perspective [20].

5.1 Reawakening of hope

The reawakening of hope, reclaiming a positive self and meaning through personal growth. Antecedents include the disruption of illness, stigmatization, internal inventory, and contemplative recovery. Identified consequences include the return to normality, reconstruction of self, and active social connection. The conceptual definition is the reawakening of hope and rediscovery of a positive sense of self through finding meaning and purpose within personal growth and connection using creative self-care coping strategies. Hope is essential in the Tidal model [19, 24]. The implication for nursing is the congruence of recovery-orientated practice with the process of recovery experienced by young adults [25].

5.2 Support from others

Young adults with mental illness need support from others. Someone who believes in their ability to regain well-being and helps them start believing in themselves. Conversation plays a significant role in recovery, giving these young adults the opportunity to open. The courage to do so exists in a non-judgmental approach where trust can be built. A changed thought pattern, where acceptance is the key factor, provides strength to young adults. To manage thoughts and emotions, to shift the focus away from distress [19].

Generating knowledge about recovery factors can equip nurses to support young adults with mental illness, ultimately promoting better mental health among young adults. The support to believe in oneself facilitated the recovery and brought them to where they are today. The significance of the social context is emphasized, as it contributes to recovery, increased quality of life, and functionality [26]. For many, the social context is their workplace, where friends and tasks can distract from issues or symptoms in young adults with mental illness. Work also provides a source of income, boosts self-esteem, and empowers. Some may view work as their contribution to society through tax payments. The society affects our health and our socioeconomic status [13, 27]. Positive relations with others and personal growth are important factors [19, 20, 24].

5.3 The importance of time

The perception of time can be deceptive or not entirely consistent with its objective nature, but it is so valuable. The core concern lies in how we opt to utilize the time at our disposal. In the end, our most essential contribution is our time. It is imperative to allocate this time generously and judiciously. The nurse plays a crucial role in making the individual cognizant that focused time is being devoted to addressing challenges in life. The nurse must express an understanding of the significance of the time the young adult is investing in the process [19, 24].

5.4 To promote nature experiences

The allocation of time in natural settings can yield health benefits by facilitating contact with natural elements, engaging in physical activity, promoting the restoration of mental and emotional well-being, and providing opportunities for social interactions. These advantages may manifest immediately, as evidenced by reductions in blood pressure and stress levels, enhanced immune system functioning, and restored attention. Alternatively, some benefits may accrue gradually over time, including weight loss, decreased symptoms of depression, and an overarching improvement in overall wellness [28]. The investment in and active interaction with nature during early life emerges as a predictive factor for later-life involvement in nature-based activities. Moreover, it is indicative of subsequent pro-environmental attitudes, with a probable correlation to pro-environmental behaviors. Consequently, fostering a connection with nature in the next generation should be regarded as a pivotal and collaborative priority in the integration of health and sustainability agendas [29]. A study reveals a significant correlation between connectedness to nature and mental well-being among psychosomatic patients, with both aspects demonstrating noteworthy improvement over time. The young adults' perspectives are reported in the study and highlight positive outcomes in terms of effectiveness, satisfaction, mood and soul-level enhancements, overall well-being, interpersonal connections, and coping mechanisms for addressing problems [30]. Consensus statements provide guidance for healthcare professionals on best-practice approaches to using physical activity to maximize benefits for mental health and well-being. Recommendations are made regarding the type, delivery, social and physical environments, and domain of physical activity to optimize mental health outcomes [31].

The nurses role is to promote health and prevent mental illness; nature experiences and outdoor life can be used as a gateway to a healthier lifestyle. By encouraging young adult to be outside more, and change negative lifestyle, the nurse can encourage young adults to have healthier lifestyle in primary care and community context. Nature can be seen as a stress-relieving factor, both to promote mental health and to treat anxiety and depression. Nature experiences not only have positive effects directly but also cause young adults with depressive symptoms to develop hope for the future and security. For young adults with mental illness, nature can be a refuge that is accessible to all without rules, requirements, and special approaches to consider. There, in the freedom and lack of negative thoughts, you do not put effort into fitting in. Instead, the focus can be on taking in nature's healing properties and not having to worry about being judged by others. Shared moments with others provided them with the opportunity to process their own challenges, but it also afforded them the chance to listen and understand the problems of others [32].

5.5 To develop awareness and motivation

Nurses need to express genuine interest in the young adult's story to create a better understanding. Genuine curiosity reflects an interest in the young adult and the young adult's unique experience. Discovering what is unique about this young adult is quite important and must be the nursing focus. Genuine curiosity is the means to realize it. The nurse shows interest in the young adult's story by asking for clarification and asking for further details. The nurse need to help the young adult to unfold the story at their own pace [19, 24].

The nurse needs to help the young adult to develop awareness of the changes in thoughts, feeling or actions. The nurse helps to develop awareness of how these subtle changes have been influenced by their own actions, the actions of others or by other circumstances. The young adult and the nurse are to become a team. Nurses are in a privileged position and should model confidence by being always transparent; helping the person understand exactly what is being done and why. By using the person's own language, and by completing all assessments and care plan records with the person, the collaborative nature of the nurse-young adult relationship becomes even more transparent. The nurse also needs to be transparent and make the young adult aware of the purpose of all processes of care. The nurse needs to help the young adults develop awareness of personal assets, strengths, or weaknesses. This helps the young adult to get a sense of autonomy or self-belief, promoting an awareness of their ability to help themselves to sustain the young adult throughout the voyage of recovery [23, 24].

5.6 Health conversations

Discussions about lifestyle habits are a crucial component of the nurse's work. These conversations are based on the patient's own perspective on their health and motivation for changing their lifestyle habits. The effects of targeted health discussions have been illuminated in numerous studies [33]. Motivational interviewing is a conversational technique that seeks to elicit the patient's reasons for change and enhance motivation to implement lifestyle changes. The methodology is evidence-based not only for discussions about lifestyle habits but also for other prevalent behavior changes [34].

6. Conclusion

There is hope for young adults' mental health if there is support from those around them and a belief in themselves. The conversation is an important part of the recovery and gives the young adult the opportunity to open. The courage to dare to do so is found in a non-judgmental approach where trust can be created. Confirmation from others through care is empowering for young adults. Acceptance is a key factor that gives strength. To be able to manage the thoughts and feelings, something is needed that can shift the focus from the troublesome. To facilitate the recovery of people with mental illness and in preventive work, the nurse has an important role. Collection of anamneses, guidance for further help and changed behavior as well as coordination of services, are parts of the nurse's work. The recovery perspectives of young adults with SUD illuminate a tapestry of experiences, challenges, and triumphs. Understanding the recovery perspectives of young adults with SUD is crucial for tailoring effective interventions that resonate with their unique challenges. Generating knowledge about factors that favor recovery can lead to the nurses getting tools to support young adults with mental illness. It enables person-centered care and strengthening of empowerment in young adults.

The young adults require support from their surroundings, positive interactions, conversations with others, validation of their feelings, the ability to change their thought patterns, and the discovery of their own methods for managing thoughts and emotions. Everyone needs to find their own motivation. With an understanding of these factors and in line with nursing theories, nurses can promote person-centered care in their interactions in primary care and community context. The responsibilities of nurses encompass the collection of comprehensive anamneses, provision of guidance for further assistance, facilitation of behavioral change, and coordination of services. The accrual of knowledge concerning factors conducive to recovery equips nurses with tools to effectively support young adults grappling with mental illness. This knowledge serves as the foundation for the implementation of person-centered care strategies, thereby fostering empowerment among young adults. Additionally, insights contribute to a ripple effect, mitigating societal stigma and fostering a more permissive environment for young adults contending with mental health challenges.

Acknowledgements

Acknowledgment is to be extended to the youth grappling with mental illness challenges, as, for the primary care nurse, it is important to implement preventive measures and promote health among young adults to establish a foundation for a sustainable society.

Conflict of interest

The author declares that there is no conflict of interest to disclose.

Acronyms and abbreviations

ASD	autism spectrum disorder
ADHD	attention deficit hyperactivity disorder
PCN	primary care nurse
SDT	self-determination theory
SUD	substance use disorder

Author details

Ulrica Lovén Wickman[1]* and Corné Coetzee[2]

1 Department of Health and Caring Sciences, Linnaeus University, Kalmar, Sweden

2 School of Health Care Sciences, Department of Pharmacy, University of Limpopo, Sovenga, South Africa

*Address all correspondence to: ulrica.lovenwickman@lnu.se

References

[1] Fyhn T, Sveinsdottir V, Reme SE, Sandal GM. A mixed methods study of employers' and employees' evaluations of job seekers with a mental illness, disability, or of a cultural minority. Work. 2021;**70**(1):235-245

[2] Goodwin J, Savage E, Horgan A. Adolescents' and young adults' beliefs about mental health services and care: A systematic review. Archives of Psychiatric Nursing. 2016;**30**(5):636-644

[3] World Health Organization (WHO). Mental health of adolescents – key facts: WHO. 2019. Available from: https://www.who.int/news-room/fact-sheets/detail/adolescent-mental-health [Accessed: February 27, 2024]

[4] Lovén Wickman U, Schmidt M. Experiences of primary care among young adults with mental illness - A systematic literature review. Scandinavian Journal of Caring Sciences. 2023;**37**(3):628-641

[5] Pop LM, Iorga M, Iurcov R. Body-esteem, self-esteem and loneliness among social media young users. International Journal of Environmental Research and Public Health. 2022;**19**(9):1-14

[6] Surkalim DL, Luo M, Eres R, Gebel K, van Buskirk J, Bauman A, et al. The prevalence of loneliness across 113 countries: Systematic review and meta-analysis. BMJ. 2022;**376**:e067068

[7] NASP. Nationellt centrum för suicidforskning och prevention – statistik. 2021. Available from: https://ki.se/nasp/statistik-0

[8] Wangensteen T, Hystad J. A comprehensive approach to understanding substance use disorder and recovery: Former patients' experiences and reflections on the recovery process four years after discharge from SUD treatment. Journal of Psychosocial Rehabilitation and Mental Health. 2022;**9**(1):45-54

[9] White WL. The mobilization of community resources to support long-term addiction recovery. Journal of Substance Abuse Treatment. 2009;**36**(2):146-158

[10] Arnett JJ. The developmental context of substance use in emerging adulthood. Journal of Drug Issues. 2005;**35**(2):235-254

[11] Laudet AB. The road to recovery: Where are we going and how do we get there? Empirically driven conclusions and future directions for service development and research. Substance Use & Misuse. 2008;**43**(12-13):2001-2020

[12] Schoenberger SF, Park TW, dellaBitta V, Hadland SE, Bagley SM. "My life Isn't defined by substance use": Recovery perspectives among young adults with substance use disorder. Journal of General Internal Medicine. 2022;**37**(4):816-822

[13] Subramaniam M, Zhang Y, Shahwan S, Vaingankar JA, Satghare P, Teh WL, et al. Employment of young people with mental health conditions: Making it work. Disability and Rehabilitation. 2022;**44**(10):2033-2043

[14] de Groot S, Veldman K, Amick Iii BC, Bültmann U. Work functioning among young adults: The role of mental health problems from childhood to young adulthood. Occupational and Environmental Medicine. 2022;**79**(4):217-223

[15] Framke E, Alexanderson K, Sørensen JK, Pedersen J, Madsen IEH, Rugulies R, et al. Emotional demands and all-cause and diagnosis-specific long-term sickness absence: A prospective cohort study in Sweden. European Journal of Public Health. 2023;**33**(3):435-441

[16] Tracy K, Wallace SP. Benefits of peer support groups in the treatment of addiction. Substance Abuse and Rehabilitation. 2016;**7**:143-154

[17] Bjorkman A, Andersson K, Bergström J, Salzmann-Erikson M. Increased mental illness and the challenges this brings for district nurses in primary care settings. Issues in Mental Health Nursing. 2018;**39**(12):1023-1030

[18] Östangård Olofsson C, Lovén WU. District nurses' experiences of giving initial health care assessment to young adults applying for mental illness in primary care: A qualitative interview study. Primary Health Care Research & Development. 2023;**24**:e27

[19] Barker P, Buchanan-Barker P. The Tidal Model: A Guide for Mental Health Professionals. London: Routledge; 2005

[20] Corey L, Keyes M. The mental health continuum: From languishing to flourishing in life. Journal of Health and Social Behavior. 2002;**43**(2):207-222

[21] Ryan RM, Deci EL. Self-determination theory and the facilitation of intrinsic motivation, social development, and well-being. The American Psychologist. 2000;**55**(1):68-78

[22] Mancini AD. Self-determination theory: A framework for the recovery paradigm. Advances in Psychiatric Treatment. 2008;**14**(5):358-365

[23] Barker P. The tidal model: Psychiatric colonization, recovery and the paradigm shift in mental health care. International Journal of Mental Health Nursing. 2003;**12**(2):96-102

[24] Buchanan-Barker P, Barker PJ. The tidal commitments: Extending the value base of mental health recovery. Journal of Psychiatric and Mental Health Nursing. 2008;**15**(2):93-100

[25] McCauley CO, McKenna HP, Keeney S, McLaughlin DF. Concept analysis of recovery in mental illness in young adulthood. Journal of Psychiatric and Mental Health Nursing. 2015;**22**(8):579-589

[26] Hovland RT, Ytrehus S, Mellor-Clark J, Moltu C. How patients and clinicians experience the utility of a personalized clinical feedback system in routine practice. Journal of Clinical Psychology. 2023;**79**(3):711-728

[27] Wang J, Geng L. Effects of socioeconomic status on physical and psychological health: Lifestyle as a mediator. International Journal of Environmental Research and Public Health. 2019;**16**(2):1-9

[28] Mitten D, Overholt JR, Haynes FI, D'Amore CC, Ady JC. Hiking:A low-cost, accessible intervention to promote health benefits. American Journal of Lifestyle Medicine. 2018;**12**(4):302-310

[29] Zelenski J, Warber S, Robinson JM, Logan AC, Prescott SL. Nature connection: Providing a pathway from personal to planetary health. Challenges. 2023;**14**(1):16

[30] Joschko L, Pálsdóttir AM, Grahn P, Hinse M. Nature-based therapy in individuals with mental health disorders, with a focus on mental well-being and connectedness to nature-a pilot study. International Journal of Environmental Research and Public Health. 2023;**20**(3):1-24

[31] Vella SA, Aidman E, Teychenne M, Smith JJ, Swann C, Rosenbaum S, et al. Optimising the effects of physical activity on mental health and wellbeing: A joint consensus statement from sports medicine Australia and the Australian Psychological Society. Journal of Science and Medicine in Sport. 2023;**26**(2):132-139

[32] Leighton J, Lopez KJ, Johnson CW. There is always Progress to be made. Therapeutic Recreation Journal. 2021;**LV**(2):185-203

[33] Lingfors H, Persson LG. All-cause mortality among young men 24-26 years after a lifestyle health dialogue in a Swedish primary care setting: A longitudinal follow-up register study. BMJ Open. 2019;**9**(1):e022474

[34] Miller WR, Rollnick S. Motivational Interviewing - Helping People Change. New York: Guilford Publications; 2012

Chapter 5

Health Issues in Nurses

Liliana David, Cristina Maria Sabo, Dorin Farcau and Dinu Iuliu Dumitrascu

Abstract

This comprehensive review delves into the intricate web of health issues affecting nurses and healthcare professionals (HCPs). The paper explores various facets of this multifaceted issue, from the historical evolution of the nursing profession to the contemporary challenges faced by nurses in their professional roles. It investigates the demanding nature of nursing duties, the often arduous working conditions nurses contend with, and the intricate interplay between health issues and the medical field. A specific focus is placed on the prevalence of medical conditions, infectious diseases, stress-related disorders, and psychological challenges that nurses commonly face. The paper also addresses the alarming issue of suicide among nurses, as well as the pervasive problem of burnout and organic diseases that afflict this essential workforce.

Keywords: nursing, women, professional duties, challenges, burnout

1. Introduction

1.1 Definition

Nursing is one of the oldest professions in the world [1] or, better, as the job or skill of caring for people who are sick or injured (Oxford Dictionary). Nurse means "a person who cares for the sick or infirm" (Merriam-Webster Dictionary). More recently, the word nurse also became a professional meaning: "a licensed health-care professional who practices independently or is supervised by a physician, surgeon, or dentist and who is skilled in promoting and maintaining health" (Merriam-Webster Dictionary).

The etymology of the word derives from the Latin word *nutricia*, meaning nourishing and was initially used for "feeding an offspring from the breast" (Merriam-Webster Dictionary). From this original use, this noun developed its meaning to the today's significance. Nursing is very largely a feminine profession; thus, the health topics presented below are mainly referred to women.

1.2 History of nursing

Although the history of nursing starts with the history of mankind and even in other species (apes), the professional nursing was established by Florence Nightingale (1820–1910) [2, 3].

After her seminal activity, nursing as healthcare professional (HCP) spread all over the world and developed training and educational premises to become indeed a profession for the benefit of those in need. Nowadays, nursing is a well-established profession, represented by 28 million persons, however 6 million less than needed worldwide, according to the World Health Organization (WHO) [4]. They are organized in every country in professional associations and own professional codes.

2. Professional duties and challenges of nurses

Nurses are healthcare providers. The main tasks of the nurses are challenging and stressful. They are listed in **Table 1**.

2.1 Working conditions in nurses

Nurses may have to practice in different settings, that is, clinical hospitals including wards, emergency rooms, and day clinics; in medical practice offices; in hospices; in rehabilitation facilities; in senior residences; in care centers for disfavored groups; in school; in dentistry practice offices; and in pharmaceutical care. Therefore, the working conditions are very variable and depend on each one particularity. Besides this, the environment is particularly important: countries or even areas in the same countries with facilities of quite different quality, the working colleagues, the terms of the working contract, etc. It means that nurses, like other HCP categories, may be exposed to deterioration of own health, caused by working conditions.

Taking care of medical records
Recording and retrieving medical data
Surveying and monitoring patients
Physical examination and observation of the patients
Collecting biological samples
Performing medical maneuvers
Performing medical investigations according to individual training and certification
Administration of oral, parenteral, and other therapy
Providing bedside care
Counseling and advising patients and relatives
Collaborating with the medical team and reporting own observations
Maintaining the medical equipment
Recording the inventory of medical equipment and drugs
Educating juniors
Self-continuous education

Table 1.
Professional tasks of the nurses.

2.2 Health issues in HCPs

The perception of health among HCPs is important. In one study [5], it has been searched for what HCPs mean by health and how this may impact on the healthcare they were providing. In a group of over 70 participants, the HCPs defined health, as expected, the physical, mental, and spiritual well-being. However, they accepted that health means not only the absence of disease but also the good functioning and keeping the chronic disease under control. According to this perception, it means that an ill HCP can fill the professional duties well not only in the absence of the disease but also in condition of psychic and somatic well-being, and even more, when chronic diseases are under control [5].

Indeed, the HCPs may themselves become patients [6]. Their diseases impact the standard of healthcare provided, and this has been obvious during the recent pandemics of COVID-19 [7, 8]. The diseases of the HCPs become relevant not only for the society but also for the patients himself/herself [9]. HCPs may consider themselves immune to disease and, therefore, expose themselves to unnecessary risks [10]. There is a need indeed to educate HCPs how to become patient. In a study, it was found out that disputing the myth of medical immunity to diseases needs not only psychological interventions for individuals but also at organizational level. HCPs should be trained to accept the possibility to become ill and to follow the road map of their own patients [11]. Even guidelines on how to manage the treating doctor-patient doctor have been proposed [11]. Given the pressure under which the HCPs work [12], it has been observed that mental illness is more common, and at risk are HCPs recently exposed to psychological challenges [13]. Indeed, not only medical doctors but also other HCPs are prone to suffer of distress and to lose the mental health [14]. They also may have problems in coping with their own disease [15]. Thus, the HCPs need to be aware of their fragility of the possibility to become themselves ill because of professional challenges and of the need to seek help when in need.

3. Medical conditions in nurses

Given the health issues that can occur in HCPs, it is necessary to evaluate the impact of nursing on the health status of nurses. The risk factors for diseases in nurses are displayed in **Table 2**.

The diseases that can be encountered in nurses belong to the types of diseases that the general population may present. These are presented in **Table 3**.

3.1 Infectious diseases in nurses

Nurses are exposed to infectious diseases as they stay, such as doctors, in the frontline of the contact with the patient. From the history of medicine, from literature or movies, we know cases of nurses who died of infectious diseases, from pests, and cholera to viral diseases [16, 17].

Nowadays, the long episode of the COVID-19 outbreak caused a lot of casualties among HCPs including nurses. Besides the death toll, many of nurses were infected with SARS-CoV-2 and suffered acute or chronic forms of the disease. This impact is due to specific working conditions [18]. Among factors predisposing to infections in nurses, one should mention the working conditions and shortage of staff [18]. Factors increasing the risk of infection spread are female sex, exhaustion, and lack of specific training, while applying clustering for nurses' care decreases spreading of infection [19]. Besides

Factors linked to the profession of nurse
Exposure to infectious agents
Stress-related conditions
Incidental trauma during the work
Injuries or accidents while working with professional equipment or devices
Working in special conditions involving health hazards
Confrontation with the assertiveness of patients or their family members
Exposure to highly emotional circumstances
Bullying or abuse
Factors not linked to the profession of nurse
Aging-related factors
Hereditary risk factors
Environmental risk factors

Table 2.
Risk factors of diseases in nurses.

Organic disease
Functional disorders
Mental diseases
Burnout
Traumatisms

Table 3.
Types of diseases in nurses.

the risks caused by the viral infection, the psychological challenge can lead during nursing care in COVID time to mental health disorders [20] or to burnout [21]. In this recent study on almost 500 respondents, there were higher scores for anxiety and depression in nurses than in the general population. Posttraumatic stress disorder was more frequent than army veterans or patients suffering injuries. Nurses working in intensive care units present the trend to leave these jobs because of the challenges caused by COVID-19 [21].

Even before the advent of COVID-19, the contact of nurses with infected patients represented a real hazard [22]. This is what can happen during flu epidemics when contact with suspects from the first visit increases the risk to get the infectious disease and leads to staff shortage when their need is highest [22]. Once the disease contracted, there is the risk to spread it among other patients who are admitted on the wards or seen in ambulatory [23]. It is therefore logical that there is a tremendous need to protect HCPs, including nurses from infectious agents [24].

3.2 Stress-related conditions in nurses

Job is an important source of stress [25, 26]. Nurses are also exposed to stress. This was emphasized after the pandemics with SARS-Cov2 [20, 21], but the facts are well known from earlier data [27–30]. This stress is related with poor health in nurses and with the intention to quit, hence the shortage of nursing staff in hospitals in many countries of the world. In an Iranian setting, the job stress in nurses was self-evaluated as medium, while in female nurses, the most common source of stress was the range of roles (48.4%), role duality (40.9%), and job environment (39.6%). Comparatively, in male nurses, the range of roles was also the most important (57.5%), followed by job environment (50%) and responsibility (45%). The disbalance between skills and training compared to job requirements was not considered stressful in all genders [27]. However, there is still a lack of consistency in this field. For instance, in another study conducted in the same country [29], many nurses perceived their stress levels as high, ranging between moderate and high. 78.4% of respondents reported that their job was stressful. Explanations were working in shifts, insufficient staff, insufficient payment, discrimination at job place, disagreement with the management, and excessive workload. Being female, married, and with lower education correlated positively with stress levels. Other sources of occupational stress were working in emergency room and working many hours in tertiary centers [29].

In a neighboring country, Saudi Arabia, on more than 400 investigated nurses, the following stress etiology was observed, in order of the importance: organizational structure and climate, job description, management, interpersonal relationships, career and achievement, and homework interface [31].

As one can see, there are several causes of stress in nurses. They are displayed in **Table 4**.

3.3 Psychological disorders in nurses

From the studies dedicated to job stress in nurses, it has been revealed that this can be associated with psychological factors [21, 29]. More recently, a large number of studies focused on this matter showed the importance of the psychological

Difficult working conditions
Critical patients
Emergencies
Work overload
Shifts working
Prolonged working hours
Insufficient staffing
Interpersonal conflicts
Lack of time
Lack of social recognition
Underpayment
Conflicts with colleagues
Conflicts with superiors
Harassment
Unpleasant administrative duties
Personal issues

Table 4.
Stress causes in nurses.

disturbances in nurses [32–35]. In a Hong Kong study, carried out on 850 nurses, history of chronic diseases and self-perception of poor health were correlated with depression, anxiety, and stress. Depression was correlated with the status of being divorced compared to married nurses. Other factors, which negatively impacted the mood of the nurses, were widowhood and separation, lack of satisfaction with the present job, conflicts, sedentarism, and sleep disturbance problems. Nurses were more depressed, anxious, and stressed than the general population [32]. Similar data were provided also in an Australian study [33]. In this study, more than one-third of study participants reported scores for depression linked to job dissatisfaction. This condition may become harmful for the patients as the professional performance diminishes in such cases. Stress is also linked with the start of the career [34] or with the beginning of another job with different responsibilities or requiring other skills than previously. In a totally different setting, Norway, similar data were reported. Besides this, nurses in night shift had insomnia, fatigue, and depression [35]. Younger nurses have higher levels of anxiety [36] as well as loss of compassion. This means that managers should take care of this aspect and organize training for nurses who are emotionally exhausted [36].

3.3.1 Suicide in nurses

Suicide is a consequence of life disbalance, depression, and loss of hope. Like in medical doctors, where suicide is relatively frequent, mainly in females [37, 38], nurses are also exposed to the risk of suicide [39]. This trend was aggravated during the pandemic, when nurses, such as other HCPs, were more to risk to commit suicide [40]. According to this paper, not only nurses but also physicians are the professional category with the highest suicidal risk in the population (therefore, it is correct to look to suicide as a professional risk in nurses), but the arrival of the SARS-COV2 epidemic led to professional risk, higher workload, fatigue, exhaustion, alcohol and substance abuse, mainly in women, all of these factors favoring the suicidal ideation [40]. Suicide in nurses is linked to smoking [41]. In female nurses surviving suicide attempts, special training programs have to be organized, in order to prevent the repetition [42].

3.3.2 Burnout

Burnout is another expression of professional risks in nurses, as for other categories of HCPs, and it is characterized by the loss of interest in filling the professional duties, fatigue, disinterest, depression, and exhaustion [43–47]. The risky nursing groups are those working in difficult conditions, mainly for intensive care units, where the rhythm of work and the difficulties of the critical patients are eroding the confidence of the nurses. Thus, nurses have a high level of burnout [48].

The main factors associated with burnout in nurses were being female, being young, marital status, having children, work in night shifts, supplementary administrative tasks, and individual psychological factors, such as neuroticism or extraversion. This means that no model of burnout in nurses should avoid the personality of the nurse [48]. Almost half of the nurses have emotional exhaustion, as reported by very recent research [49]. Working on weekends favored the emotional exhaustion, as well as low collaboration with the job mates; emotional exhaustion is correlated with more days of working incapacity in nurses [49]. Incivility at working place is an important cause of burnout, and this applies also to nurses [50, 51]. Preventing

Disease	Professional risk factor
Cardiovascular	Stress, sedentarism
Metabolic syndrome	Stress, sedentarism, unhealthy eating
Gastroesophageal reflux disease	Night shift, smoking, unhealthy eating
Dyspepsia	Stress, smoking, unhealthy eating
Irritable bowel syndrome	Stress, contact with intestinal infections
Inflammatory bowel disease	Stress
Chronic liver disease	Exposure to infected blood; alcohol, drugs
Breast cancer	Stress
Dermatological	Contact allergy, skin exposure
Musculoskeletal	Physical activity, position

Table 5.
Organic diseases presented by nurses.

burnout in such cases requires solving the social problems linked with incivility vents at working place. It is expected that different degrees of burnout are detected between different categories of HCPs [52].

3.4 Organic diseases

The nurses may present organic diseases. Some diseases have a prevalence and incidence like in the general population, and others have an association with the job of nurse. The main organic diseases encountered in nurses are presented in **Table 5** [53–68].

There are an increasing number of studies emphasizing the professional risk of female nurses and recommending prevention programs.

4. Nurses and morphological sciences

There are trained nurses working also in morphological laboratories: pathology, histology, anatomy, embryology, etc. These are at risk to develop allergic asthma or skin diseases from the inhalation or contact with aggressive chemical compounds. Despite the paucity of the literature data on this topic, it is to recommend to ladies exposed to such professional toxic compounds, mainly during the fertility period, to respect all the indications and procedures to avoid professional diseases in laboratories of morphological sciences.

Another aspect related to this working place is represented by the sight problems that can occur in people working all the time with classical optic microscopes. New technology created the conditions to improve the health of women working in pathology or anatomy labs.

One can see nowadays that, compared with the state 30 years ago, when the professional health problems of women nurses, caused by their occupation, could simply be divided into four main chapters: biological, chemical, physiological, and psychosocial hazards by Tan in 1991, and now, the landscape of occupational hazards in this category of HCPs is more complex [69]. In other aspects, the risks perpetuated but working conditions and preventive procedures changed also [66].

5. Social image of female nurses and its impact on their occupation

Recent decades contributed to change of the social perception of the nurse as she is perceived in cultural products or in mass media. From the image of a nurse at the beginning, or of a dedicated, virtuous, and very engaged woman, it shifted toward a beautiful assistant of the male physician. This can be reflected by the plethora of cartoons, movies, plays, video clips, etc. These contributed to the erroneous presentation of the nurse of a frivol person, always submitted to her male boss. Besides the caricatural image, the lack of reality and even of political correctness is obvious.

There is a general impression that this perspective is a handicap for the profession of nursing, mainly female nurses [70].

In an Internet survey, it has been observed that in interval of few years, the image of the nurse improved from the caricatural one into a balanced and realistic one [71]. Indeed, after screening about 150 Internet sites where the image of nurses was promoted, one could find out that nowadays the emphasis is put on the professional skills and the scientific activity (even doctoral studies being reflected on the websites) [71, 72]. Therefore, one should use the social media to improve and spread the positive image of the nurses. Indeed, a bad image or reputation is a cause of stress and burnout in HCPs [43]. The job dress, that is, the uniform worn by nurses at work, contributes as well to the image of nurses, as well as in the case of physicians [73].

Due to the representation of the beautiful nurse, many women want to become nurses for plastic or esthetic surgery [74, 75]. In this position, they assist physicians of therapeutics in improving the self-image of their patients, thus harmonizing their profession with their vocation.

6. Conclusions

The nurses have a professional pathology caused by their working conditions. Medical conditions associated with the profession of nurse are organic or functional, somatic, and psychological. These diseases have to be recognized in time and prevented, in order to improve the health of the nurses. Besides this, social and administrative measures have to be taken by managers in respect to the work organization and staffing.

Funding sources

The authors have no sources of funding to declare.

Conflict of interest

The authors have no conflicts of interest to declare.

DOI: http://dx.doi.org/10.5772/intechopen.1005248

Author details

Liliana David[1], Cristina Maria Sabo[1]*, Dorin Farcau[2] and Dinu Iuliu Dumitrascu[3]

1 2nd Medical Department, "Iuliu Hațieganu" University of Medicine and Pharmacy, Cluj-Napoca, Romania

2 Clinic of Pediatrics II, "Iuliu Hațieganu" University of Medicine and Pharmacy, Cluj-Napoca, Romania

3 Department of Anatomy, "Iuliu Hațieganu" University of Medicine and Pharmacy, Cluj-Napoca, Romania

*Address all correspondence to: cristina.marica90@yahoo.com

References

[1] Buhler-Wilkerson K, D'Antonio P. Nursing. Encyclopedia Britannica; 2022. Available from: https://www.britannica.com/science/nursing [Accessed: 4 January 2023]

[2] Dumitrascu DI, David L, Dumitrascu DL, Rogozea L. Florence nightingale bicentennial: 1820-2020. Her contributions to health care improvement. Medicine and Pharmacy Reports. 2020;**93**(4):428-430. DOI: 10.15386/mpr-1799

[3] David L, Farcau D, Dumitrascu DL, Rogozea L. Florence Nightingale (1820-1910), întemeietoarea nursingului, la bicentenar | [Florence Nightingale (1820-1910), the founder of nursing, at the bicentenary]. Jurnal Medical Brașovean. 2019;**2**:73-77. DOI: 10.31926/jmb.2019.2.1

[4] Lovelace B Jr. WHO Says There's a Global Shortfall of 5.9 Million Nurses as World Battles Coronavirus Pandemic [Internet]. 2020. Available from: https://www.cnbc.com/2020/04/06/who-says-theres-a-global-shortfall-of-5point9-million-nurses-as-world-battles-coronavirus-pandemic.html [Accessed: 4 January 2023]

[5] Julliard K, Klimenko E, Jacob MS. Definitions of health among healthcare providers. Nursing Science Quarterly. 2006;**19**(3):265-271. DOI: 10.1177/0894318406289575

[6] Illich I. Medical Nemesis. Pantheon: Australian Broadcasting Commission, Science Programmes Unit;

[7] Daher-Nashif S. Doctors' challenges during infectious disease outbreaks: Medical education insights from realistic fiction movies. Advances in Medical Education and Practice. 2021;**12**:265-272. DOI: 10.2147/AMEP.S297427

[8] Saracoglu KT, Simsek T, Kahraman S, Bombaci E, Sezen Ö, Saracoglu A, et al. The psychological impact of COVID-19 disease is more severe on intensive care unit healthcare providers: A cross-sectional study. Clinical Psychopharmacology and Neuroscience. 2020;**18**(4):607-615. DOI: 10.9758/cpn.2020.18.4.607

[9] Klitzman R. When Doctors Become Patients. New York: Oxford University Press; 2008. 344 p

[10] Donaldson LJ. Sick doctors. BMJ. 1994;**309**(6954):557-558. DOI: 10.1136/bmj.309.6954.557

[11] Fox F, Harris M, Taylor G, Rodham K, Sutton J, Robinson B, et al. What happens when doctors are patients? Qualitative study of GPs. The British Journal of General Practice. 2009;**59**(568):811-818. DOI: 10.3399/bjgp09X472872

[12] Carrieri D, Briscoe S, Jackson M, Mattick K, Papoutsi C, Pearson M, et al. Care under pressure': A realist review of interventions to tackle doctors' mental ill-health and its impacts on the clinical workforce and patient care. BMJ Open. 2018;**8**(2):e021273. DOI: 10.1136/bmjopen-2017-021273

[13] Bugaj TJ, Valentini J, Miksch A, Schwill S. Work strain and burnout risk in postgraduate trainees in general practice: An overview. Postgraduate Medicine. 2020;**132**(1):7-16. DOI: 10.1080/00325481.2019.1675361

[14] Wistrand JEG. Distressed doctors: A narrative and historical study of work-related mental discomfort among practising physicians. Medical Humanities. 2020;**46**(3):250-256. DOI: 10.1136/medhum-2018-011525

[15] Wistrand J. When doctors are patients: A narrative study of help-seeking behaviour among addicted physicians. Medical Humanities. 2017;**43**(1):19-23. DOI: 10.1136/medhum-2016-011002

[16] Thomas AJ. Cholera: The Victorian Plague. Barnsley: Pen & Sword History; 2015. Hardcover. 248 pp

[17] Honigsbaum M. The Pandemic Century: A History of Global Contagion from the Spanish Flu to COVID-19. UK: Penguin Random House; 2020. 357 pp

[18] Stone PW, Clarke SP, Cimiotti J, Correa-de-Araujo R. Nurses' working conditions: Implications for infectious disease. Emerging Infectious Diseases. 2004;**10**(11):1984-1989. DOI: 10.3201/eid1011.040253

[19] Hendy A, Soliman SM, Al-Sharkawi SS, Alruwaili MF, Hassani R, Reshia FAA. Effect of clustering nursing care on spreading COVID-19 infection among nurses: A retrospective study. International Journal of General Medicine. 2022;**15**:6801-6809. DOI: 10.2147/IJGM.S376726

[20] Maben J, Conolly A, Abrams R, Rowland E, Harris R, Kelly D, et al. 'You can't walk through water without getting wet' UK nurses' distress and psychological health needs during the Covid-19 pandemic: A longitudinal interview study. International Journal of Nursing Studies. 2022;**131**:104242. DOI: 10.1016/j.ijnurstu.2022.104242

[21] Guttormson JL, Calkins K, McAndrew N, Fitzgerald J, Losurdo H, Loonsfoot D. Critical care nurse burnout, moral distress, and mental health during the COVID-19 pandemic: A United States survey. Heart & Lung. 2022;**55**:127-133. DOI: 10.1016/j.hrtlng.2022.04.015

[22] Bernard H, Fischer R, Mikolajczyk RT, Kretzschmar M, Wildner M. Nurses' contacts and potential for infectious disease transmission. Emerging Infectious Diseases. 2009;**15**(9):1438-1444. DOI: 10.3201/eid1509.081475

[23] Huttunen R, Syrjänen J. Healthcare workers as vectors of infectious diseases. European Journal of Clinical Microbiology & Infectious Diseases. 2014;**33**(9):1477-1488. DOI: 10.1007/s10096-014-2119-6

[24] Weber DJ, Rutala WA, Schaffner W. Lessons learned: Protection of healthcare workers from infectious disease risks. Critical Care Medicine. 2010;**38**(8 Suppl):S306-S314. DOI: 10.1097/CCM.0b013e3181e69ebd

[25] Lamontagne AD, Keegel T, Louie AM, Ostry A, Landsbergis PA. A systematic review of the job-stress intervention evaluation literature, 1990-2005. International Journal of Occupational and Environmental Health. 2007;**13**(3):268-280. DOI: 10.1179/oeh.2007.13.3.268. Erratum in: International Journal of Occupational and Environmental Health 2008; 14(1):24

[26] Semmer NK. Job stress interventions and organization of work. In: Quick JC, Tetrick LE, editors. Handbook of Occupational Health Psychology. American Psychological Association; 2003. pp. 325-353

[27] Najimi A, Goudarzi AM, Sharifirad G. Causes of job stress in nurses: A cross-sectional study. Iranian Journal of Nursing and Midwifery Research. 2012;**17**(4):301-305

[28] Ghawadra SF, Abdullah KL, Choo WY, Phang CK. Psychological distress and its association with job satisfaction among nurses in a teaching

hospital. Journal of Clinical Nursing. 2019;**28**(21-22):4087-4097. DOI: 10.1111/jocn.14993

[29] Kakemam E, Raeissi P, Raoofi S, Soltani A, Sokhanvar M, Visentin D, et al. Occupational stress and associated risk factors among nurses: A cross-sectional study. Contemporary Nurse. 2019;**55**(2-3):237-249. DOI: 10.1080/10376178.2019.1647791

[30] Yeh MC, Yu S. Job stress and intention to quit in newly-graduated nurses during the first three months of work in Taiwan. Journal of Clinical Nursing. 2009;**18**(24):3450-3460. DOI: 10.1111/j.1365-2702.2009.02941.x

[31] Al-Aameri AS. Source of job stress for nurses in public hospitals. Saudi Medical Journal. 2003;**24**(11):1183-1187

[32] Cheung T, Yip PS. Depression, anxiety and symptoms of stress among Hong Kong nurses: A cross-sectional study. International Journal of Environmental Research and Public Health. 2015;**12**(9):11072-11100. DOI: 10.3390/ijerph120911072

[33] Maharaj S, Lees T, Lal S. Prevalence and risk factors of depression, anxiety, and stress in a cohort of Australian nurses. International Journal of Environmental Research and Public Health. 2018;**16**(1):61. DOI: 10.3390/ijerph16010061

[34] Alhroub A, Albakri H, Al-Awaysheh H, Alloubani A. Anxiety level among newly hired nurse in a specialized oncology hospital: An observational study. F1000Res. 2022;**11**:162. DOI: 10.12688/f1000research.74420.1

[35] Øyane NM, Pallesen S, Moen BE, Akerstedt T, Bjorvatn B. Associations between night work and anxiety, depression, insomnia, sleepiness and fatigue in a sample of Norwegian nurses. PLoS ONE. 2013;**8**(8):e70228. DOI: 10.1371/journal.pone.0070228

[36] Hegney DG, Craigie M, Hemsworth D, Osseiran-Moisson R, Aoun S, Francis K, et al. Compassion satisfaction, compassion fatigue, anxiety, depression and stress in registered nurses in Australia: Study 1 results. Journal of Nursing Management. 2014;**22**(4):506-518. DOI: 10.1111/jonm.12160

[37] Esmail A, Everington S. GMC needs to take a more proactive role in preventing harm and suicide in doctors under investigation. BMJ. 2022;**379**:o2883. DOI: 10.1136/bmj.o2883

[38] Okawara M, Ishimaru T, Yoshikawa T, Kido M, Nakashima Y, Nakayasu A, et al. Working hours, side work, and depressive symptoms in physicians: A nationwide cross-sectional study in Japan. Journal of Occupational Health. 2022;**64**(1):e12377. DOI: 10.1002/1348-9585.12377

[39] Hawton K, Vislisel L. Suicide in nurses. Suicide & Life-Threatening Behavior. 1999;**29**(1):86-95. DOI: 10.1111/j.1943-278X.1999.tb00765.x

[40] Awan S, Diwan MN, Aamir A, Allahuddin Z, Irfan M, Carano A, et al. Suicide in healthcare workers: Determinants, challenges, and the impact of COVID-19. Frontiers in Psychiatry. 2022;**12**:792925. DOI: 10.3389/fpsyt.2021.792925

[41] Hemenway D, Solnick SJ, Colditz GA. Smoking and suicide among nurses. American Journal of Public Health. 1993;**83**(2):249-251. DOI: 10.2105/ajph.83.2.249

[42] Samuelsson M, Asberg M. Training program in suicide prevention for

psychiatric nursing personnel enhance attitudes to attempted suicide patients. International Journal of Nursing Studies. 2002;**39**(1):115-121. DOI: 10.1016/s0020-7489(00)00110-3

[43] Bria M, Spânu F, Baban A, Dumitrascu DL. Maslach burnout inventory—General survey: Factorial validity and invariance among Romanian healthcare professionals. Burnout Research. 2014;**1**:103-111. DOI: 10.1016/j.burn.2014.09.001

[44] Bria M, Băban A, Dumitrascu DL. Systematic review of burnout risk factors among European healthcare professionals. Cognition, Brain, Behavior: An Interdisciplinary Journal. 2012;**16**(3):423-452

[45] Bria M, Spânu F, Băban A, Dumitrașcu DL. Burnout among Romanian healthcare professionals: The role of work–home interference. Revista Sociologie Românească. 2013;**11**(3):83-96

[46] Bria M, Băban A, Andreica S, Dumitraşcu DL. Burnout and turnover intentions among Romanian ambulance personnel. Procedia - Social and Behavioral Sciences. 2013;**84**(9):801-805. DOI: 10.1016/j.sbspro.2013.06.650

[47] Browning SG. Burnout in critical care nurses. Critical Care Nursing Clinics of North America. 2019;**31**(4):527-536. DOI: 10.1016/j.cnc.2019.07.008

[48] Cañadas-De la Fuente GA, Vargas C, San Luis C, García I, Cañadas GR, De la Fuente EI. Risk factors and prevalence of burnout syndrome in the nursing profession. International Journal of Nursing Studies. 2015;**52**(1):240-249. DOI: 10.1016/j.ijnurstu.2014.07.001

[49] Petersen J, Wendsche J, Melzer M. Nurses' emotional exhaustion: Prevalence, psychosocial risk factors and association to sick leave depending on care setting—A quantitative secondary analysis. Journal of Advanced Nursing. 2023;**79**(1):182-193. DOI: 10.1111/jan.15471

[50] Hur WM, Kim BS, Park SJ. The relationship between coworker incivility, emotional exhaustion, and organizational outcomes: The mediating role of emotional exhaustion. Human Factors and Ergonomics in Manufacturing & Service Industries. 2015;**25**(6):701-712. DOI: 10.1002/hfm.20587

[51] Schilpzand P, De Pater IE, Erez A. Workplace incivility: A review of the literature and agenda for future research. Journal of Organizational Behavior. 2016;**37**:S57-S88. DOI: 10.1002/job.197626

[52] Lucas G, Colson S, Boyer L, Inthavong K, Haller PH, Lancon C, et al. Risk factors for burnout and depression in healthcare workers: The national AMADEUS study protocol. Encephale. 2022;**48**(3):247-253. DOI: 10.1016/j.encep.2021.06.001

[53] Larese F, Fiorito A. Musculoskeletal disorders in hospital nurses: A comparison between two hospitals. Ergonomics. 1994;**37**(7):1205-1211. DOI: 10.1080/00140139408964898

[54] Telksniene R, Januskevicius V. Occupational skin diseases in nurses. International Journal of Occupational Medicine and Environmental Health. 2003;**16**(3):241-247

[55] Kim O, Jang HJ, Kim S, Lee HY, Cho E, Lee JE, et al. Gastroesophageal reflux disease and its related factors among women of reproductive age: Korea Nurses' Health Study. BMC Public Health. 2018;**18**(1):1133. DOI: 10.1186/s12889-018-6031-3

[56] Bitwayiki R, Orikiiriza JT, Kateera F, Bihizimana P, Karenzi B, Kyamanywa P, et al. Dyspepsia prevalence and impact on quality of life among Rwandan healthcare workers: A cross-sectional survey. South African Medical Journal. 2015;**105**(12):1064-1069. DOI: 10.7196/SAMJ.2015.v105i12.9482

[57] Jung HS, Lee B. Factors associated with the occurrence of functional dyspepsia and insomnia in shift-working nurses. Work. 2016;**54**(1):93-101. DOI: 10.3233/WOR-162283

[58] Nojkov B, Rubenstein JH, Chey WD, Hoogerwerf WA. The impact of rotating shift work on the prevalence of irritable bowel syndrome in nurses. The American Journal of Gastroenterology. 2010;**105**(4):842-847. DOI: 10.1038/ajg.2010.48

[59] Liu L, Xiao QF, Zhang YL, Yao SK. A cross-sectional study of irritable bowel syndrome in nurses in China: Prevalence and associated psychological and lifestyle factors. Journal of Zhejiang University. Science. B. 2014;**15**(6):590-597. DOI: 10.1631/jzus.B1300159

[60] Okami Y, Kato T, Nin G, Harada K, Aoi W, Wada S, et al. Lifestyle and psychological factors related to irritable bowel syndrome in nursing and medical school students. Journal of Gastroenterology. 2011;**46**(12):1403-1410. DOI: 10.1007/s00535-011-0454-2

[61] Ananthakrishnan AN, Khalili H, Pan A, Higuchi LM, de Silva P, Richter JM, et al. Association between depressive symptoms and incidence of Crohn's disease and ulcerative colitis: Results from the Nurses' Health Study. Clinical Gastroenterology and Hepatology. 2013;**11**(1):57-62. DOI: 10.1016/j.cgh.2012.08.032

[62] Colditz GA. Epidemiology of breast cancer. Findings from the nurses' health study. Cancer. 1993;**71**(4 Suppl):1480-1489. DOI: 10.1002/cncr.2820710413

[63] Chico-Barba G, Jiménez-Limas K, Sánchez-Jiménez B, Sámano R, Rodríguez-Ventura AL, Castillo-Pérez R, et al. Burnout and metabolic syndrome in female nurses: An observational study. International Journal of Environmental Research and Public Health. 2019;**16**(11):1993. DOI: 10.3390/ijerph16111993

[64] Bartosiewicz A, Łuszczki E, Nagórska M, Oleksy Ł, Stolarczyk A, Dereń K. Risk factors of metabolic syndrome among polish nurses. Metabolites. 2021;**11**(5):267. DOI: 10.3390/metabo11050267

[65] Yu E, Rimm E, Qi L, Rexrode K, Albert CM, Sun Q, et al. Diet, lifestyle, biomarkers, genetic factors, and risk of cardiovascular disease in the nurses' health studies. American Journal of Public Health. 2016;**106**(9):1616-1623. DOI: 10.2105/AJPH.2016.303316

[66] Williamson KM, Turner JG, Brown KC, Newman KD, Sirles AT, Selleck CS. Occupational health hazards for nurses—Part II. Image – the Journal of Nursing Scholarship. 1988;**20**(3):162-168. DOI: 10.1111/j.1547-5069.1988.tb00059.x

[67] Coppola N, De Pascalis S, Onorato L, Calò F, Sagnelli C, Sagnelli E. Hepatitis B virus and hepatitis C virus infection in healthcare workers. World Journal of Hepatology. 2016;**8**(5):273-281. DOI: 10.4254/wjh.v8.i5.273

[68] Sotaniemi EA, Sutinen S, Arranto AJ, Sutinen S, Sotaniemi KA, Lehtola J, et al. Liver damage in nurses handling cytostatic agents. Acta Medica Scandinavica. 1983;**214**(3):181-189. DOI: 10.1111/j.0954-6820.1983.tb08593.x

[69] Tan CC. Occupational health problems among nurses. Scandinavian Journal of Work, Environment & Health. 1991;**17**(4):221-230. DOI: 10.5271/sjweh.1709

[70] Courtois AC, Courtois R, Cuminet L, Grandsire A. Quelle est l'image de l'infirmière aujourd'hui? [What is the image of nurses today?]. Soins. 2005;**700**(700):41-46. French

[71] Kalisch BJ, Begeny S, Neumann S. The image of the nurse on the internet. Nursing Outlook. 2007;**55**(4):182-188. DOI: 10.1016/j.outlook.2006.09.002

[72] Tzeng HM. Testing a conceptual model of the image of nursing in Taiwan. International Journal of Nursing Studies. 2006;**43**(6):755-765. DOI: 10.1016/j.ijnurstu.2005.10.004

[73] Shaw K, Timmons S. Exploring how nursing uniforms influence self image and professional identity. Nursing Times. 2010;**106**(10):21-23

[74] Moncada G. Why certification for plastic surgery nurses? The Journal of Plastic and Reconstructive Surgical Nursing. 1981;**1**(4):107

[75] Williams T. Addressing body image after reconstructive surgery in adult patients with cancer. Plastic and Aesthetic Nursing. 2022;**42**(4):217-225. DOI: 10.1097/PSN.0000000000000478

Chapter 6

Work-Related Musculoskeletal Disorders in Nurses: Still an Unsolved Problem in Reality (Narrative Literature Review)

Miroljub Jakovljević

Abstract

Work-related musculoskeletal disorders are a major cause of morbidity in nursing. They include a range of signs and symptoms that can affect the quality of performance of work tasks and quality of life. Workplace risk factors can generally be divided into biomechanical (physical), psychosocial, sociocultural, individual (personal), organisational, and environmental risk factors. The risk factors are numerous and interact positively and negatively with each other. There are various methods and tools for assessing work-related risk exposure or risk factors in the workplace. In general, the methods for risk assessment of work-related musculoskeletal disorders can be categorised as self-report, (expert) observation, direct measurement, and remote sensing. When selecting assessment tools, we must consider their measurement characteristics as well as financial and time constraints, the characteristics of the researchers, the clients, and the environment. The assessment of risk factors forms the basis for the development of intervention measures to reduce and/or prevent work-related musculoskeletal disorders. The intervention framework usually consists of a sequence of several steps. Given the dynamic nature of change in work-related musculoskeletal disorders, this process is iterative and continuous and is likely to be most effective when individualised. Healthy employees in a well-functioning work environment should be the goal in every workplace in the healthcare system.

Keywords: work-related musculoskeletal disorders, nursing, risk factors, intervention, prevention

1. Introduction

Musculoskeletal health refers to the performance of the musculoskeletal system, which consists of intact muscles, bones, joints, and neighbouring connective tissue [1]. Musculoskeletal disorders (injuries or disorders of the muscles, nerves, tendons, joints, cartilage, and spinal discs) are the most common causes of disability and limitations in daily life and employment [2]. Around 1.7 billion people on the planet suffer from musculoskeletal disorders, such as back pain, neck pain, fractures, and

IntechOpen

other injuries, as well as osteoarthritis, rheumatoid arthritis, and amputations [3]. The prevalence of musculoskeletal disorders in the general population varies considerably depending on country, occupation, and sociodemographic factors [4, 5]. Work-related musculoskeletal disorders (WRMSDs) are conditions in which the work environment and work performance contribute significantly to the condition and/or the condition is exacerbated or prolonged by working conditions [6]. The definition of WRMSDs is any musculoskeletal problem that occurs at work and causes discomfort, difficulty, or pain in performing the job [7]. It refers to muscle, nerve, or other soft tissue injuries or disorders caused by workplace-related risk factors [8]. The term refers not only to medically based periarticular disorders of the limbs and spine (specific WRMSDs) but also to multiple or localised pain syndromes (non-specific WRMSDs) [9]. WRMSDs are the largest contributor to the work-related burden of disease and are largely related to ergonomic factors in the workplace [4]. WRMSDs are sometimes referred to as cumulative trauma disorder or disease, repetitive strain injuries, overuse syndromes, regional musculoskeletal disorders, repetitive motion injuries, and soft tissue disorders [10]. The aetiology of WRMSD is complex as it encompasses physical, psychological, social, and spiritual aspects of the work environment.

2. Methods

This narrative literature review is intended to discuss the relevant literature that has studied work-related musculoskeletal disorders in nursing, their prevalence, risk factors for occurrence, and interventions for their reduction and/or prevention. Narrative literature review covered a broad range of topics by using studies of various complexity and design. A search was conducted in December 2023 in the databases PubMed, Google Scholar, and ScienceDirect. The search terms were "work-related musculoskeletal disorders AND nursing". Inclusion criteria were the empirical research and review articles to contextualise the findings and freely available articles in their entirety.

3. Results

A total of 200 articles were initially identified to be potentially relevant for the review. A total of 150 articles were included, and they were found to match the inclusion criteria.

3.1 Prevalence of work-related musculoskeletal disorders in nurses

WRMDs are very common among healthcare professionals. Nursing is at the top of all professions, with the potential to develop WRMSDs [11]. A prevalence of over 80% was found in physiotherapists [12], masseurs [13], dentists [14], surgeons [15], midwives [16], and nurses [17]. The prevalence of WRMSDs among nurses is in some cases higher than in other occupations, such as production workers and doctors [18, 19], ranging from 60 to 98% [20, 21], and varies widely due to the more or less complex work in primary, secondary, and tertiary healthcare, depending on the departments, the hospital, and even the countries in which they work [22, 23], which seems to be related to many different occupational exposures of nurses to WRMSDs [24]. The high exposure to WMSDs is directly related to their job, which requires multiple tasks and high physical exertion [25]. They affect the quality of life [26] and lead to varying degrees of long-term illness, work restrictions, high treatment costs, absenteeism, disability [27], patient safety issues, and reduced quality of care [28, 29]. Nurses with WRMSDs have a higher risk of depression [30] and a higher tendency to turnover [31]. In this population, compensation payments, diagnostic testing, and medical services can cost between $50,000 and $100,000 per musculoskeletal injury [32], and WRMSDs are also a major cause of sick leave.

The prevalence of WRMSDs can vary from 33.0% to 88.0% among nurses around the world [33, 34] or from 60–95% [35, 36].

3.2 Prevalence of work-related musculoskeletal disorders by body region

The neck and lower back were the most afflicted regions across all health-care occupations, with an average frequency of between 26.7% and 70.1% [25]. Compared to dentists and surgeons, nurses had a lower average prevalence for the neck (33.1%) [37]. The most common complaints among nurses are lower back, shoulder, neck [38–40], hands, and legs (**Figure 1**) [38, 39]. The prevalence of WRMSDs on the feet and the whole body was higher in developed areas than in developing areas. Conversely, the prevalence of WRMSDs at other anatomical sites was higher in developing areas than in developed areas [33]. WRMSDs in the neck, upper back, and other anatomical sites decreased over time, while the prevalence of WRMSDs in the shoulder and knee showed an increasing trend [33].

3.3 Risk factors

WRMSD is a multifactorial phenomenon influenced by various [41] direct and indirect risk factors (**Figure 2**). The nursing profession is a very demanding occupation (physically, psychologically, socially, and mentally), which makes nurses more

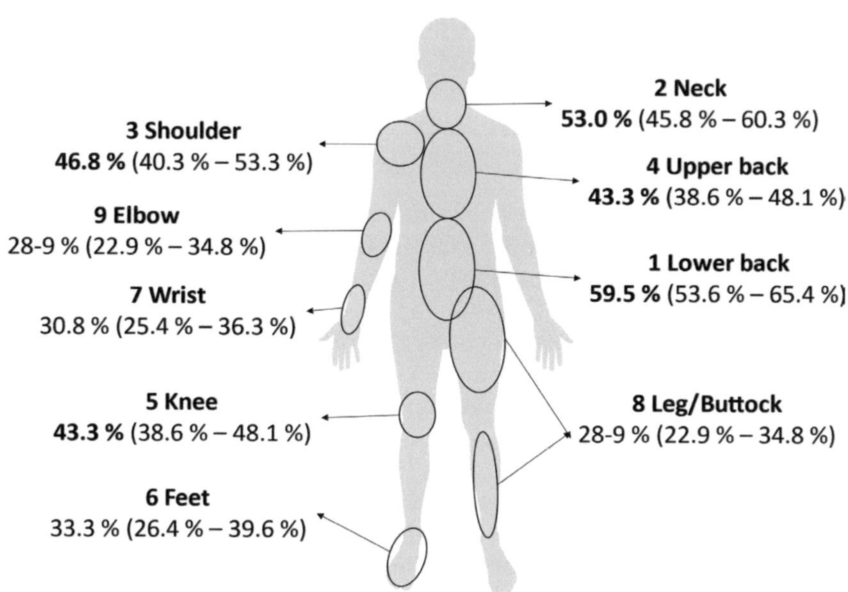

Figure 1.
Annual prevalence of WMSDs in different anatomical sites by prevalence rate (adopted from ref. [33]).

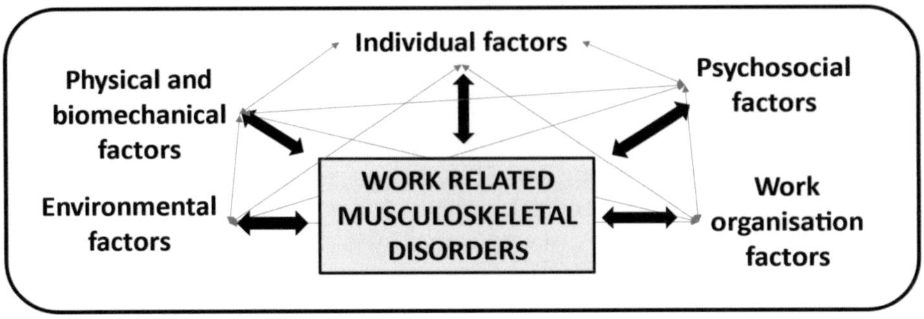

Figure 2.
Dynamic relationship between workplace risk factors for WRMSDs. All risk factors influence each other, either inhibitory or facilitative.

vulnerable to WRMSD. Due to the complexity and abundance of risk factors, researchers usually opt for a framework that narrows the field and facilitates understanding of their interplay. In the workplace, these factors can generally be divided into biomechanical (physical), psychosocial, sociocultural, individual (personal) [42, 43], organisational, and environmental risk factors.

3.3.1 Physical and biomechanical factors

Physical and biomechanical risk factors include repetitive movements, carrying heavy objects, unfavourable postures [44], patient handling, and long working hours [45–47]. Patient handling tasks were documented as the main factors for WRMSD in nursing staff. Perceived physical demands that carers are frequently exposed to include moving objects, pulling/pushing machines, lifting patients, repetitive movements, and extreme bending, bending, twisting, and sudden movements [48]. Highly repetitive activities on a continuous basis can trigger WRMSDs [49]. These physical demands increase the risk of complaints in various parts of the body [50, 51]. WMSDs have been shown to be associated with patient-handling tasks in nurses [52, 53].

3.3.2 Psychological and social factors

The interactions between the work environment, job content, organisational conditions and skills, needs, and personal considerations outside of work that can affect relationships with patients (clients), job performance, and health are referred to as psychosocial factors at work [24]. Nurses who have at least one WRMSD in one body segment have expressed dissatisfaction with their profession, citing poor nurse-physician contact, staff disengagement, and lack of support from immediate superiors [54]. Nurses may face various types of difficulties during their work that contribute to WRMSDs [55], including psychological distress [46, 47], problems with patients, problems with management and physicians [55], lack of support from others, lack of decision-making power [56], anxiety, and depression [46, 47]. Unfavourable psychological and social factors led to an unfavourable work attitude, shortened time interval between rest and activity, and possibly reduced cooperation with colleagues, thereby reducing workers' ability to resist WMSD [57].

Spirituality refers to a sense of connection between the individual and the universe, the meaning of life, purpose, integration, growth, truth, and mindfulness [58].

Today, more and more organisations are recognising the importance of spirituality in the workplace. It is about finding meaning, value, and motivation in one's work to achieve better performance and care outcomes [59]. Spirituality in the workplace is becoming an essential aspect of healthcare. It has numerous benefits, such as improved overall employee well-being, higher employee productivity, increased motivation and job satisfaction, engagement and team effectiveness, and team cohesion [60]. Spiritual stress can also have a direct impact on health. Research indicates that those exhibiting comparatively elevated levels of spiritual distress are more prone to experiencing pain, depression [61–64], suicide risk [62–64], higher levels of clinically effective anxiety [63, 64], and a higher resting heart rate [64]. Spirituality in the workplace has integrated some spiritual concepts such as inner connection, sense of community, connectedness, compassion, transcendence, and mindfulness in the workplace to improve employees' mental health and well-being, increase their engagement and motivation, and improve organisational outcomes of companies [65]. It has been demonstrated that workplace programmes rooted in spirituality offer a multitude of advantages to both workers and employers. These advantages include heightened creativity and revenue, elevated productivity and performance, decreased absenteeism, and elevated levels of intrinsic motivation and job satisfaction [66]. By incorporating spirituality into workplace health promotion programmes, employees can be supported by their organisations in managing burnout, work-related stress, and violence, as well as other psychosocial risk factors in the workplace [67].

3.3.3 Factors in the organisation of work

There is evidence that the development of WRMSD is highly related to work organisational factors, including problems with scheduling [68, 69], shift work, staff shortages, poor working conditions [46, 47], and extended working hours [17, 70], which may be risk factors contributing to the development of WRMSD in nurses. Nurses are at very high risk for WMSD due to the shift-heavy culture and long working hours in this field [71, 72]. Hale and Hovden [73] have identified three stages in the development of occupational health and safety management, with the third stage characterised by the consideration of organisational and management issues as fundamental factors in improving safety. This suggests that what matters is how well an organisation's culture is established and communicated to employees to facilitate their working relationships. The term "organisational factors" encompasses all the elements that influence the way the organisation and each individual within it behaves. Typically, these elements include:

- formal management systems (e.g., safety and competence management),
- assurance processes (monitoring, audit, and review),
- work practises, regardless of whether they are formally documented or not,
- risk awareness,
- how the organisation has learned from experience,
- safety culture of the organisation.

There is a direct, significant relationship between organisational culture and job performance, and a strong, employee-friendly organisational culture can lead to effective employee performance [74]. Organisational culture and performance are two variables that are significantly correlated [75, 76].

3.3.4 Environmental factors

As the authors of [77] previously explained, the idea of healthy buildings is a biopsychosocial framework that focuses on redesigning the built environment to promote and improve occupants' health, well-being, performance, productivity, and quality of life. The interior design of medical facilities is unique. Interior design aims to create a therapeutic environment for patients and make their stay in a facility as non-threatening, comfortable, and stress-free as possible. However, the needs of patients are often at odds with the needs of staff in medical facilities [78].

Environmental influences include light sources and levels that deliver too much or too little light, cold or too warm temperatures, noise levels [79], humidity, and biochemical dangers. These conditions have a negative impact on employee health. Research indicates that environmental variables, like uncomfortable temperatures, can play a major role in the onset and aggravation of WRMSDs [80, 81]. In addition to having a negative impact on workers' health (including musculoskeletal symptoms) and job performance, heat stress [82] and cold stress [80, 81] can also increase psychological distress and mental health issues [83, 84], lower key human psychological performance variables [85], and cause irritability, inattention, a sense of exhaustion, and mood swings. Current findings suggest that hot and cold temperature exposure negatively affects performance and that other variables (e.g., duration of temperature exposure or task duration) can alter this relationship [86]. Increased noise in the workplace [87], insufficient availability of light [88], dry air, and temperature fluctuations [89] were also significantly associated with an increased risk of WRMSD. Biological (experience with cuts/wounds/injuries, airborne infections, physical contact with retroviral patients and specimens, and exposure to blood-borne specimens), chemical, and radiation hazards to which nurses are exposed and their association with WRMSD have not been adequately studied.

3.3.5 Individual factors

Individual (personal) factors include age, gender, body mass index, lifestyle issues, and living conditions [90]. WRMSDs are common among nurses and primarily affect the lower back. The likelihood of developing WRMSDs is high with increasing age, BMI, and work experience, as well as among nurses working in intensive care units and public hospitals. Some studies confirm such an association between nurses' age and WRMSDs (especially neck, arms, and lower back) [91, 92], while others contradict these findings [93, 94]. It was not age but rather high physical job demands that significantly increased the risk of WRMSD in all age groups [95]. Differences in workload, biological status, and body size between men and women may be connected to the correlation between gender and musculoskeletal discomfort [96, 97]. Compared to normal-weight workers, obese workers had a higher risk of developing WRMSDs and a lower recovery from symptoms [98]. The rate of WRMSDs increases significantly with increasing work experience [96, 99]. The physical abilities (muscle strength) that enable people to cope with physical job demands naturally decline over time due to age [100]. Physically demanding nursing professions with long working hours and shift work can contribute to nurses being less physically active in their free time [101]. Studies suggest that physical activity at work and in leisure time may not have the same health benefits, although the results vary [102, 103]. Given their strong correlation with six of the seven factors contributing to early death [104], physical exercise at the proper degree and intensity, as well as a nutritious diet are regarded as the most significant positive health behaviours in preventive healthcare [105]. It is very likely that physical activity during leisure time, with appropriate parameters, can prevent musculoskeletal disorders, especially in nurses with long work experience [106].

3.4 Risk factors assessment

There are various methods and tools for assessing work-related risk exposure or for identifying potentially hazardous workplaces or risk factors in the workplace. In general, WRMSD risk assessment methods can be categorised as self-reporting, (expert) observation, direct measurement, and remote sensing (**Figure 3**). Risk assessments should be carried out using methods that are objective and accurate, that is, reliable and valid. Risk analyses can also be carried out when evaluating the effect of a measure in the workplace.

Self-report was originally developed to assess WRMSD problems and is widely used in epidemiological and ergonomic studies [114, 115]. Sometimes, it is a face-to-face interview between the workers and an investigator. This method is easy to use with large groups of workers and allows comparisons over time and between groups. However, self-reporting takes time and interrupts employees' ongoing work. Internet surveys, video recordings, and video conferencing have also been used to improve the efficiency and accuracy of the self-reporting process. Self-reporting has the benefit of allowing many employees to report on concerns and difficulties that are challenging to see (such as pain and perceived workload), and it is an economical and flexible strategy that can be used in a variety of work environments. Self-reporting has the

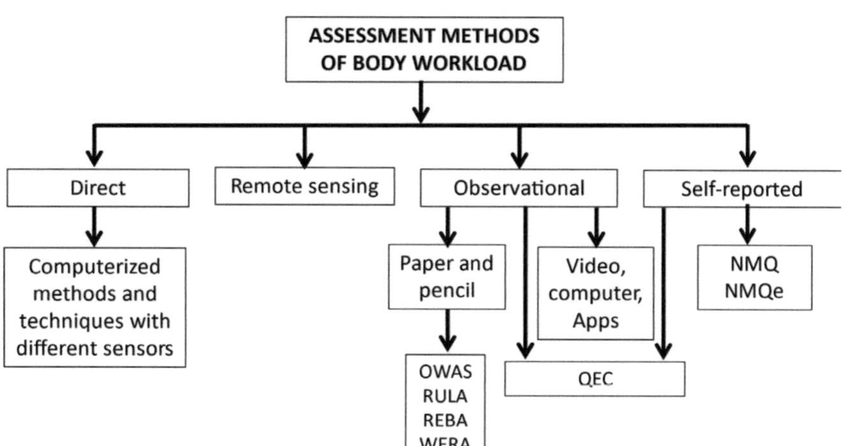

Figure 3.
Schematic presentation of the assessment methods of body workload (OWAS – Ovako Working Posture Analysing System [107]; RULA – Rapid Upper Limb Assessment [108]; REBA – Rapid Upper Limb Assessment [109]; QEC – Quick Exposure Check [110]; WERA – Workplace Ergonomic Risk Assessment [111]; NMQ – Nordic Musculoskeletal Questionnaire [112]; NMQe – Nordic Musculoskeletal Questionnaire-Extended [113]).

drawback that as the results are dependent on subjective assessments, they can differ greatly between individuals. Furthermore, survey replies may be skewed because of personal ramifications, which calls into question the validity of this approach, considering alternative approaches like direct measurement and sophisticated sensing techniques [116].

The methodical documentation of postures during work, including location, frequency, intensity, and duration, is called observation [115]. WRMSD hazards for a possible job or work environment redesign are normally measured by specialists using assessment forms and an experienced observer. Although these techniques take longer, their validity and reliability have been determined to be acceptable [117].

Direct measurements are more objective than expert views and self-reports. In order to analyse biomechanics and tissue and joint loads, common direct measurements include electromyography, optical markers, goniometers, inclinometers, optical scanners, and sound sensors. Recently, numerous new technical methods for observing postures, movements, and loads have been developed. These instruments are generally very accurate but also have some disadvantages. They are more expensive than observation methods, need to be operated by experts, and interfere with the organisation's work.

Modern remote sensing methods use distance or image/video sensors to record human motions using marker-less sensor-based biomechanics. Motion or kinematic data can be gathered and used as input for biomechanical modelling, which computes joint or tissue loading – a factor that is strongly correlated with WRMSD risks – as well as for the observational risk assessment techniques already in use to establish the degree of risk in the field. These methods can be utilised for assessments in actual workplaces because they do not require human participants to be directly attached to markers or signal receivers [118]. Because sensor-based approaches can record objective, precise movement data that may be used to predict joint loads, they have an advantage over self-assessment and observational methods.

When selecting assessment tools, we need to consider not only their measurement properties but also the financial and time constraints, the characteristics of the researchers, the clients, and the environment (**Figure 4**).

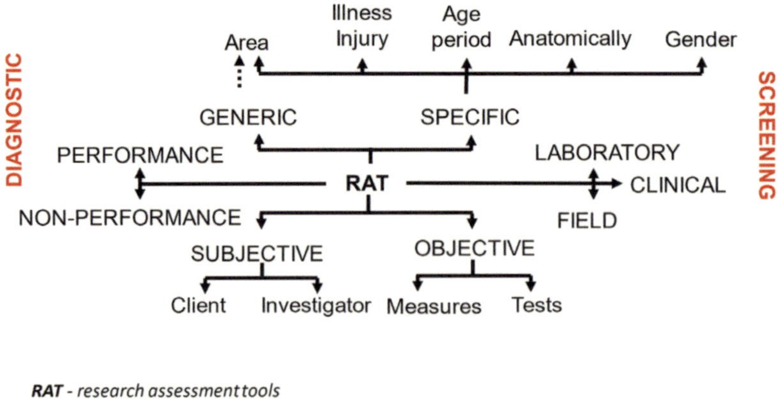

Figure 4.
Graphic representation of guidelines for decision-making on the selection of assessment tools.

3.4.1 Interventions to reduce work-related musculoskeletal disorders

Four categories (specialised equipment, staff training, policies and procedures to reduce work-related musculoskeletal illnesses, and support and follow-up) can be used to categorise the interventions documented in the literature [119].

The introduction of handling equipment, also known as specialised equipment, lifting devices, repositioning devices, and handling equipment, was a prominent trend among the treatments. These included fast-ascending electric beds, sliding boards, overhead lifts (also known as mechanical lifts) [120, 121], and overhead lifts [122]. Positive results from all of these various tactics included a decrease in injuries [119].

The staff training programmes with the most positive outcomes were designed and delivered by care facility management [120, 122]. Conversely, Peterson et al. [123] found no significant reduction in pain, discomfort, or the general physical and mental health of participants after training.

Training programmes for correct posture, physical exercise, and redesign of the work environment by staff were also used to reduce stressful boot postures [124]. Gold et al. [121] also supported physical exercise training to improve flexibility and prevent or reduce low back pain, particularly in individuals with a history of low back pain.

Adherence to specific policies and procedures guiding mobility interventions in care homes reduced work-related musculoskeletal disorders [120, 121]. The introduction of these guidelines took into account the availability of specialised equipment and centred on its appropriate use and maintenance, such as the prompt cleaning of slings and battery recharging. These measures significantly impacted the correct use of specialised equipment and further decreased the rate of injuries [119].

To promote compliance with the use of specialised equipment, measures were initiated to comply with training programmes, implement guidelines as a follow-up, and support staff in a multidimensional environment [119]. The utilisation of therapy sessions as a follow-up technique to avoid musculoskeletal diseases connected to employment was another supportive intervention [125, 126].

Workplace physical activity, or physical activity at work, is a form of organised physical exercise that tries to establish areas where employees can spontaneously take a break from their monotonous schedule to exercise their body and mind and grow in self-awareness, which can enhance their connection with the workplace [127]. The main goal of physical activity in the workplace is to improve performance during the working day and prevent musculoskeletal disorders. Depending on the time of day or purpose, different physical activity modalities can be used in the workplace [128]. Physical exercise can be performed at the beginning of work and is referred to as preparatory, as its main purpose is to warm up the whole body before starting the job tasks [129–131]. Because compensatory movement in the workplace entails stopping work duties to move around, it is often referred to as a short active break [132]. These pauses are intended to alleviate tension in the musculoskeletal system (joints and muscles) brought on by task-related variables and to make up for bad posture. Workers' physical and emotional well-being depends on this kind of mobility [133]. At the conclusion of the workday, employees should practice relaxation techniques [134]. It can also be used in conjunction with mind-body interventions, such as progressive muscle relaxation, acupuncture, yoga, Pilates, and meditation, as complementary therapies [135]. There is consistent evidence that physical activity in the workplace significantly reduces general musculoskeletal pain and neck and shoulder pain [136].

3.4.2 Prevention of work-related musculoskeletal disorders

In many countries, the population is ageing, and the retirement age of the labour force is increasing [137]. There is a general tendency for the incidence of WRMSDs to increase with age [138], but work-related hazard exposures significantly accelerate this age-related increase [139].

There is a growing urgency for workplaces to adopt evidence-based risk management practices that more effectively reduce WRMSD risk [140]. Given the influence of multiple risk factors on the occurrence of WRMSDs, the implementation of prevention and control programmes and measures requires the simultaneous identification and control of a range of risk factors [44]. Hazards are best eliminated at the source. This is a fundamental principle of occupational health and safety. Despite knowledge of the factors associated with WRMSDs, primary prevention measures for WRMSDs through changes in work-related physical factors, such as manual handling advice [141] and ergonomic workplace design [142], have not been shown to be effective or too successful in preventing WRMSDs. In addition, the global burden of WRMSDs appears to have increased rather than decreased in recent years [143], although many preventive measures and strategies exist (e.g., workplace measures or ergonomic guidelines). The latter does not apply to all topographical areas [144]. Theories and/or programme failures, such as inadequate translation of information about aetiological mechanisms into well-crafted intervention programmes, may be to blame for the failure of WRMSD prevention efforts [145]. For these reasons, a framework for WRMSD prevention research using a repeated sequencing approach was proposed by van der Beek et al. [146]. It is based on the "risk identification, assessment, control and evaluation framework", which serves as a foundation for

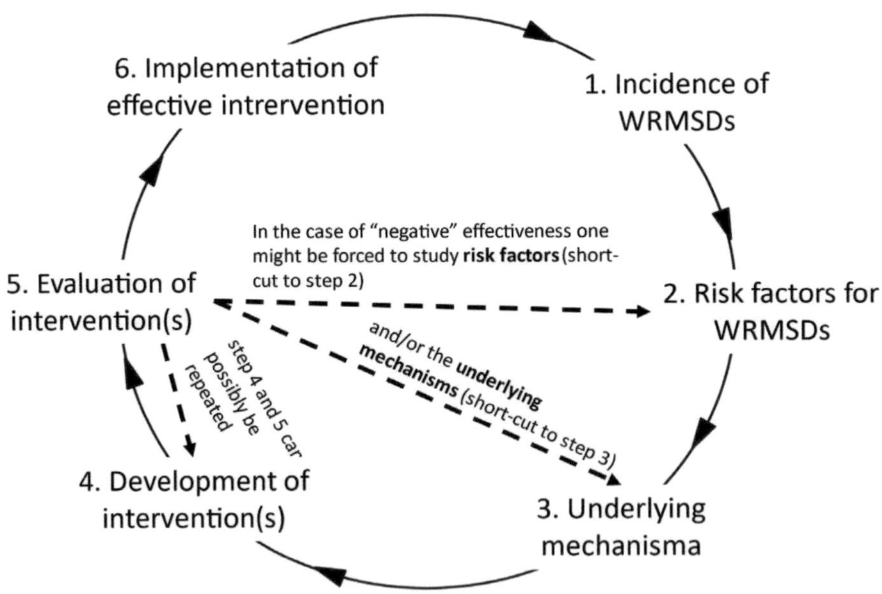

Figure 5.
Suggested a recurring protocol to prevent musculoskeletal diseases associated with the workplace. The steps should ideally be followed in order, beginning with step 1 and concluding with step 6 (solid lines), after which it can be repeated. As an alternative, one could go back to steps 2, 3, or 4 (dashed lines) if interventions in step 5 have not shown to be successful (adapted from [146]).

international labour policy and practise [147], as well as similar frameworks from other research fields [148–150]. There are six steps in the suggested framework (**Figure 5**).

In line with the authors' findings [146], this framework has the potential to enhance existing theories and bolster the creation and execution of preventive measures for WRMSDs. The development of interventions in research based on an identified problem (step 1) and targeting risk factors that seem to be associated with a WRMSDs problem (step 2), possibly with a solid understanding of the underlying mechanisms and pathogenesis (step 3), is necessary to achieve the best possible outcome in the prevention of WRMSDs [146]. A demonstrated effective preventive intervention (step 5) should be fully implemented using evidence-based implementation strategies (step 6), while the intervention should also be optimally targeted to the particular occupational population and work environment (step 4) [146]. In order to successfully execute changes in the workplace, it is crucial.

4. Discussion

Numerous studies have been conducted on WRMSD in workers across a range of industries, including the nursing field. The majority of cross-sectional, retrospective, or prospective investigations have shown that WRMSD is quite prevalent in nurses. Studies on the incidence are scarcer. Numerous risk factors for the development of WRMSDs are present in nurses. Most research focuses on physical stress at work as one of the primary risk factors; however, social, psychological, and spiritual elements – especially the ways in which they interact with one another – are sometimes overlooked. There are many programmes aimed at lowering the incidence and primary prevention of WRMSD; nevertheless, their effectiveness is frequently minimal or transitory. The majority of these interventions overlook the individuality of each worker in favour of targeting a larger group of workers, or average workers, and they disregard each person's individuality. Like diseases, WRMDs are a dynamic process. To lessen their impact on society at large and on healthcare workers specifically, regular interventions based on frequently repeated analyses of the work organisation, the demands of work processes, and the worker—who also changes over time—are likely to be most effective.

5. Conclusions

With low back pain and ankle/foot pain having the greatest prevalence rates, neck and shoulder pain following, and elbow pain having the lowest prevalence rate among the 13 body locations included in the study, WRMSD is highly prevalent among nurses. The primary risk variables for WRMSD were age, gender (female), high body mass index, and length of employment. These association patterns also provide insight into potential intervention tactics to enhance a positive psychosocial work environment and encourage a healthy lifestyle. Appropriate screening programmes for musculoskeletal pain risk factors among nurses should be implemented, and prevention, early diagnosis, treatment, rehabilitation, and counselling are needed. Solutions could also include increasing staff numbers and rescheduling working hours by the health manager or senior management. Healthy employees in a well-functioning work environment should be the goal in every workplace in the health care system.

Author details

Miroljub Jakovljević
Faculty of Health Sciences, University of Ljubljana, Ljubljana, Slovenia

*Address all correspondence to: miroljub.jakovljevic@zf.uni-lj.si

References

[1] World Health Organisation – WHO. Musculoskeletal Health. 2022. Available from: https://www.who.int/news-room/fact-sheets/detail/musculoskeletal-conditions

[2] Briggs AM, Woolf AD, Dreinhöfer K, Homb N, Hoy DG, Kopansky-Giles D, et al. Reducing the global burden of musculoskeletal conditions. Bulletin of the World Health Organization. 2018;**96**(5):366-368. DOI: 10.2471/BLT.17.204891

[3] Cieza A, Causey K, Kamenov K, Hanson SW, Chatterji S, Vos T. Global estimates of the need for rehabilitation based on the global burden of disease study 2019: A systematic analysis for the global burden of disease study 2019. The Lancet. 2021;**396**(10267):2006-2017

[4] de Kok J, Vroonhof P, Snijders J, Roullis G, Clarke M, Peereboom K, et al. Work-related musculoskeletal disorders: Prevalence, costs and demographics in the EU. European Risk Observatory Report. European Agency for Safety and Health at Work. Luxembourg: Publications Office of the European Union; 2019

[5] Parno A, Sayehmiri K, Parno M, Khandan M, Poursadeghiyan M, Maghsoudipour M, et al. The prevalence of occupational musculoskeletal disorders in Iran: A meta-analysis study. Work (Reading, Mass.). 2017;**58**(2):203-214. DOI: 10.3233/WOR-172619

[6] Bernard BP. Musculoskeletal Disorders and Workplace Factors: A Critical Review of Epidemiologic Evidence for Work-Related Musculoskeletal Disorders of the Neck, Upper Extremity, and Low Back. DHHS Publication; no. (NIOSH). National Institute for Occupational Safety and Health. 1997. pp. 1-14. Available from: https://stacks.cdc.gov/view/cdc/21745

[7] Gauthy R, Vrbinc M, Vrbinc A, Sapir M, Bohm L. Mišično-kostne bolezni: slabo razumljena pandemija. Ljubljana: Zveza Svobodnih SindikatovSlovenije; 2007

[8] Guifan S. Occupational Health and Occupational Medicine. 7th ed. Beijing: People's Health Publishing House; 2012

[9] Roquelaure Y. Musculoskeletal Disorders and Psychosocial Factors at Work ETUI Research Paper – Report 142. 2018. Available from: https://ssrn.com/abstract=3316143

[10] Nur Azma BA, Rusli BN, Oxley JA, Quek KF. Work related musculoskeletal disorders in female nursing personnel: Prevalence and impact. International Journal Collaborative Research of Internal Medicine and Public Health. 2016;**8**:294-298

[11] Mailutha J. Prevalence of musculoskeletal disorders among nurses in Kenya: Part 1, anthropometric data and MSDS. International Journal of Emerging Technology and Advanced Engineering. 2020;**10**:158-163

[12] Kinaci E, Ataoğlu S. Work related musculoskeletal disorders among the physiotherapists: Sample of a region in Turkey. Turkish Journal of Medical Sciences. 2020;**5**:495-502. DOI: 10.5336/healthsci.2019-71762

[13] Glowinski S, Bryndal A, Grochulska A. Prevalence and risk of spinal pain among physiotherapists in Poland. PeerJ. 2021;**9**:e11715. DOI: 10.7717/peerj.11715

[14] Anton D, Rosecrance J, Merlino L, Cook TM. Prevalence of musculoskeletal symptoms and carpal tunnel syndrome among dental hygienists. American Journal of Industrial Medicine. 2002;**42**:248-257. DOI: 10.1002/ajim.10110

[15] Liang CA, Levine VJ, Dusza SW, Hale EK, Nehal KS. Musculoskeletal disorders and ergonomics in dermatologic surgery: A survey of Mohs surgeons in 2010. Dermatologic Surgery: Official Publication for American Society for Dermatologic Surgery [et al.]. 2012;**38**(2):240-248. DOI: 10.1111/j.1524-4725.2011.02237.x

[16] Arslan Okuyucu K, Jeve Y, Doshani A. Work-related musculoskeletal injuries amongst obstetrics and gynaecology trainees in East Midland region of the UK. Archives of Gynecology and Obstetrics. 2017;**296**(3):489-494. DOI: 10.1007/s00404-017-4449-y

[17] Munabi IG, Buwembo W, Kitara DL, Ochieng J, Mwaka ES. Musculoskeletal disorder risk factors among nursing professionals in low resource settings: A cross-sectional study in Uganda. BMC Nursing. 2014;**13**(1):7. DOI: 10.1186/1472-6955-13-7

[18] Xu Q, Ling R, Liu Y, Zhang H, Li G, Wang R, et al. Incidence patterns and risk factors of work-related musculoskeletal disorders in medical industry in China. Chinese Journal of Disease Control & Prevention. 2022;**26**(8):888-896

[19] Alnaser MZ, Aljadi SH. Physical therapists with work-related musculoskeletal disorders in the State of Kuwait: A comparison across countries and health care professions. Work. 2019;**63**(2):261-268

[20] Nguyen TH, Hoang DL, Hoang TG, et al. Prevalence and characteristics of multisite musculoskeletal symptoms among district hospital nurses in Haiphong, Vietnam. BioMed Research International. 2020;**2020**:3254605

[21] Passali C, Maniopoulou D, Apostolakis I, Varlamis I. Work-related musculoskeletal disorders among Greek hospital nursing professionals: A cross-sectional observational study. Work (Reading, Mass.). 2018;**61**(3):489-498. DOI: 10.3233/WOR-182812

[22] Ribeiro T, Serranheira F, Loureiro H. Work related musculoskeletal disorders in primary health care nurses. Applied Nursing Research. 2017;**33**:72-77. DOI: 10.1016/j.apnr.2016.09.003

[23] Serranheira F, Sousa-Uva M, Sousa-Uva A. Hospital nurses tasks and work-related musculoskeletal disorders symptoms: A detailed analysis. Work (Reading, Mass.). 2015;**51**(3):401-409. DOI: 10.3233/WOR-141939

[24] Krishnan KS, Raju G, Shawkataly O. Prevalence of work-related musculoskeletal disorders: Psychological and physical risk factors. International Journal of Environmental Research and Public Health. 2021;**18**(17):9361. DOI: 10.3390/ijerph18179361

[25] Jacquier-Bret J, Gorce P. Prevalence of body area work-related musculoskeletal disorders among healthcare professionals: A systematic review. International Journal of Environmental Research and Public Health. 2023;**20**(1):841. DOI: 10.3390/ijerph20010841

[26] Kumagai G, Wada K, Kudo H, Tanaka S, Asari T, Chiba D, et al. The effect of low back pain and neck-shoulder stiffness on health-related quality of life: A cross-sectional population-based study. BMC Musculoskeletal Disorders.

2021;**22**(1):14. DOI: 10.1186/s12891-020-03871-5

[27] Hartvigsen J, Hancock MJ, Kongsted A, Louw Q, Ferreira ML, Genevay S, et al. What low back pain is and why we need to pay attention. Lancet (London, England). 2018;**391**(10137):2356-2367. DOI: 10.1016/S0140-6736(18)30480-X

[28] Ping Y, Li Z, Yi Y, et al. Absenteeism caused by work-related musculoskeletal disorders among nurses in Xinjiang. Journal of Nursing Science. 2017;**32**(21):60-63

[29] Thinkhamrop W, Sawaengdee K, Tangcharoensathien V, Theerawit T, Laohasiriwong W, Saengsuwan J, et al. Burden of musculoskeletal disorders among registered nurses: Evidence from the Thai nurse cohort study. BMC Nursing. 2017;**16**:68. DOI: 10.1186/s12912-017-0263-x

[30] Zhang Y, ElGhaziri M, Nasuti S, Duffy JF. The comorbidity of musculoskeletal disorders and depression: Associations with working conditions among hospital nurses. Workplace Health & Safety. 2020;**68**(7):346-354. DOI: 10.1177/2165079919897285

[31] Fochsen G, Josephson M, Hagberg M, Toomingas A, Lagerström M. Predictors of leaving nursing care: A longitudinal study among Swedish nursing personnel. Occupational and Environmental Medicine. 2006;**63**(3):198-201. DOI: 10.1136/oem.2005.021956

[32] Gershon RR, Stone PW, Zeltser M, Faucett J, MacDavitt K, Chou SS. Organizational climate and nurse health outcomes in the United States: A systematic review. Industrial Health. 2007;**45**(5):622-636. DOI: 10.2486/indhealth.45.622

[33] Sun W, Yin L, Zhang T, Zhang H, Zhang R, Cai W. Prevalence of work-related musculoskeletal disorders among nurses: A meta-analysis. Iranian Journal of Public Health. 2023;**52**(3):463-475. DOI: 10.18502/ijph.v52i3.12130

[34] Choi SD, Brings K. Work-related musculoskeletal risks associated with nurses and nursing assistants handling overweight and obese patients: A literature review. Work (Reading, Mass.). 2015;**53**(2):439-448. DOI: 10.3233/WOR-152222

[35] Cheung K, Szeto G, Lai GKB, Ching SSY. Prevalence of and factors associated with work-related musculoskeletal symptoms in nursing assistants working in nursing homes. International Journal of Environmental Research and Public Health. 2018;**15**(2):265. DOI: 10.3390/ijerph15020265

[36] Soylar P, Ozer A. Evaluation of the prevalence of musculoskeletal disorders in nurses: A systematic review. Medicine Science International Medical Journal. 2018;**7**(3):479-488

[37] Kee D, Seo SR. Musculoskeletal disorders among nursing personnel in Korea. International Journal of Industrial Ergonomics. 2007;**37**:207-212. DOI: 10.1016/j.ergon.2006.10.020

[38] Wang SY, Liu LC, Lu MC, Koo M. Comparisons of musculoskeletal disorders among ten different medical professions in Taiwan: A nationwide, population-based study. PLoS One. 2015;**10**(4):e0123750. DOI: 10.1371/journal.pone.0123750

[39] Freimann T, Coggon D, Merisalu E, Animägi L, Pääsuke M. Risk factors for musculoskeletal pain amongst nurses in Estonia: A cross-sectional study. BMC

Musculoskeletal Disorders. 2013;**14**:334. DOI: 10.1186/1471-2474-14-334

[40] Carugno M, Pesatori AC, Ferrario MM, Ferrari AL, Silva FJ, Martins AC, et al. Physical and psychosocial risk factors for musculoskeletal disorders in Brazilian and Italian nurses. Cadernos De Saude Publica. 2012;**28**(9):1632-1642. DOI: 10.1590/s0102-311x2012000900003

[41] Buckle P. Ergonomics and musculoskeletal disorders: Overview. Occupational Medicine (Oxford, England). 2005;**55**(3):164-167. DOI: 10.1093/occmed/kqi081

[42] Lim MC, Lukman KA, Giloi N, Lim JF, Avoi R, Rahim SA, et al. Prevalence of upper limb musculoskeletal disorders and its associated risk factors among janitorial workers: A cross-sectional study. Annals of Medicine and Surgery. 2021;**73**:103201. DOI: 10.1016/j.amsu.2021.103201

[43] Norouzi S, Tavafian SS, Cousins R, Mokarami H. Study protocol for a randomized controlled trial to improve the quality of life of housewives with musculoskeletal disorders: A health promotion intervention based on a participatory ergonomic approach-the housewives ergonomic intervention (HEI) trial. Trials. 2021;**22**(1):490. DOI: 10.1186/s13063-021-05436-w

[44] Tang KHD. The prevalence, causes, and prevention of occupational musculoskeletal disorders. Global Academic Journal of Medical Sciences. 2022;**4**:56-68. DOI: 10.36348/gajms.2022.v04i02.004

[45] Singh LP. Prevalence of MSDs among nurses: A study in Indian health care industry. Ergonomics International Journal. 2018;**2**:10

[46] Rathore FA, Attique R, Asmaa Y. Prevalence and perceptions of musculoskeletal disorders among hospital nurses in Pakistan: A Cross-sectional survey. Cureus. 2017;**9**(1):e1001. DOI: 10.7759/cureus.1001

[47] Tinubu BM, Mbada CE, Oyeyemi AL, Fabunmi AA. Work-related musculoskeletal disorders among nurses in Ibadan, south-West Nigeria: A cross-sectional survey. BMC Musculoskeletal Disorders. 2010;**11**:12. DOI: 10.1186/1471-2474-11-12

[48] Khudhir KM, Saleh KK, Qadir MS, Mahmood KA, Ariffin AA. Association between work-relate musculoskeletal disorder and ergonomic risk factors among nursing professionals in Ranya and Qaladiza districts. Kurdistan Journal of Applied Research. 2017;**2**:65-70

[49] Malchaire J, Cock N, Vergracht S. Review of the factors associated with musculoskeletal problems in epidemiological studies. International Archives of Occupational and Environmental Health. 2001;**74**(2):79-90. DOI: 10.1007/s004200000212

[50] Yang S, Lu J, Zeng J, Wang L, Li Y. Prevalence and risk factors of work-related musculoskeletal disorders among intensive care unit nurses in China. Workplace Health & Safety. 2019;**67**(6):275-287. DOI: 10.1177/2165079918809107

[51] Chiwaridzo M, Makotore V, Dambi JM, Munambah N, Mhlanga M. Work-related musculoskeletal disorders among registered general nurses: A case of a large central hospital in Harare, Zimbabwe. BMC Research Notes. 2018;**11**(1):315. DOI: 10.1186/s13104-018-3412-8

[52] Alperovitch-Najenson D, Treger I, Kalichman L. Physical therapists versus

nurses in a rehabilitation hospital: Comparing prevalence of work-related musculoskeletal complaints and working conditions. Archives of Environmental & Occupational Health. 2014;**69**(1):33-39. DOI: 10.1080/19338244.2012.719555

[53] Pompeii LA, Lipscomb HJ, Schoenfisch AL, Dement JM. Musculoskeletal injuries resulting from patient handling tasks among hospital workers. American Journal of Industrial Medicine. 2009;**52**(7):571-578. DOI: 10.1002/ajim.20704

[54] Yitayeh A, Mekonnen S, Fasika S, Gizachew M. Annual prevalence of self-reported work-related musculoskeletal disorders and associated factors among nurses working at Gondar town governmental health institutions, Northwest Ethiopia. Emergency Medicine Australasia. 2015;**5**:1-7

[55] Yasobant S, Rajkumar P. Work-related musculoskeletal disorders among health care professionals: A cross-sectional assessment of risk factors in a tertiary hospital, India. Indian Journal Of Occupational And Environmental Medicine. 2014;**18**(2):75-81. DOI: 10.4103/0019-5278.146896

[56] Keyaerts S, Godderis L, Delvaux E, Daenen L. The association between work-related physical and psychosocial factors and musculoskeletal disorders in healthcare workers: Moderating role of fear of movement. Journal of Occupational Health. 2022;**2022**(64):e12314. DOI: 10.1002/1348-9585.12314

[57] Josephson M. Work Factors and Musculoskeletal Disorders-an Epidemiological Approach Focusing on Female Nursing Personnel (Thesis). Stockholm, Sweden: Karolinska Institute; 1998. pp. 5-6

[58] Harrington WJ, Preziosi RC, Gooden DJ. Worldview resiliency of business degree graduate students – An examination of spiritual experiences and psychological attitudes. In: Parris MA, Barnes B, Vickers MH, editors. Proceedings of the 12th Annual International Conference 2004: Leadership in the 21st Century: Working, Living, and Surviving Organizational Life. Association on Employment Practices and Principles. New York City, New York: Manhattan College; 2004

[59] Hall E, Hughes B, Handzo G. Spiritual Care: What it Means, Why it Matters in Health Care. 2016. Available from: https://www.researchgate.net/publication/309346734_Spiritual_Care_What_It_Means_Why_It_Matters_in_Health_Care

[60] Pradhan RK, Jena LK. Workplace spirituality and employee job behaviour: An empirical investigation in Indian manufacturing organizations. Paradigm. 2016;**20**(2):1-17

[61] Hui D, de la Cruz M, Thorney S, Parsons HA, Delgado-Guay M, Bruera E. The frequency and correlates of spiritual distress among patients with advanced cancer admitted to an acute palliative care unit. The American Journal of Hospice & Palliative Care. 2011;**28**(4):264-270. DOI: 10.1177/1049909110385917

[62] Kopacz MS, Hoffmire CA, Morley SW, Vance GC. Using a spiritual distress scale to assess suicide risk in veterans: An exploratory study. Pastoral Psychology. 2015;**64**(3):381-390

[63] Abu-Raiya H, Pargament KI, Krause N, Ironson G. Robust links between religious/spiritual struggles, psychological distress, and well-being in a national sample of American adults. The American Journal of

Orthopsychiatry. 2015;**85**(6):565-575. DOI: 10.1037/ort0000084

[64] Krause N, Ironson G, Pargament KI. Spiritual struggles and resting pulse rates: Does strong distress tolerance promote more effective coping? Personality and Individual Differences. 2016;**98**:261-265

[65] Beheshtifar M, Zare E. Effect of spirituality in workplace on job performance. Interdisciplinary Journal of Contemporary Research in Business. 2013;**5**:248-254. DOI: 10.3389/fpsyg.2022.881675

[66] Pouragha B, Sheikhbardsiri H, Asgharnezhad M, Abdolahi M, Sahebi A, Amiri H. Does workplace spirituality enhance motivation of hospitals social workers? The scrutiny in Iran. The International Journal of Social Psychiatry. 2022;**68**(5):1135-1140. DOI: 10.1177/00207640211023081

[67] Chirico F, Acquadro Maran D, Sharma M. Editorial: Spirituality in the workplace. Frontiers in Psychology. 2023;**14**:1162716. DOI: 10.3389/fpsyg.2023.1162716

[68] Long MH, Johnston V, Bogossian F. Work-related upper quadrant musculoskeletal disorders in midwives, nurses and physicians: A systematic review of risk factors and functional consequences. Applied Ergonomics. 2012;**43**(3):455-467. DOI: 10.1016/j.apergo.2011.07.002

[69] Caruso CC, Waters TR. A review of work schedule issues and musculoskeletal disorders with an emphasis on the healthcare sector. Industrial Health. 2008;**46**(6):523-534. DOI: 10.2486/indhealth.46.523

[70] Deepti KC, Nirupa T. Prevalence and risk factors of musculoskeletal pain among nurses in selected hospitals of Kaski, Nepal. IOSR Journal of Nursing and Health Science. 2019;**8**(6):57-66

[71] Takahashi M, Iwakiri K, Sotoyama M, Hirata M, Hisanaga N. Musculoskeletal pain and night-shift naps in nursing home care workers. Occupational medicine (Oxford, England). 2009;**59**(3):197-200. DOI: 10.1093/occmed/kqp029

[72] Trinkoff AM, Le R, Geiger-Brown J, Lipscomb J, Lang G. Longitudinal relationship of work hours, mandatory overtime, and on-call to musculoskeletal problems in nurses. American Journal of Industrial Medicine. 2006;**49**(11):964-971. DOI: 10.1002/ajim.20330

[73] Hale AR, Hovden J. Management and culture: The third age of safety. A review of approaches to organizational aspects of safety, health and environment. In: Hale AR, Hovden J, editors. Occupational Injury: Risk, Prevention and Intervention. Boca Raton, FL: CRC Press; 1998. pp. 129-165

[74] Ojo O. Organisational culture and performance: Empirical investigation of Nigerian insurance companies. Manager Journal. 2008;**8**:118-127

[75] Ogiamien L, Izuagbe R. Impact of organisational and psychological factors on the job performance of personnel in private university libraries in south-South Nigeria. Open Access Library Journal. 2016;**3**:1-14. DOI: 10.4236/oalib.1102419

[76] Imam A, Abbasi AS, Muneer S, Qadri MM. Organizational culture and performance of higher educational institutions: The mediating role of individual readiness for change. European Journal of Business and Management. 2013;**5**:23-34

[77] Gherscovici ED, Mayer JM. Relationship of healthy building determinants with Back and neck pain: A systematic review. American Journal of Health Promotion: AJHP. 2023;**37**(1):103-131. DOI: 10.1177/08901171221112571

[78] Magnavita N, Elovainio M, De Nardis I, Heponiemi T, Bergamaschi A. Environmental discomfort and musculoskeletal disorders. Occupational Medicine (Oxford, England). 2011;**61**(3):196-201. DOI: 10.1093/occmed/kqr024

[79] David G, Woods V, Li G, Buckle P. The development of the quick exposure check (QEC) for assessing exposure to risk factors for work-related musculoskeletal disorders. Applied Ergonomics. 2008;**39**(1):57-69. DOI: 10.1016/j.apergo.2007.03.002

[80] Bang BE, Aasmoe L, Aardal L, Andorsen GS, Bjørnbakk AK, Egeness C, et al. Feeling cold at work increases the risk of symptoms from muscles, skin, and airways in seafood industry workers. American Journal of Industrial Medicine. 2005;**47**(1):65-71. DOI: 10.1002/ajim.20109

[81] Chiang HC, Ko YC, Chen SS, Yu HS, Wu TN, Chang PY. Prevalence of shoulder and upper-limb disorders among workers in the fish-processing industry. Scandinavian Journal of Work, Environment & Health. 1993;**19**(2):126-131. DOI: 10.5271/sjweh.1496

[82] Chad KE, Brown JM. Climatic stress in the workplace: Its effect on thermoregulatory responses and muscle fatigue in female workers. Applied Ergonomics. 1995;**26**(1):29-34. DOI: 10.1016/0003-6870(95)95749-p

[83] Berry HL, Bowen K, Kjellstrom T. Climate change and mental health: A causal pathways framework. International Journal of Public Health. 2010;**55**(2):123-132. DOI: 10.1007/s00038-009-0112-0

[84] Tawatsupa B, Lim LL, Kjellstrom T, Seubsman SA, Sleigh A, The Thai Cohort Study Team. The association between overall health, psychological distress, and occupational heat stress among a large national cohort of 40,913 Thai workers. Global Health Action. May 2010;**13**:3. DOI: 10.3402/gha.v3i0.5034. PMID: 20485479; PMCID: PMC2871739

[85] Hancock PA, Ross JM, Szalma JL. A meta-analysis of performance response under thermal stressors. Human Factors. 2007;**49**(5):851-877. DOI: 10.1518/001872007X230226

[86] Pilcher JJ, Nadler E, Busch C. Effects of hot and cold temperature exposure on performance: A meta-analytic review. Ergonomics. 2002;**45**(10):682-698. DOI: 10.1080/00140130210158419

[87] Abaraogu UO, Ezema CI, Igwe SE, Egwuonwu AV, Okafor UC. Work-related back discomfort and associated factors among automotive maintenance mechanics in eastern Nigeria: A cross sectional study. Work (Reading, Mass.). 2016;**53**(4):813-823. DOI: 10.3233/WOR-162247

[88] Abraha TH, Demoz AT, Moges HG, Ahmmed AN. Predictors of back disorder among Almeda textile factory workers, North Ethiopia. BMC Research Notes. 2018;**11**(1):304. DOI: 10.1186/s13104-018-3440-4

[89] Cagnie B, Danneels L, Van Tiggelen D, De Loose V, Cambier D. Individual and work related risk factors for neck pain among office workers: A cross sectional study. European Spine Journal: Official Publication of the European Spine Society, the European

Spinal Deformity Society, and the European Section of the Cervical Spine Research Society. 2007;**16**(5):679-686. DOI: 10.1007/s00586-006-0269-7

[90] Tang DKH, Leiliabadi F, Olugu EU. Factors affecting the safety of processes in the Malaysian oil and gas industry. Safety Science. 2017;**92**:44-52. DOI: 10.1016/j.ssci.2016.09.017

[91] Alexopoulos EC, Burdorf A, Kalokerinou A. Risk factors for musculoskeletal disorders among nursing personnel in Greek hospitals. International Archives of Occupational and Environmental Health. 2003;**76**(4):289-294. DOI: 10.1007/s00420-003-0442-9

[92] Trinkoff AM, Lipscomb JA, Geiger-Brown J, Storr CL, Brady BA. Perceived physical demands and reported musculoskeletal problems in registered nurses. American Journal of Preventive Medicine. 2003;**24**(3):270-275. DOI: 10.1016/s0749-3797(02)00639-6

[93] Daraiseh NM, Cronin SN, Davis LS, Shell RL, Karwowski W. Low back symptoms among hospital nurses, associations to individual factors and pain in multiple body regions. International Journal of Industrial Ergonomics. 2010;**19**:14e24

[94] Menzel NN, Brooks SM, Bernard TE, Nelson A. The physical workload of nursing personnel: Association with musculoskeletal discomfort. International Journal of Nursing Studies. 2004;**41**(8):859-867. DOI: 10.1016/j.ijnurstu.2004.03.012

[95] Heiden B, Weigl M, Angerer P, Müller A. Association of age and physical job demands with musculoskeletal disorders in nurses. Applied Ergonomics. 2013;**44**(4):652-658. DOI: 10.1016/j.apergo.2013.01.001

[96] Heidari M, Borujeni MG, Rezaei P, Kabirian Abyaneh S. Work-related musculoskeletal disorders and their associated factors in nurses: A Cross-sectional study in Iran. The Malaysian Journal of Medical Sciences: MJMS. 2019;**26**(2):122-130. DOI: 10.21315/mjms2019.26.2.13

[97] Akrouf QA, Crawford JO, Al-Shatti AS, Kamel MI. Musculoskeletal disorders among bank office workers in Kuwait. Eastern Mediterranean Health Journal = La revue de sante de la Mediterranee orientale = al-Majallah al-sihhiyah li-sharq al-mutawassit. 2010;**16**(1):94-100

[98] Viester L, Verhagen EA, Oude Hengel KM, Koppes LL, van der Beek AJ, Bongers PM. The relation between body mass index and musculoskeletal symptoms in the working population. BMC Musculoskeletal Disorders. 2013;**14**:238. DOI: 10.1186/1471-2474-14-238

[99] Gorgi Z, Assadollahi Z, Ghaffarian A, Rezaeian M. The prevalence of musculoskeletal disorders in the employees of office systems at Rafsanjan University of Medical Sciences in 2012. Journal of Rafsanjan University of Medical Sciences. 2012;**12**(12):991-1002

[100] Voorbij AI, Steenbekkers LP. The composition of a graph on the decline of total body strength with age based on pushing, pulling, twisting and gripping force. Applied Ergonomics. 2001;**32**(3):287-292. DOI: 10.1016/s0003-6870(00)00068-5

[101] Chin DL, Nam S, Lee SJ. Occupational factors associated with obesity and leisure-time physical

activity among nurses: A cross sectional study. International Journal of Nursing Studies. 2016;**57**:60-69. DOI: 10.1016/j.ijnurstu.2016.01.009

[102] Allman-Farinelli MA, Chey T, Merom D, Bauman AE. Occupational risk of overweight and obesity: An analysis of the Australian health survey. Journal of Occupational Medicine and Toxicology (London, England). 2010;**5**:14. DOI: 10.1186/1745-6673-5-14

[103] Martín AR, Nieto JM, Ruiz JP, Jiménez LE. Overweight and obesity: The role of education, employment and income in Spanish adults. Appetite. 2008;**51**(2):266-272. DOI: 10.1016/j.appet.2008.02.021

[104] World Cancer Research Fund – WCRF. The Link between Food, Nutrition, Diet and Non-Communicable Diseases. London, UK: WCRF; 2021

[105] World Health Organization – WHO. World Health Organization Global Status Report on Noncommunicable Diseases 2014. Geneva, Switzerland: WHO Library Cataloguing in-Publication Data; 2014

[106] Mynarski W, Grabara M, Nawrocka A, Niestrój-Jaworska M, Wołkowycka B, Cholewa J. Rekreacyjna aktywność fizyczna i dolegliwości mięśniowo-szkieletowe pielęgniarek [Physical recreational activity and musculoskeletal disorders in nurses]. Medycyna Pracy. 2014;**65**(2):181-188

[107] Karhu O, Kansi P, Kuorinka I. Correcting working postures in industry: A practical method for analysis. Appled Ergonomics. 1977;**8**:199-201

[108] McAtamney L, Nigel Corlett E. RULA: A survey method for the investigation of work-related upper limb disorders. Applied Ergonomics. 1993;**24**(2):91-99. DOI: 10.1016/0003-6870(93)90080-s

[109] Hignett S, McAtamney L. Rapid entire body assessment (REBA). Appled Ergonomics. 2003;**31**:201-205

[110] Li G, Buckle P. Evaluating Change in Exposure to Risk forMusculoskeletal Disorders—A Practical Tool. Suffolk: HSE Books; 1999

[111] Abd Rahman MN, Abdul Rani MR, Rohani JM. WERA: An observational tool develop to investigate the physical risk factor associated with WMSDs. Journal of Human Ergology. 2011;**40**(1-2):19-36

[112] Kuorinka I, Jonsson B, Kilbom A, Vinterberg H, Biering-Sørensen F, Andersson G, et al. Standardised Nordic questionnaires for the analysis of musculoskeletal symptoms. Applied Ergonomics. 1987;**18**(3):233-237. DOI: 10.1016/0003-6870(87)90010-x

[113] Dawson AP, Steele EJ, Hodges PW, Stewart S. Development and test–retest reliability of an extended version of the Nordic musculoskeletal questionnaire (NMQ-E): A screening instrument for musculoskeletal pain. The Journal of Pain. 2009;**10**(5):517-526. DOI: 10.1016/j.jpain.2008.11.008

[114] Inyang N, Al-Hussein M, El-Rich M, Al-Jibouri S. Ergonomic analysis and the need for its integration for planning and assessing construction tasks. Journal of Construction Engineering Management. 2012;**138**(12):1370-1376. DOI: 10.1061/(ASCE)CO.1943-7862.0000556

[115] David GC. Ergonomic methods for assessing exposure to risk factors for work-related musculoskeletal disorders. Occupational Medicine (Oxford, England). 2005;**55**(3):190-199. DOI: 10.1093/occmed/kqi082

[116] Jones T, Kumar S. Comparison of ergonomic risk assessment output in four sawmill jobs. International Journal of Occupational Safety and Ergonomics: JOSE. 2010;**16**(1):105-111. DOI: 10.1080/10803548.2010.11076834

[117] Takala EP, Pehkonen I, Forsman M, Hansson GÅ, Mathiassen SE, Neumann WP, et al. Systematic evaluation of observational methods assessing biomechanical exposures at work. Scandinavian Journal of Work, Environment & Health. 2010;**36**(1):3-24. DOI: 10.5271/sjweh.2876

[118] Coenen P, Kingma I, Boot CR, Faber GS, Xu X, Bongers PM, et al. Estimation of low back moments from video analysis: A validation study. Journal of Biomechanics. 2011;**44**(13):2369-2375. DOI: 10.1016/j.jbiomech.2011.07.005

[119] Asuquo EG, Murphy Tighe S, Bradshaw C. Interventions to reduce work-related musculoskeletal disorders among healthcare staff in nursing homes; an integrative literature review. International Journal of Nursing Studies Advances. 2021;**3**:100033

[120] Kurowski A, Gore R, Roberts Y, Kincaid KR, Punnett L. Injury rates before and after the implementation of a safe resident handling program in the long-term care sector. Safety Science. 2017;**92**:217-224. DOI: 10.1016/j.ssci.2016.10.012

[121] Gold JE, Punnett L, Gore RJ, ProCare Research Team. Predictors of low back pain in nursing home workers after implementation of a safe resident handling programme. Occupational and Environmental Medicine. 2017;**74**(6):389-395. DOI: 10.1136/oemed-2016-103930

[122] Tompa E, Dolinschi R, Alamgir H, Sarnocinska-Hart A, Guzman J. A cost-benefit analysis of peer coaching for overhead lift use in the long-term care sector in Canada. Occupational and Environmental Medicine. 2016;**73**(5):308-314. DOI: 10.1136/oemed-2015-103134

[123] Peterson EL, McGlothlin JD, Blue CL. The development of an ergonomics training program to identify, evaluate, and control musculoskeletal disorders among nursing assistants at a state-run veterans' home. Journal of Occupational and Environmental Hygiene. 2004;**1**(1):D10-D16. DOI: 10.1080/15459620490264427

[124] Kozak A, Freitag S, Nienhaus A. Evaluation of a training program to reduce stressful trunk postures in the nursing professions: A pilot study. Annals of Work Exposures and Health. 2017;**61**(1):22-32. DOI: 10.1093/annweh/wxw002

[125] Larsen AK, Thygesen LC, Mortensen OS, Punnett L, Jørgensen MB. The effect of strengthening health literacy in nursing homes on employee pain and consequences of pain – A stepped-wedge intervention trial. Scandinavian Journal of Work, Environment & Health. 2019;**45**(4):386-395. DOI: 10.5271/sjweh.3801

[126] O'Brien WH, Singh RS, Horan K, Moeller MT, Wasson R, Jex SM. Group-based acceptance and commitment therapy for nurses and nurse aides working in Long-term care residential settings. Journal of Alternative and Complementary Medicine (New York, N.Y.). 2019;**25**(7):753-761. DOI: 10.1089/acm.2019.0087

[127] Martinez VML. The importance of workplace exercise. Revista brasileira de medicina do trabalho: publicacao oficial

da Associacao Nacional de Medicina do Trabalho-ANAMT. 2021;**19**(4):523-528. DOI: 10.47626/1679-4435-2021-666

[128] Maciel R, Albuquerque A, Melzer A, Leônidas S. Quem se beneficia dos programas de ginástica laboral? Cad Psicologia Social Trabalho. 2005;**8**:71-86. DOI: 10.11606/issn.1981-0490.v8i0p71-86

[129] Park HK, Jung MK, Park E, Lee CY, Jee YS, Eun D, et al. The effect of warm-ups with stretching on the isokinetic moments of collegiate men. Journal of Exercise Rehabilitation. 2018;**14**(1):78-82. DOI: 10.12965/jer.1835210.605

[130] Shariat A, Cleland JA, Danaee M, Kargarfard M, Sangelaji B, Tamrin SBM. Effects of stretching exercise training and ergonomic modifications on musculoskeletal discomforts of office workers: A randomized controlled trial. Brazilian Journal of Physical Therapy. 2018;**22**(2):144-153. DOI: 10.1016/j.bjpt.2017.09.003

[131] Tsang SMH, So BCL, Lau RWL, Dai J, Szeto GPY. Effects of combining ergonomic interventions and motor control exercises on muscle activity and kinematics in people with work-related neck-shoulder pain. European Journal of Applied Physiology. 2018;**118**(4):751-765. DOI: 10.1007/s00421-018-3802-6

[132] Serra MVGB, Pimenta LC, Quemelo PRV. Efeitos da ginástica laboral na saúde do trabalhador: uma revisão da literatura. Revista Pesquisa em Fisioterapia. 2014;**4**(3):197-205. DOI: 10.17267/2238-2704rpf.v4i3.436

[133] de Freitas-Swerts FC, Robazzi ML. The effects of compensatory workplace exercises to reduce work-related stress and musculoskeletal pain. Revista Latino-Americana de Enfermagem. 2014;**22**(4):629-636. DOI: 10.1590/0104-1169.3222.2461

[134] Bernardes JM. Ginástica laboral e prática de atividades físicas de lazer: uma revisão bibliográfica. Revista de Educação Física. 2011;**2**(1):71-81

[135] Gok Metin Z, Ejem D, Dionne-Odom JN, Turkman Y, Salvador C, Pamboukian S, et al. Mind-body interventions for individuals with heart failure: A systematic review of randomized trials. Journal of Cardiac Failure. 2018;**24**(3):186-201. DOI: 10.1016/j.cardfail.2017.09.008

[136] Moreira-Silva I, Teixeira PM, Santos R, Abreu S, Moreira C, Mota J. The effects of workplace physical activity programs on musculoskeletal pain: A systematic review and meta-analysis. Workplace Health & Safety. 2016;**64**(5):210-222. DOI: 10.1177/2165079916629688

[137] Bloom DE, Canning D, Fink D. Implications of population ageing fo reconomic growth. Oxford Review of Economic Policy. 2010;**26**(4):583-612

[138] March L, Smith EU, Hoy DG, Cross MJ, Sanchez-Riera L, Blyth F, et al. Burden of disability due to musculoskeletal (MSK) disorders. Best practice & research. Clinical Rheumatology. 2014;**28**(3):353-366. DOI: 10.1016/j.berh.2014.08.002

[139] von Bonsdorff ME, Huuhtanen P, Tuomi K, Seitsamo J. Predictors of employees' early retirement intentions: An 11-year longitudinal study. Occupational Medicine (Oxford, England). 2010;**60**(2):94-100. DOI: 10.1093/occmed/kqp126

[140] Macdonald W, Oakman J. Requirements for more effective prevention of work-related

musculoskeletal disorders. BMC Musculoskeletal Disorders. 2015;**16**:293. DOI: 10.1186/s12891-015-0750-8

[141] Verbeek JH, Martimo KP, Karppinen J, Kuijer PP, Viikari-Juntura E, Takala EP. Manual material handling advice and assistive devices for preventing and treating back pain in workers. The Cochrane Database of Systematic Reviews. 2011;**6**:CD005958. DOI: 10.1002/14651858.CD005958.pub3

[142] Hoe VC, Urquhart DM, Kelsall HL, Sim MR. Ergonomic design and training for preventing work-related musculoskeletal disorders of the upper limb and neck in adults. The Cochrane Database of Systematic Reviews. 2012;**2012**(8):CD008570. DOI: 10.1002/14651858.CD008570.pub2

[143] Global Burden of Disease Study 2013 Collaborators. Global, regional, and national incidence, prevalence, and years lived with disability for 301 acute and chronic diseases and injuries in 188 countries, 1990-2013: A systematic analysis for the global burden of disease study 2013. Lancet (London, England). 2015;**386**(9995):743-800. DOI: 10.1016/S0140-6736(15)60692-427

[144] Cattrell A, Harris EC, Palmer KT, Kim M, Aylward M, Coggon D. Regional trends in awards of incapacity benefit by cause. Occupational Medicine (Oxford, England). 2011;**61**(3):148-151. DOI: 10.1093/occmed/kqr008

[145] Wells R. Why have we not solved the MSD problem? Work (Reading, Mass.). 2009;**34**(1):117-121. DOI: 10.3233/WOR-2009-0937

[146] van der Beek AJ, Dennerlein JT, Huysmans MA, Mathiassen SE, Burdorf A, van Mechelen W, et al. A research framework for the development and implementation of interventions preventing work-related musculoskeletal disorders. Scandinavian Journal of Work, Environment & Health. 2017;**43**(6):526-539. DOI: 10.5271/sjweh.3671

[147] ISO 31000. Risk management. Geneva, Switzerland: International Organization for Standardization; 2015

[148] Finch C. A new framework for research leading to sports injury prevention. Journal of Science and Medicine in Sport. 2006;**9**(1-2):3-10. DOI: 10.1016/j.jsams.2006.02.009

[149] Sallis JF, Owen N, Fotheringham MJ. Behavioral epidemiology: A systematic framework to classify phases of research on health promotion and disease prevention. Annals of Behavioral Medicine: A Publication of the Society of Behavioral Medicine. 2000;**22**(4):294-298. DOI: 10.1007/BF02895665

[150] van Mechelen W, Hlobil H, Kemper HC. Incidence, severity, aetiology and prevention of sports injuries. A review of concepts. Sports Medicine (Auckland, N.Z.). 1992;**14**(2):82-99. DOI: 10.2165/00007256-199214020-00002

Section 2

Education and Training of Nurses

Chapter 7

Perspective Chapter: Clinical Competency Framework – Standardized Nurse Competence Development

Susan Boyer and Miriam Chickering

Abstract

A regional nurse leadership group established the Clinical Competency Framework with representation from academic, regulation, and practice-based settings. The framework provides structures, tools and workplace systems that address the full continuum of care. It is the only competency framework that: 1) integrates evidence-based preceptor support systems, 2) standardizes competency and coaching tools, 3) addresses all levels of nurse hires with a universal set of competencies, and 4) offers shared ownership for program dissemination. The Framework supports clinical preceptors, orientees, students, and transition into new specialties. It addresses issues of competency validation for nurses in multiple settings and the same templates/guidelines are used for settings across the continuum of care. The competency-based orientation is achieved through a preceptorship model, emphasizing the need for preceptor development. Allied healthcare partners have adapted the tools for their use and the model is shared via a membership venue that invites educators to 'share and share back.'

Keywords: nurse competence, preceptor development, clinical competencies, nurse professional development, academic-practice clinical development

1. Introduction

The Clinical Competency Framework (CCF) was established by a state-wide nurse leadership group with members from academia, regulation and practice-based roles and settings. The project sought to bridge the transition to practice gap experienced by new graduate nurses. Currently, the model provides supporting structures, tools, and workplace support systems for a transition framework that addresses the full continuum of care within a single competency framework [1]. The CCF is the only competency framework that a) integrates evidence-based preceptor development/support systems, b) standardizes competency and clinical coaching tools, c) addresses all levels of nurse hires with a universal set of competency expectations, and d) offers a shared ownership model for program dissemination.

The framework delivers a competency-based orientation process supported by clinical preceptors. Fundamental model concepts include evidence-based practice,

IntechOpen

sampling, accountability, high-end apprenticeships, coaching plans, concept-based development, reflective learning, and patient-centric practice [2–6]. The concepts within the model are constantly evolving, but users must comprehend the role of each framework element before recommendations for change are reliable.

Conducting research validity and reliability analysis is not a sufficient measure to validate a competency-based orientation tool that must adapt to diverse care settings and evolving healthcare practice [7]. The core measure of a successful tool is whether the collected data reveals an accurate portrayal of the ability of the employee to provide safe, effective care; based on agency protocol. Another important measure is whether the regulatory surveyors accept the contents and process as addressing their core requirements [8]. These measures of reliability are met by the CCF as adapted and used in multiple settings – both urban and rural, from trauma center to critical access hospital, and across the continuum of care.

The initial literature search led to the realization that foundational orientation tools focused on tasks, procedures, and equipment; but overlooked the role of critical thinking, reasoning, clinical analysis, and nursing judgement within professional practice. When this competency requirement gap is combined with the need for preceptor development systems, the team recognized that three subsets of response were required. First, our orientation, internship, and competency tools need to detail what critical thinking and clinical judgement looks like within our care settings. Secondly, essential instruction must occur to establish critical thinking (CT) development within the preceptor's role and responsibilities. And thirdly, the competency or transition tools must state specific strategies for developing reasoning skills in the newly hired nurse. These framework components were addressed along with updates in the identified roles of the preceptor to increase focus on the roles of protection and evaluation.

2. Benefits and measures

Patient care outcomes are significantly impacted by new graduate preparation for practice. Del Bueno [9] reported in 2005 that new graduate nurses met entry level expectations only 35% of the time. A follow-up study conducted 10 years later, revealed a drop to 28% meeting expectations [10]. This presents a serious concern with the ever- increasing complexity of healthcare environments and interventions. One component of the problem is development of clinical judgement and the importance of teaching nurses how to think like a nurse [11].

Multiple research and quality improvement projects have applied the CCF tools and processes. The Nebraska Center for Nursing project [12] included specific data collection regarding cost of orientation. CCF resources were used to modify how preceptors are taught and utilized in both urban and rural settings across Nebraska. Managers reported significant reduction in estimated orientation costs between the control and treatment periods. Baseline orientation costs were reported at $7,028 per new graduate, with reduction to $4,961 with CCF implementation. Outcomes also revealed a reduction in incidence of errors or near misses. The study concluded that new nursing graduates were more satisfied, better prepared, and had fewer errors.

Robbins [13] reported that nurse employment turn-over rate decreased from 33.6% (prior to program) to 16.5% in the year following completion of the program, a 50% decrease ($p < 0.1$). He averaged the cost of $85,000/nurse oriented to the Burn ICU specialty, thus retention results in significant cost savings. Data analysis validated both efficacy and improved staff satisfaction resulting from model use. The success within the

Burn Unit was demonstrated as replicable in other specialties and further work within the military medical system ensued [14]. Currently the CCF tools and process are being adapted for both military nurse competency and combat casualty care development.

Multiple studies, performance and quality improvement projects have utilized CCF components. Program outcomes show a reduction in incidence of patient errors/near misses, lowered orientation costs, and improvements on factors of satisfaction, retention, and positive workplace culture [12, 14, 15].

3. Program overview

The CCF is a 'best practice' clinical transition program that has been in place for over two decades and has seen annual growth, expansion, evaluation, and advancement. The preceptor supported design provides experience and deliberate practice to support learning and successful transition into clinical practice. The experiential learning within the CCF occurs synergistically with individual studies, staff development courses, clinical conferences, and one-on-one support and instruction from a preceptor. The program advances clinical practice skills needed to deliver safe, comprehensive care in existing and emerging organized health care systems. Collaborative resource development, ongoing research, and evidence-based preceptor support systems are featured within the framework. The model is suitable for new hire orientation, transition of new graduates (or new to specialty), nurse residency programs, and/or competency validation for contractors or travelers.

The CCF is built upon prominent nursing theories which include, Benner's novice to expert model, her more recent call for three high-end apprenticeships, and the Competency Outcomes Performance Assessment (COPA) model [16, 17]. Core concepts related to teaching and learning, emotional intelligence, team process, systems thinking, transition shock, reflective learning, professional accountability, and sampling theory are incorporated within the framework. The COPA model works synergistically with Quality and Safety Education for Nurses (QSEN) [17, 18] as displayed within the competency tools and process. While addressing the same core performance focus of QSEN knowledge, skills, and attitudes, the CCF shifts the goals to target the manner in which nurses provide clinical care. Specific skills identified within the competency tools emphasize nursing clinical practice, clinical reasoning, and professional judgement. CCF performance criteria reflect the need to view the patient in a holistic manner and consider the possibility of differential diagnoses or related issues. The nurse development targets a concept-based approach to learning and to competence development.

Reflective learning theory integrates with competency validation work to ensure current practice capability while developing reasoning and judgment skills. Both reflective and experiential learning strategies are employed within clinical coaching plans that guide the preceptor in their crucial role [19–21]. The preceptor fosters reflection within the clinical learning environment, provides deliberate practice to enhance both skill development and professional practice confidence, and documents achievement of specific competency requirements [21].

4. Core concepts integrated within the CCF

The *Competence Outcomes Performance Assessment (COPA) model sets* format and content considerations for competency tools within the CCF [16]. Lenburg identified eight essential competencies of: assessment and intervention, communication, critical thinking, teaching, human caring relationships, management, leadership, and knowledge integration. All the specific skills. actions, and judgement that nurses engage can be listed under one of these categories. This model initiated a complete re-thinking of new hire orientation tools [22]. Previously, most agencies used diverse sets of checklists detailing the tasks and procedures pertaining to the nurse's role. The COPA model caused a shift in thinking to quantify and prioritize aspects of critical thinking and knowledge integration; while focusing energy and evaluation on aspects of leadership and management within our direct care roles. With Dr. Lenburg's help, the competency criteria address high-level performance expectations within clear, concrete, and concise statements. Performance criteria address the top levels of Bloom's pyramid of action verbs [19, 23], rather than the bottom.

The Clinical Transition Framework uses COPA because it is a model that also fits for the full interdisciplinary team. The universal competencies for nurses are easily adaptable for Rehabilitation, Respiratory, and other direct care personnel [24]. The COPA model establishes the performance outcomes focus of the assessment process. It targets critical thinking and clinical judgement, as crucial aspects of professional practice and goes a step further in its focus on action statements that reveal actions, reflection, reasoning, and clinical judgement. Core strengths of the COPA model include the focus on practice-based outcomes that are integral to actual practice.

The CCF uses the COPA model in both universal and unit specific CBO tools. The Universal Competency tool is outlined by the eight core competencies and offers aspects of practice that are engaged in all clinical care settings [24]. The Unit-Specific tools build upon the foundation presented within the Universal tool and present performance goal statements in the manner in which we provide care, or within goals related to specific aspects of patient presentation and clinical practice. Integration of the COPA model ensures that the Competency Based Orientation tools extend beyond the commonly seen lists of tasks, procedures, equipment, and documentation issues. Dr Lenburg provided guidance in how to write specific statements to achieve clear, concise, and concrete criteria that are observed within clinical practice. The resulting documents provide a systematic standardized approach to competency development and validation.

Professional accountability is a core function that requires commitment from every licensed care provider [5, 6, 25]. Inclusion of the accountability statement within the orientation form defines what accountability looks like in this setting and provides a specific testimony from the orientee. Each universal and unit specific tool concludes orientation with a 'summary statement' within the signature page for completion of the onboarding program. This summary statement is introduced by the preceptor at the start of the preceptor/preceptee relationship. The statement starts the new hire with specific directions related to their professional practice expectations. It then becomes part of the signed form attesting to clinical competence validation for the individual [22, 26].

Summary statement signature attests to individual accountability for:

- recognizing the limits of their capability or knowledge base
- seeking assistance to meet professional performance criteria
- using learning modules to meet individual knowledge base needs
- accepting personal obligation to maintain practice capability, knowledge base, and patient safety

The orientee accepts responsibility for their practice by signing the accountability statement on completion of orientation. The signature indicates personal responsibility for their actions and inaction, as well as their knowledge base. As a professional care provider, each licensed nurse is responsible and accountable for both their practice and the ongoing capability development. Our profession requires continuous professional development to ensure that we maintain capability and can provide competent patient care. Without ongoing development, the practice of any nurse is outdated within months of completing their coursework and orientation.

Ensuring *nursing and patient centric goal statements* is essential to professional practice. When questioned about "How do we know what they know?" leadership response has often entailed building systems that attempt to address every detail of practice. This response leaves us bogged down in the minutiae of nursing, instead of focusing on professionalism. Orientation and competency tools often present extensive lists of the tasks and procedures that are completed, but these lists do not describe professional nursing practice. What makes nursing care unique and valuable is the clinical reasoning and nursing judgement skills integrated with delivery of tasks, procedures, assessment, and care. The nursing unique parts of our practice apply clinical reasoning and judgement skills within care delivery. Individual tasks are inherent to achieving goals that are patient focused and nursing centric. The 'medical model' of knowledge and skills development approaches learning and competency from a system perspective – as in body systems, or a set of tasks and procedures that are components of care. Many of us continue to follow the patterns with in the medical model due to our prior experience with learning and competency systems. But our prior experience was often not based in evidence or theory, which calls for re- evaluation of those aspects within further development.

Documentation is easier when we use statements that are shaped by the manner in which patients present. The preceptor can sign off on observations of care within a specific patient assignment instead of searching for scattered elements of care in extensive lists of tasks and procedures.

The nurse and patient centric model of developing competencies portray the relationship between tasks, procedures, equipment, tools, assessments, and nursing judgement. Assessment skills are empty and incomplete if a conclusion is not determined and then acted on. The judgement call comes before implementing the plan and is a fundamental responsibility of the clinical nurse.

Competency and coaching goal statements should target aspects of nursing care, while keeping the patient at the center of that care. When goal statements present in the manner in which we provide patient care, they follow the pattern of patient assignments and nursing practice. This presentation makes the preceptor's competency verification and documentation requirements easier, as the aspects of care that are performed are directly linked with the goal statement which was the center of the performance development and/or validation.

Wording does make a difference in how we interpret our role. The shift to a nursing focus is represented in the competency statements listed below in **Table 1.**

In the first statement, the work of the nurse targets the physician and patient care is a by- product. In reality, our work is patient centric and engages nursing unique aspects of practice, thus the second statement better identifies the role and function of nursing. The third competency reveals the traditional, medical view of targeting the heart instead of considering and treating the patient as a whole. The nursing and patient centric statement reflects the manner in which patients present. This presentation guides our practice to start with the presenting problem, and then continue care in a manner that considers differential diagnoses as well as any urgent interventions.

Medical model		Nurse and patient centric
1. Assists the ED physician in the minor procedure room	vs.	2. Ensures patient well-being with minor procedures with/without sedation
3. Determines hemodynamic effects of cardiac dysfunction	vs.	4. Manages care of the patient presenting with 'complaints of chest pain'

Table 1.
Nursing focused competencies vs. those based on the medical model [20].

Sampling theory serves a crucial goal of the model – to ensure a process that remains as clear, concrete, and concise as possible. With this goal in mind, competency validation engages sampling theory to reduce the volume of practice observations [2, 27, 28].

Addressing every possible procedure, task, and care issue is not possible in the medical field as our practice changes weekly with advances in medical technology and health management. With that in mind, sampling methodology provides the most effective approach in selecting the required elements for orientation and competence validation data. Sampling also reduces the workload of the educator, preceptor, and manager.

The concept of sampling allows a selection of specific performance elements to be validated within orientation, and that overall competence can be extrapolated based on this sample. Sampling concepts are used consistently in research, pharmaceutical studies, testing for knowledge base, the assessment that NCLEX uses for licensing, and Joint Commission surveys.

The directions for the form and process need to detail how sampling is applied within the program. Form directions should remain with the documentation files to answer any questions posed by reviewers or surveyors. Having the directions remain with the form is also helpful to the preceptor/orientee team as they complete the tools and revisit the scoring key for accuracy.

Sample selection is impacted by the capabilities that the learner brings to the clinical setting. The performance criteria that are validated can remain the same, even when the patient assignment is modified to the user's capability. For example: the preceptor will want to see a significant amount of clinical practice by a new graduate before signing them off, whereas they might be able to validate performance for a traveler within a single assignment. In the CCF the required elements are highlighted in bold print and the form directions indicate the minimum requirements for completion of competency validation within a competency-based orientation.

It is important that we identify both the initial and ongoing performance expectations for the new hire. By communicating this within orientation, each individual can establish an ongoing performance improvement plan that evolves beyond the basic expectations and carries them into proficient/expert practice. Without this presented on initial orientation, the question remains as to when and how this information is communicated to the new hire. With ongoing expectations identified within orientation documents, everyone is aware of practice expectations at the start of employment. Both high-level, complex performance criteria and the scoring key elements of proficient and expert are used to indicate further advancement of clinical practice. Preceptors and educators involved in learner development support concepts of continuous development within role modeling and discussions of professional goals. Yet the orientation process and preceptor roles remain the same for each direct care provider.

Determining competency validation requirements entails identifying the high risk, high frequency aspects of nursing care that occur on your unit, in your agency. In the process of selecting elements to be included in the sample, the experienced nurse educators and managers consider what clinical care and level of practice is a reasonable expectation for new graduate achievement within an orientation period. The selected sample is then evaluated with consideration of whether it is feasible to achieve within a few days of patient assignments for the traveling nurse. Within the CCF process we have identified these elements in bold script with the directions stating specifically that the bolded items indicate the selected sample for orientation competency validation.

Deliberate practice can bridge the gap between didactic knowledge and clinical application in those engaged with their first nursing position or a new specialty practice. Instead of challenging the orientee with a new and more complex assignment each day, concepts of deliberate practice encourage repeating a same or similar assignment for enough times for the learner to develop dexterity and some level of automaticity in care delivery. Preceptors allow deliberate practice by the newly hired nurse, which results in growth of confidence along with clinical competence [21, 29–31]. This practice establishes a foundation of clinical capability that supports new challenges within later assignments.

There are four core tenets within Deliberate Practice:

1. motivation to attend to task and exert effort,

2. tasks that are outside of a learner's comfort zone,

3. opportunity for immediate feedback, and

4. repeated performance.

Deliberate Practice (DP) allows integration of thinking and skills in a controlled environment, through repeated opportunities to practice skill performance [21]. The repeated practice provides an opportunity to develop automaticity and dexterity with manual skills. With the technical skills becoming habitual, the care provider gains time for thinking through the process to determine its impact and the data that is forthcoming from ongoing assessment and clinical reasoning.

Integrating three high-end apprenticeships – The CCF responds to the 'call for radical transformation in Educating Nurses' as proposed by Benner et al. [3]. Based on her research, Benner calls for three high end apprenticeships as part of the education and development of nurses.

The apprenticeships include stages of:

1. Developing the nursing education, science, and specialty knowledge required as a foundation for safe practice

2. Engaging in deliberate clinical practice to enhance skilled know-how, dexterity, and reflective learning

3. Professional Formation – An apprenticeship in ethical affect, demeanor, and professional formation as a healthcare professional.

These apprenticeships are deliberately integrated within the CCF with coaching plans which provide specific, standardized knowledge content and guidance for the preceptor/new hire team.

Professional Formation is the third essential apprenticeship identified by Benner [3]. Competency within professional practice is an elusive concept that is based in attributes required to act effectively in a healthcare setting. True clinical competency is much more than skills proficiency and requires blended aspects of reasoning, judgement, and decision-making [2, 21].

Reflective and concept-based learning strategies – True clinical competency is much more than skills proficiency and requires blended aspects of reasoning, judgement, and decision-making [21, 29, 32]. Within the CCF, specific strategies target development of clinical reasoning and nursing judgment. The original CCF coaching plans addressed reflective learning strategies with specific questions related to success, challenges and alternative responses to issues that occurred during the week. Weekly conference time is factored into the preceptor's role and responsibilities in pursuit of fostering critical thinking development in the new hire. Reflective questions within the coaching plans start the conversation and assist preceptors in accomplishing this role component. Teaching about how to support reflection learning and clinical reasoning strategies are part of core instructional needs of preceptors.

Concept based learning is engaged within the CCF model of development. It is a concept-based process which views each patient holistically, from a nursing perspective. The forms, format and preceptor development promote replacing traditional 'systems-based' instruction with concept-based learning. This approach engages reflective learning in that the preceptor is encouraged to query "what is the same, what is different" to highlight how aspects of care are related within different diagnosis or issues. Concept-based learning in academia utilizes authentic learning opportunities that mirror actual practice. It also shifts from a focus on task to emphasizing reasoning skills and this shift requires specific instruction and guidance for preceptors. The preceptor needs to target an organizing principle, or a classification of information, and emphasize how aspects of nursing care are related. Preceptors learn new ways to present concepts and exemplars that require problem-solving, and learners strive to understand how to connect facts and concepts within actual patient care for in-depth understanding. The process encourages nurses to use effective thinking skills, promoting safety and quality of care for their patients.

KISS principle represents the phrase, *Keep It Short & Simple*! With adherence to this principle, educators strive to eliminate extraneous verbiage and multi-faceted scoring keys as they develop tools and process for transition into clinical practice. Within the CCF tools and model, we strive to simplify – to make the form and process as easy to use as possible. The tools within the framework focus on clear, concrete, and concise statements and work expectations. The scoring key identifies observed performance or explanations and targets only the aspects pertinent to the clinical preceptor's role and responsibilities. For example, the preceptor should not be expected to document attendance in general orientation, computer training or other elements that are tracked elsewhere. If they are not part of the preceptor's role to deliver, it should not be an element on their documentation tools.

The KISS principle is a key concept applied to preceptor expectations. Traditionally, agencies and schools of nursing have engaged preceptors for work with students and new hires without planning for the additional time required for effective teaching, deliberate practice by the learner, and the time needed for performance validation. VNIP chooses to look at all expectations for the clinical preceptor and evaluate whether the work and timing is feasible for clinical application. With that in mind, courses, tests, education classes, and simulation do not appear on the preceptor's documentation tool, as participation in those events is managed and documented elsewhere. The CCF limits tool contents to aspects of learning or validation that are clearly under the preceptor's jurisdiction. The scoring key is structured in the simplest manner possible with reminders inserted wherever suitable. Time for teaching is factored within policy statements and considered as an essential aspect of developing assignments. Formative evaluation of the program is constantly considering whether the KISS principle is being met to the greatest extent possible. As new tools or concepts are added or evaluated, a key question is its fit with the KISS principle.

Standardized knowledge is outlined within the coaching plans. These tools identify the knowledge that is inherent to practice in a specialty setting or is needed to achieve a specific clinical care goal. Within the coaching plan, this knowledge is identified and linked with the specific performance goal and may be indicated by titles of policy statements, standards of practice, clinical practice guidelines, specialty practice texts, and/or and specific learning modules. With expert published resources available from specialty practice organizations, the educator and preceptor can simply refer to the text, rather than creating, listing, and updating individual resource materials.

Administrative workload reduction within a planned assignment is essential for protecting the role and efficacy of preceptors. As tools and process are established, those developing documentation forms and model requirements must consider who will be responsible for completion of the model or tools. Line by line analysis of orientation tools must include identifying the number of times a preceptor, educator or manager must sign off on elements of competent practice, and how easy it is to find the correct line for documentation. One major health system was able to reduce the required lines for signing with date and preceptor name/initials from 682 to 124 [33]. This workload issue must be considered when planning the assignment of those responsible for guiding the new hire, student, or new graduate nurse.

Administrative workload is a crucial consideration when writing guidelines or policy documents regarding the competency validation process. Asking the clinical care provider to precept, is asking them to complete another task within their workday. Those additional tasks need to be planned into the assignment – with consideration of how the provider will find time to ensure that the task is completed in a safe, effective, and efficient manner.

Program success measures are crucial concepts within the model. A comprehensive competency program provides documentation of performance-based, evidence to validate that requirements were met and/or gaps in capability identified. Performance issues may indicate a need for further development or termination.

A successful competency framework clinical competency framework tracks and documents:

1. Achievement of clearly defined performance expectations, or

2. Early identification of when the new hire is a 'wrong fit' for the unit or role

3. Early identification of when new hire is a potential threat to safe, effective care

All participants must keep these aspects in mind as new staff members are developed. If we are unable to identify early when there is a 'wrong fit' for the novice, the individual's self-esteem and potential are reduced due to inability to meet competency requirements. With early identification of barriers, a remediation plan can be developed, whether it provides additional learning/practice support or recommends a move to a different practice area.

Identifying a potential threat to safe care is core to protecting our patients from potential harm. Making this determination early decreases the potential for a clinical error or harm to the patient. Educators and preceptors must consider these measures of success as they guide the new nurse to a specialty area or aspect of practice where they may flourish. The competency program should be structured to assist educators, managers, and preceptors in identifying those who may succeed, while guiding those that are not doing well to a more suitable practice setting.

Documentation identified as the learner's responsibility. Some preceptors have reported leaving gaps in competency documentation due to the demands and complexity of their dual roles as care provider and preceptor. The complications of the added role can be eased by establishing appropriate expectations. The learner is in orientation for the sake of learning and/or competency validation. They are being paid to complete orientation process and documentation, thus need to take responsibility for both clinical performance and documentation follow-through.

The orientee or student can review the documents and identify which elements might be 'signed off' each day or week. Making this request of the preceptor can assist in completing documentation, while leaving the decision of sufficient evidence to the preceptor. The process may also foster specific discussions about performance accomplishments and needs. To achieve these results, learners must be guided and directed to routinely review and request documentation of the day's accomplishments. This shift in responsibility requires that both preceptors and new hires are instructed and guided in the process change.

Rapid cycle quality improvement process is utilized to ensure that the tools, teaching, and framework are effective [27, 28]. Within this approach to evaluation, changes in content and format occur in an ongoing manner of prompt response to concerns, issues, and environmental influences. The tools and model remain evidence based, as the changes and adaptations are based on the current evolving evidence within clinical practice.

To establish a sampling strategy for Rapid Cycle Quality Improvement, Etchells & Woodcock recommend two useful guiding principles for sampling. "1. obtain just enough data to guide next steps 2. make full use of local subject matter expertise in selecting the most appropriate samples" [34, p. 63].

The rapid cycle quality improvement process reflects the execution of plan-do-study-act cycles as detailed by Taylor et al. [30]. "The PDSA cycle presents a pragmatic scientific method for testing changes in complex systems. The four stages mirror the scientific experimental method of formulating a hypothesis, collecting data to test this hypothesis, analyzing, and interpreting the results and making inferences to iterate the hypothesis. The pragmatic principles of PDSA cycles promote the use of a small-scale, iterative approach to test interventions, as this enables rapid assessment and provides flexibility to adapt the change according to feedback to ensure fit-for-purpose solutions are developed. Starting with small-scale tests provides users with freedom to act and learn; minimizing risk to patients, the organization and resources required and providing the opportunity to build evidence for change and engage stakeholders as confidence in the intervention increases" [30, p. 29].

Within the CCF, the local subject matter experts are the clinical care providers within each unit or specialty. The framework collects data in an ongoing manner to evolve the model for optimal engagement of both new and experienced staff members. These experts provide the necessary data to ensure that changes in the delivery model produce safe and effective care that adheres to protocols as established by the agency and specialty practice organizations.

Identifying core elements of nursing practice must be a first priority. A crucial goal of the CCF is to establish evidence that the individual is competent to engage in independent nursing practice. With the assistance of competency assessment tools, evidence collection within orientation or transition programs seeks to determine if the new hire consistently engages four elements of professional practice.

The program is successful and effective if it ensures that the new hire can meet four practice elements:

1. Provide safe and effective care as per protocol

2. Adapt plan of care to patient's changing needs & priorities

3. Identify the limits of capability

4. Seek assistance appropriately

Consider your current program tools, documentation, and reflective learning strategies to support nurse development. Are the tools complete and are they completed fully/correctly by the preceptors? Do they support the development of preceptors as clinical educators? Are preceptors able to engage strategies that foster critical thinking, reasoning skills, and clinical judgement? If those aspects of practice are important in our clinical settings, the agency needs to invest in instruction, resources, tools, and preceptor support systems to ensure that they are communicated, tracked, and developed.

Core questions for nurse leadership include: "Which clinical performance elements portray nursing practice in your agency and how are the elements prioritized within the orientation and/or competency validation system?" The answer to these questions establishes our focus for nurse performance development and competency data collection.

When line by line content itemization was completed on previously used orientation and competency validation tools, the practice elements identified within a specific *"Agency"* tool produced the chart displayed in **Figure 1**.

The same itemization of content for the CCF Universal Competency tool reveals a different picture of nursing practice. Within this chart, CCF Universal the practice elements were re-sorted in order of percentages, **Figure 2** shows how the tool prioritizes elements of nurse practice. Within the Universal tool, a single performance criteria statement may pertain to multiple elements as listed. In this case, wording makes a significant difference in what is communicated about our practice.

From the practice elements listed in, which 'non-task elements' should be included within your orientation and/or competency validation tool? And what percentage of practice should they represent?

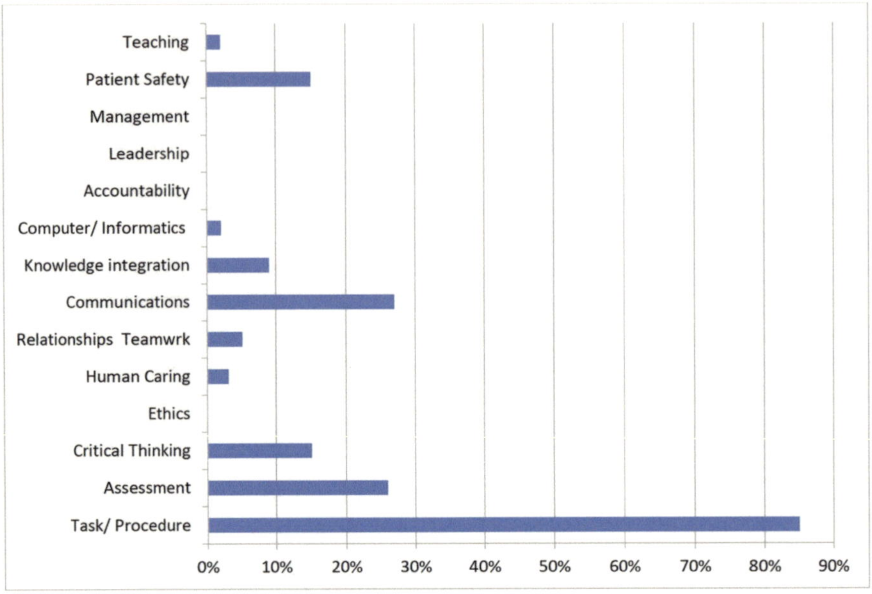

Figure 1.
Percentage of "Agency" RN orientation/competency items addressing elements of nursing practice as listed in the documentation tool.

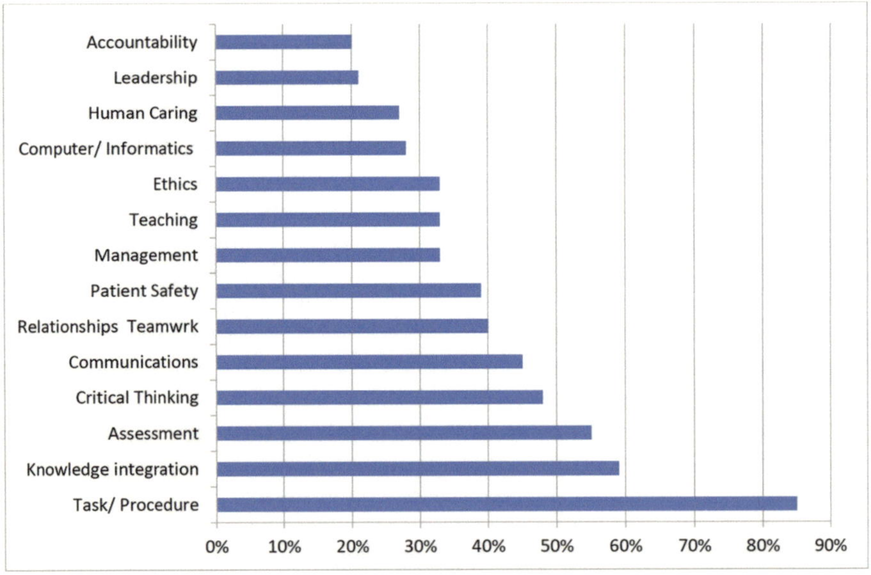

Figure 2.
Percentage of CCF Universal RN orientation/competency items that addressed identified practice elements as listed in the documentation tool.

5. Tools and templates for competency development and validation

The CCF uses a Universal Competency Tool to track performance expectations that are engaged in all settings. The performance criteria listed herein address universal aspects of professional practice as outlined by the essential elements within the COPA model. With these common aspects of clinical practice outlined herein, the unit specific tools may focus on aspects that are unique to specialty practice settings.

Competency tools include both 1) Universal and 2) unit specific performance expectations. These are valid and reliable tools for competency verification that identify specific, measurable performance-based criteria for assessment. Competency criteria include aspects of caring, leadership, management, teaching, safety, accountability, knowledge integration, critical thinking, reasoning, and clinical judgment capability.

The framework of the COPA model essential practice competencies provides the categories within the Universal competency form. Performance criteria address elements of nurse practice that are used in all healthcare settings, rather than breaking down to specialty- specific content. Unit specific tools outline clinical performance in practice-based statements that reveal the manner in which care is provided or a practice component that is unique to the specialty.

Within this division of skills sets, the common criteria lay the foundation for performance and the unit specific address the specialty-unique knowledge and skills. The initial completion of the universal tool is the basis for cross training that focuses on elements within specialty practice.

Both universal and unit-specific CBOs are used for competency development and validation. The Universal CBO tool is outlined with the COPA model core elements of practice. Under each of the eight categories, specific sub-skills and tasks are detailed. Specific documentation directions guide the preceptor in validating a sample of skills that give evidence of overall capability and clinical competence.

Important features of the universal CBO tool include that it:

- Addresses skills and practice that nurses apply in all settings, all specialties

- Specifies practice categories of: Communication, Leadership, Management, Critical Thinking, Teaching, Human relationships/ethics, and Knowledge integration to be combined within completion of Assessment and Interventions as essential nursing practice components

- Provides detailed performance criteria and sub-skills that give evidence of the above list of essential elements of practice

- Communicates that these elements are threaded through all that we do as professional care providers

- Identifies the required sample of skills that must be validated

- Introduces a specific description of accountability expectations

Unit specific competencies address nursing care as applied for specialty practice settings. Herein you will find the elements of patient care and nursing practice that are unique to the setting, rather than universal in all settings. By separating the Universal and unit specific tools, care providers do not need to repeat universal competency validation when they change specialties. Instead, they can immediately focus on what is unique to the new practice setting. Unit specific competencies can be presented as a set of complete coaching plans, or may be condensed to offer only the performance criteria statements.

Form directions and scoring key apply documentation at the *Advanced Beginner* or *Capable* level (see **Table 2.**) as evidence that the individual not only meets the specific performance criteria that is being signed off, but also identifies the limits of their capability and seeks assistance appropriately (see definition of 2 Capable). That assistance is detailed further within the accountability or summary statement at the end of the competency assessment tool.

While the tools and process make use of Benner's model for skills acquisition, the scoring key uses different titles from those used by Benner and Dreyfus for the first three levels [35, p. 19]. The terms selected for the scoring key deliberately focus on performance enhancement instead of words indicating *failure, or not able to achieve*.

In clinical practice, it may take 2–3 years for a new graduate to achieve the competent level as defined by Dreyfus [19] and Benner [35]. Yet the new nurse is a safe and effective practitioner prior to this level of experience, so long as he/she recognizes the limits of their own capability and seeks assistance appropriately. These aspects of practice are inherent to the explanation of the codes in **Table 2**.

The description of the numerical code of 2 is: "*Capable* – familiar with skill/ equipment, but may need assistance, seeks support when unfamiliar with process/ skill". Your policy statement and/or the directions for the form reinforce this statement as the 'passing' requirements to complete basic orientation. "A score of 2 = capable, matches with the *Advanced Beginner* level within Benner's model for development of clinical skills. The achievement of this level of practice is linked with the accountability statement that is included in the sign-off process for completing orientation.

The response outlined in the CCF targets the scoring key and accountability. With a score of 2 being addressed within initial competency validation, the preceptor is validating that the orientee consistently recognizes when they are unfamiliar with an aspect of care and that they seek appropriate assistance, resources, or guidance.

With the use of Benner's model and this scoring key, a crucial need to teach preceptors about the Novice to Expert continuum was experienced. Additional supporting documents may be indicated to help clinical staff understand the concepts and what they are looking for within competence validation.

CCF competency tool scoring key	Novice to expert
1. *Identified limitation* – requires direct guidance & support, little or no experience with skill	*Novice* = Inflexible, rule-based. Little or no background understanding of why and how to apply or adapt the 'rules'
2. *Capable* – familiar with skill/equipment, but may need assistance, seeks support when unfamiliar with process/skill	*Advanced beginner* = starting to use and make sense of situational elements & depend on the context. Temporal focus is immediate & present
3. *Performs independently* – knowledgeable to perform tasks safely as a result of training & experience	*Competent* = Increased efficiency; planning is still conscious, abstract, analytic, and deliberate.
4. *Proficient* – extensive experience in this area/ skill, able to teach and mentor others	*Proficient* = situations are perceived as a whole rather than as unconnected aspects
5. *Expert* – all of the above; fluid performance; ensures evidence-based practice for clients and agency	*Expert* = Understanding of task, as well as the decision of what to do next, performance is intuitive and fluid

Table 2.
Scoring key matched with Benner's Novice to Expert definitions [28].

At the beginning of each Competency Assessment Tool there are specific directions on how to complete the tool, where to document, and what the observer's initials/date indicate within the tool. It is intended that the directions remain with the tool, ensuring readily available clarification when a surveyor or reviewer asks questions specific to an individual's orientation and/or competency evidence.

Self assessment of capability - At the start of orientation, the new hire will use the scoring key to self-assess their capability and skills. *Self -assessment is not a valid or acceptable method of competency validation.* Instead, this information is used to build an individualized learning plan for each new hire, with a focus on validation of core competencies in a timely manner. The directions also provide an ongoing reminder of how to document within the form and what is communicated within specific locations on the form.

Clinical coaching plans are a single page tool that provides an outline of specific expectations, resources, achievements, reflections, and what practice (competence validation) gaps remain. When documentation is kept current and complete, the tools function as a safety guide and ensure continuous development for the learner. These individualized teaching plans are developed to support clinical and experiential learning with preceptor supervision. Each plan addresses a specific goal as listed for the specialty practice or developmental process. The coaching plan is a single page tool that adds details about both learning activities and measurable performance outcomes. The tools include a nurse-focused, patient centered goal statement, standardized knowledge required to meet the goal, performance criteria that show achieving the goal outcome, and a specific reflective learning activity. These tools assist the preceptor and new hire by providing an outline of learning resources and clinical expectations, along with preceptor 'hand-off' communications. The tools move us towards viewing both patient care and the learning process in a holistic, evaluative manner. That evaluation continues to improve care quality and professionalism through rapid cycle quality improvement.

While providing a learning/teaching guide, coaching plans ensure a venue for documentation of the learner's progress, needs, and achievements. Coaching plans are a single page tool that provides an outline of specific expectations, resources, achievements, reflections, and what practice (competence validation) gaps remain. When documentation is kept current and complete, the tools function as a safety guide and ensure continuous development for the learner.

The coaching plans are concrete, concise, and current tools that support both experiential learning and performance validation. CCF resources include more than 200 individual coaching plans to support development of work organization skills and clinical expertise in multiple specialties from across the continuum of care. The plans are written and used to support development of the nurse new to an aspect of healthcare. Preceptors and educators determine which plans best serve the new nurse's learning needs, and then customize the plan to match the individual.

Coaching plans follow principles of teaching/learning while they foster progression of the novice through competency/orientation requirements. Coaching plans outline the core knowledge related to the goal statement and guide reflective learning strategies for fostering critical thinking development.

These standardized plans serve multiple functions. When used effectively, they can:

- Outline the standardized knowledge required for a specific aspect of patient care
- Establish clearly defined expectations in measurable, observable performance terms

- Track completion of critical elements of performance – with opportunity for positive feedback as the learner progresses through, and completes each tool
- Document progression – and lack thereof – to clarify and ease the process of difficult communications pertaining to performance issues
- Offer specific questions for fostering critical thinking development
- Direct discussion and reflective learning
- Ensure accurate, complete, and concise 'hand-off communications' from one preceptor to the next (or from preceptor to manager or educator).
- Be adapted for use as an action plan or performance improvement tool by adding a time frame requirement for meeting specific goals
- Provide effective, legal documentation of both the learning process and competency validation within the domain of a specialty practice

CCF coaching plans and competency tools address acute, long term, clinic, and home care settings. Currently validated tools include target groups of RNs and LPNs, with some tools for respiratory therapy, rehabilitation professionals, medical assistants, and nurse aides. Others may be developed in collaboration with content experts

Hand-off communications are a core function of the plans. The tools ensure communication of progress, challenges, and achievements from one preceptor to another. Without this vital 'hand-off' communication, progress of the learner may be hampered by each preceptor taking the learner, student, or orientee back to prior steps or expectations.

Orientees can maintain their documentation tools within a folder that is present in the clinical setting or compiled within an electronic data management system. Having this information available in the practice area ensures that changes in preceptor, educator, or manager include a fluid transition of clinical learning. The tools track evidence of capability that supports patient care and task assignments that build progressively more complex, while recognizing the foundational skills and evidence already accomplished. The assignments consider appropriateness based on prior experience and demonstrated capability. The documented observations also determine whether supervision of clinical performance is appropriate and required, or not.

6. Integrated preceptor development and support

A unique feature of the CCF is integration of preceptor development and support as a crucial component of the competency program. Agencies have often implemented nurse residencies or new orientation programs without quantifying the challenges placed upon the shoulders of preceptors. Through 20 years of work with preceptors, students, and newly hired nurses, the CCF team learned that preceptors require basic development related to: Communication, Competency Assessment, Critical Thinking skills, Delegation/Liability, Interpersonal Issues, Roles/Responsibilities, Teaching/learning styles, Novice to Expert Continuum, Challenging Experiences, and Documentation. This content is taught using multiple media to ensure addressing all learning styles and time constraints. Preceptor texts and workbooks have been developed for collaborative learning experiences. The full allied healthcare team has benefited from the instruction and courses have included participants from across the continuum of care.

For success of the overall program, preceptors require specialized education related to their roles as preceptors along with focused instruction that addresses the unique challenges presented by the CCF. Defining clinical competence for preceptors is core to the issue, as preceptors are called upon to create meta-cognitive knowledge through reflective practice and reflective learning [26, 29, 30].

Specific planning for critical thinking development is engaged. Critical thinking and reasoning lead to clinical judgement and decisions regarding optimal nursing care. To develop this judgement in others, a preceptor must engage core competencies in: higher-order thinking; conducting assessment in a reliable, valid manner; effective communication; and supporting learners in evidence- based practice. Preceptors are the essential partners who facilitate the development of practical skills, communication, professional socialization, documentation, prioritization, and planning of daily activities. They fill a crucial role in bridging the nurse education theory-practice gap when they have preparation and supporting structures for their specialized role.

Preceptor roles and responsibilities have been defined and researched for the CCF model with emphasis on roles of Protector, Educator, Competency Validator, and Facilitator. The CCF engages preceptors with specific instruction related to roles and the skills required to fulfill the roles. Preceptors must also strive to foster development of clinical judgement in the new nurse – whether a new graduate or an experienced nurse transitioning into a new workplace.

There are many elements within each role component and all must be integrated effectively to support both students and new hires. When the Educator role is engaged by the preceptor, one of the most important aspects is that of fostering critical thinking development and reflective practice. Development of the nurse's skills and capability in reasoning leads to improved Clinical Judgment skills [21].

Preceptors engage specific strategies for fostering reflective learning and development of clinical judgment [19, 29]. Critical thinking provides the foundation for clinical reasoning, which leads to decision-making – or the application of Clinical Judgment to the patient's unique issues and needs. The preceptor uses weekly meetings, case scenarios, documentation tools, discussion, and/or problem solving to foster critical thinking development. Discussion, dialogue, constructive feedback, and reflections contribute to the "thought development' of the novice nurse.

7. Membership venue

Clinical Alliance (Alliance) membership with annual renewal requirements created a venue to share, sustain, grow, improve, and disseminate the model. Alliance members gain proprietary rights to all CCF resources and contribute to ongoing development of best practices in clinical competency and preceptor development. The Alliance provides an innovative means for sharing proprietary rights for the competency framework components, tools, instruction, and resources. The shared templates and model are systematic, standardized, evidence-based and readily available in commonly used formats. The practice-based concepts and tools provide a foundation for competency validation in more than 700 healthcare agencies across the nation. Starting in 2000, the CCF innovation developed from a local initiative, to statewide implementation, to national influence, and now global linkages; creating a solid foundation upon which others build. The membership venue is managed by Nurses International, a non-profit organization that is creating affordable, technologically savvy nursing curriculum for developing countries, thus empowering nurses to change their world [36].

8. Conclusion

The CCF engages core theories and concepts to establish a comprehensive, evidence-based approach for supporting students, new graduates, and experienced nurses as they undergo transitions within healthcare. The engages universal and unit specific competency tools to detail the clinical performance requirements. Sampling theory is engaged to gather evidence of capability.

The American Nurse Association believes that competence is situational, dynamic, and is both an outcome and an ongoing process [4]. The situation, setting and challenges determine what competencies are necessary. With a focus on the dynamic, situational nature of competence; the CCF tools, documentation, and model focus on care of the patient instead of targeting equipment, skills, and completion of procedures. The performance criteria within the CCF specifically outline the way in which professional practice incorporates clinical reasoning, judgment, and decision-making within serious situations [17, 33]. In clinical practice, skills and tasks are incorporated as part of the larger picture identifying the multiple attributes leading to effective action. Transitional evaluation is not complete until an accountability statement summarizes the professional responsibilities and ongoing learning needs of each care provider.

Preceptor education and support is a crucial element of the successful transition system [37]. Preceptors apply concepts pertaining to communication skills, giving feedback, conflict management, teamwork, competency validation, sampling theory, accountability, novice to expert, and fostering critical thinking development. Use of coaching plans in the clinical setting is a new and unique challenge for preceptors which has proven a positive experience with projects implemented to date [2].

Unique aspects within the framework include: an emphasis on fostering critical thinking development; integrating professional accountability; role development related to gathering evidence of competence; and both introduction to, and practice with, the CCF unique tools. A comprehensive competency development framework also requires supporting the structures such as policies, standards of practice, survey or evaluation tools, and rapid cycle quality improvement process.

The CCF supports safe transition within healthcare roles, experiential learning, and competence validation in the clinical setting. This type of competency-directed framework requires specific protections to ensure safe, effective patient care and a supportive learning environment. Preceptors protect both patients and learners, while collecting evidence related to clinical competence. CCF resources include curriculum outlines for preparing preceptors, policy templates, and evaluative survey tools; as well as competency tools and clinical teaching plans used to support learners within the practice setting.

A membership venue is used to share the resources, model, templates, and instructional tools. This approach ensures sustainability of the work, continues the evidence-based development, and allows nurse educators to start their work from established templates, instead of 're-inventing the wheel' of orientation and competency model development.

Author details

Susan Boyer[1]* and Miriam Chickering[2]

1 Nurses International, Weathersfield, VT, USA

2 Nurses International, Bethel, MN, USA

*Address all correspondence to: susanb@nursesinternational.org; sb.vnip@gmail.com

References

[1] Boyer S. Clinical transition framework: Nurse competence and preceptor development. Academia Letters. 2021:1-8. Article 4425. DOI: 10.20935/AL4425

[2] Boyer SA, Mann-Salinas EA, Valdez-Delgado KK. Clinical transition framework: Integrating accountability, sampling and coaching plans in professional practice development. Journal for Nurses in Professional Development. 2018;**34**(2):84-91

[3] Benner P, Sutphen M, Leonard V, Day L. Educating Nurses: A Call for Radical Transformation. San Francisco, CA: Jossey-Bass; 2010

[4] Laibhen-Parkes N. Evidence-based practice competence: A concept analysis. International Journal of Nursing Knowledge. 2014;**25**(3):173-182

[5] Krautscheid LC. Defining professional nursing accountability: A literature review. Journal of Professional Nursing. 2014;**30**(1):43-47. Available from: https://www.sciencedirect.com/science/article/abs/pii/S8755722313000860

[6] Zittel B, Moss E, O'Sullivan A, Siek T. Registered nurses as professionals: Accountability for education and practice. Online Journal of Issues in Nursing. 2016;**21**(3):1. Available from: https://www.ncbi.nlm.nih.gov/pubmed/27856083

[7] Beaver C, Magnan MA, Henderson D, DeRose P, Carolin K, Bepler G. Standardizing assessment of competences and competencies of oncology nurses working in ambulatory care. Journal for Nurses in Professional Development. 2016;**32**(2):64-73

[8] Despotou G, Her J, Avanitis T. Nurses' perceptions of joint commission international accreditation on patient safety in tertiary care in South Korea: A Pilot Study. Journal of Nursing Regulation. 2020;**10**(4):30-36. Available from: https://www.sciencedirect.com/science/article/pii/S2155825620300119

[9] Del Bueno D. A crisis in critical thinking. Nursing Education Perspectives. 2005;**26**(5):278-282

[10] Kavanagh JM, Szweda C. A crisis in competency: The strategic and ethical imperative to assessing new graduate nurses' clinical reasoning. Nursing Education Perspectives. 2017;**38**(2):57-62

[11] Caputi LJ, Kavanagh JM. Want your graduates to succeed? Teach Them to Think! Nursing Education Perspectives. 2018;**39**(1):2-3. Available from: https://journals.lww.com/neponline/Pages/articleviewer.aspx?year=2018&issue=01000&article=00002&type=Fulltext

[12] Hawkins P, Exstrom S. Adaptation of a Transition to Practice Program for New Graduates in Acute and Long-term Care Facilities in Urban and Rural Nebraska: A Pilot Study. Chicago, IL: National Council of Nurse State Board of Nursing; 2014. Available from: https://www.ncsbn.org/1527.htm

[13] Robbins JR. Implementation and Outcomes of an Evidence-based Precepting Program for Burn Nurses. Vol. 43. Bethseda, MD: Tri-Service Nursing Research Program; 2014

[14] Robbins JR, Valdez-Delgado KK, Caldwell NW, Yoder LH, Hayes EJ, Barba MG, et al. Implementation and outcomes of an evidence-based precepting program for burn nurses. Burns. 2017;**43**(7):1441-1448

[15] Delfino P, Williams J, Wegener J, Homel P. The preceptor experience: The impact of the vermont nurse internship project/partnership model on nursing orientation. Journal for Nurses in Professional Development. 2014;**30**(3):122-126

[16] Lenburg C. Teaching Nursing: The Art and Science. 2nd ed. Vol. 2. Glen Ellyn, IL: College of Dupage Press; 2010

[17] Lenburg C, Abdur-Rahman V, Spencer T, Boyer S, Klein C. Implementing the COPA model in nursing education and practice settings: Promoting competence, quality care, and patient safety. Nursing Education Perspectives. 2011;**32**(5):290-296

[18] Olds D, Dolansky MA. Quality and safety research: Recommendations from the Quality and Safety Education for Nursing (QSEN) Institute. Applied Nursing Research. 2017;**35**:126-127

[19] Dreyfus HL, Dreyfus SE. The ethical implications of the five-stage skill-acquisition model. Bulletin of Science Technology Society. 2004;**24**(3):251-264

[20] Ericsson KA. Acquisition and maintenance of medical expertise. Academic Medicine. 2015;**90**(11):1471-1486

[21] Ross JG. Repetitive practice with peer mentoring to foster skill competence and retention in baccalaureate nursing students. Nursing Education Perspectives. 2019;**40**(1):48-49

[22] Windsor C, Douglas C, Harvey T. Nursing and competencies – A natural fit: The politics of skill/competency formation in nursing. Nursing Inquiry. 2011;**19**(3):213-222. Available from: http://eprints.qut.edu.au/42326/1/42326.pdf?origin=publicationdetail,%202012

[23] Forehand M. Bloom's Taxonomy [Internet] [cited December 9, 2023]. 2012. Available from: http://www4.edumoodle.at/gwk/pluginfile.php/109/mod_resource/content/5/forehand_bloomschetaxonomie02.pdf

[24] Boyer S. Clinical transition framework: Efficient solutions for transitional support systems. Nurse Leader. 20171;**15**:425-428

[25] Oyetunde MO, Brown VB. Professional accountability. JONA'S Healthcare Law, Ethics and Regulation. 2012;**14**(4):109-114

[26] Zigmont JJ, Wade A, Edwards T, Hayes K, Mitchell J, Oocumma N. Utilization of experiential learning, and the learning outcomes model reduces RN orientation time by more than 35%. Clinical Simulation in Nursing. 2015;**11**(2):79-94. Available from: https://www.nursingsimulation.org/article/S1876-1399(14)00214-X/fulltext

[27] Perla RJ, Provost LP, Murray SK. Sampling considerations for health care improvement. Quality Management in Health Care. 2013;**22**(1):36-47

[28] Etchells E, Ho M, Shojania KG. Value of small sample sizes in rapid-cycle quality improvement projects: Table 1. BMJ Quality and Safety. 2015;**25**(3):202-206

[29] Miraglia R, Asselin ME. Reflection as an educational strategy in nursing professional development. Journal for Nurses in Professional Development. 2015;**31**(2):62-72

[30] Taylor MJ, McNicholas C, Nicolay C, Darzi A, Bell D, Reed JE. Systematic review of the application of the Plan–do–study–act method to improve quality in healthcare. BMJ Quality &

Safety. 2014;**23**(4):290-298. Available from: https://qualitysafety.bmj.com/content/23/4/290

[31] Botma Y. Suggested competencies for a preceptor training programme. Trends in Nursing. 25 Nov 2016;**3**(1):1-12. DOI: 10.14804/3-1-16

[32] Boyer S. Preceptorship: Pathway to safe practice and clinical reasoning. In: Feldman H et al., editors. Nursing Leadership: A Concise Encyclopedia. 2nd ed. New York: Springer Publishing Company; 2011. pp. 29-31

[33] Boyer S et al. Impact of a nurse residency program on transition to specialty practice. Journal for Nurses in Professional Development. 2017;**5**:220-227. DOI: 10.1097/NND.0000000000000384

[34] Etchells E, Woodcock T. Value of small sample sizes in rapid-cycle quality improvement projects 2: Assessing fidelity of implementation for improvement interventions. BMJ Quality and Safety. 2017;**27**(1):61-65

[35] Benner PE. From Novice to Expert: Excellence and Power in Clinical Nursing Practice. Upper Saddle River, NJ: Prentice Hall; 2001

[36] Chickering M. Nurses International – Learn about the Mission, the Vision and the People [Internet]. Nurses International. 2023. Available from: https://nursesinternational.org/about/

[37] Goss CR. Systematic review building a preceptor support system. Journal for Nurses in Professional Development. 2015;**31**(1):E7-E14

Chapter 8

Perspective Chapter: Ubuntu Model of Health Care – Re-Envisioning Nursing Practice in the Digital Era

Fhumulani Mulaudzi and Rodwell Gundo

Abstract

Ubuntu is an African philosophy that emphasizes the importance of care, concern, and interconnectedness between people. During the period of the COVID-19 pandemic, nurse practitioners and nurse educators were forced to rely on digital technology, but many faced challenges due to a lack of resources and skills. To adapt to global changes, nurses need to embrace digital transformation and be involved in the design and implementation of digital technology. Unfortunately, nurses' voices are often unheard in this process. The Ubuntu philosophy can offer valuable insights, reflecting the African continent's ethos and social wisdom, to promote digital inclusion. In this chapter, we will delve into the significance of an African voice in digital governance through the lens of the Ubuntu community model of nursing.

Keywords: COVID-19, digital technology, nurse practitioners, pandemics, philosophy

1. Introduction

The rapid integration of digital technology into professions and personal lives has also influenced the role of nursing, which is to provide compassionate and humanistic care to patients [1]. The COVID-19 pandemic has presented unprecedented challenges for healthcare workers, especially those in nursing. However, it has also created opportunities for integrating digital technology in healthcare and education [2]. To adapt to new ways of providing services, healthcare professionals and educators have turned to digital tools such as telehealth, online communication platforms like Zoom and Google Meet, and even artificial intelligence. These digital methods of care have expanded and improved access to care for many patients, and reduced per capita health costs [3].

Healthcare professionals have successfully embraced the opportunities presented by the digital age, using technology to enhance their practices and elevate the quality of patient care [4]. With cutting-edge technology, healthcare professionals can now use electronic medical records, and diagnose and treat patients in novel ways, by using diagnostic tools such as mobile ultrasound machines and 3D printing. Hospitals have also introduced robots to serve as supplemental healthcare workers and assist with other tasks that require less human intervention [5]. These tools are used to identify patient needs, diagnose, and treat patients early, prevent medication errors, and improve compliance with practice guidelines thereby improving patient safety [4, 6]. In addition, simulation methods are used in nursing education to teach student nurses [7].

However, innovations in digital technology have posed ethical challenges in many fields including nursing practice. Some scholars argue that ethical principles such as compassion and caring which are the core of nursing and healthcare practice cannot be replaced by robots and machines with automated decision-making systems [5]. Nurses provide compassionate care and uphold ethical values such as respect, beneficence, justice, and non-maleficence. Compassion is a crucial element of the healing process, as it directly impacts the quality of healthcare outcomes. Nursing with compassion entails placing the patients at the core of care. The same sentiments are expressed in the Chinese culture in Confucianism. Based on Confucian approaches, all people are social beings and relational. The core beliefs are respect for elders, harmony between individuals, justice, loyalty to family and friends, and filial piety which is viewed as respect for one's parents [8]. However, nursing is not limited to this aspect; it combines both an art and a science [9].

Robots may not be able to provide the relational ways, humanization, and values expected in nurse-patient relationships. Similarly, the use of simulation techniques in nursing education has been questioned as nursing students are not given opportunities to practice on real patients. However, Samani et al. [10], observed that cultural values can influence the development of robotics and that robotics can create its values and cultures. Furthermore, Mhlambi [5] has also proposed using the values of the African philosophy of Ubuntu to create a more relational framework for governing artificial intelligence. They propose that robotics should focus on enabling virtues and the social and relational aspects of robots. While embracing technology in healthcare, it is crucial to be mindful of the caring aspects. The chapter proposes the application of the African philosophy of Ubuntu as a foundation of caring and the basis for the Ubuntu model of healthcare in the digital era.

2. Lessons from the COVID-19 pandemic that should make us re-envision healthcare and nursing practice

At the peak of the COVID-19 pandemic, the global health workforce was called upon to lean on technology more than ever to support their practice. The pandemic highlighted the need for telemedicine or telehealth, the provision of health services through telephone, email, and videoconferencing. It is a health-related service which relies on telecommunicating and electronic information technologies to facilitate consultation, screening, health education, and information-sharing [11]. Telemedicine became necessary for triaging and screening for COVID-19 symptoms, deployment of services, collaboration between the multidisciplinary team, and continuation of care provision while reducing the in-patient burden [12]. It also helped to promote social distance between the healthcare providers and their patients. However, many struggled for a timely and coordinated telehealth response due to the lack of skills [13]. Since then, digital health has been transforming healthcare provision and is strongly recommended by the World Health Organization to improve healthcare and nursing practice [14].

In addition, the global pandemic brought a silver lining by shining a spotlight on the exceptional work done by nurses worldwide [15]. People are now more aware of the advanced clinical skills that nurses possess, the complexity of their job, their unwavering commitment to patient care, and the critical role they play in providing comfort and compassion to patients in their last moments [16]. Despite the challenges such as workload and stress [17], the nurses felt like superheroes due to the responsibilities that they shouldered during the pandemic [18]. It is expected that the nurses' previous experiences in handling difficult situations during the pandemic will make them more confident in dealing with stressful situations [17].

The pandemic must be a catalyst for fundamental and systemic change in preparedness for future global outbreaks [19]. Nurses are at the frontline of healthcare, representing more than 59% of the world's healthcare workforce. As such, the effectiveness of health service delivery is influenced by the state of the nursing profession [16]. They have first-hand knowledge of the challenges and barriers to health [12]. They play a central role in efforts to achieve universal health coverage and the global Sustainable Development Goals (SDGs). Some of the challenges that were exposed by the pandemic can be addressed by investing in nursing education and enabling nurses to be empowered in digital technology and artificial intelligence. There is a need to provide ICT training, IT support, computer accessibility, and social media access to equip nurses with digital technology [20].

Nurses must also consider the pandemic as an opportunity to reflect, learn, and grow [16]. Renewed awareness of digital technology offers an impetus for change that nurses should embrace. Nurses must radically reframe their relationship with digital technology to achieve universal health coverage by 2030. They also need to learn to engage relevant stakeholders, provide leadership, and champion such initiatives. Unfortunately, the nurses' voices are absent in the design and implementation of digital technology although they constitute most of the healthcare workforce. Promoting the nurses' digital literacy and involvement has the potential to improve health outcomes. A digitally enabled nursing profession will also attract the youth into the profession. Ultimately, this will help to curb the global shortage of nurses. On the other hand, failure to involve nurses will lead to a lack of trust in the technology, reluctance towards its use, and pose a risk to cyber security issues [12]. Lastly, health professionals including nurses are challenged to navigate the new models of care in this digital era.

3. Ubuntu in nursing

Ubuntu is a term that is expressed in different languages but means the same thing in African countries. For example, it is called *gimuntu* in Angola, *muthu* in Botswana, *umunthu* in Malawi and *bantu* in Rwanda [21, 22]. In South Africa, Ubuntu is a Nguni word that is expressed in the idiom, *muthu ndi muthu nga vhathu* and loosely translated as *I am because* you are [23]. Similarly, in Malawi, the relational aspect of Ubuntu is expressed in the saying, a loner is a beast, those in the company of each other are humans [24]. The black African people believe Ubuntu is a collection of values that make a human being authentic. It emphasizes interdependence and interconnectedness among people such that a person is perceived as authentic when they belong to a larger and more significant relational, communal, societal, environmental, and spiritual world [21]. Ubuntu is also perceived as a caring ethic and a core of nursing as it promotes care, respect, concern, and engagement for one another [22, 23].

The Ubuntu model of healthcare is a new approach to nursing practice that seeks to re-envision the role of nurses in the digital era. It aims to incorporate technology to enhance the delivery of healthcare services while maintaining a human-centered approach to care [25]. This is consistent with Coeckelberg [26] recommendation for an Ubuntu social robot that will be able to accommodate the values of Africans as the current social robots are based on Western individualism. However, Mhlambi [5] argues that automated decision-making machines and robotics cannot replace personhood. Nurses are a connection point between innovations and patients [12] therefore they have a critical role in collaborating with engineers, researchers, and technologists to ensure that the human part and the cultural aspects are embedded in shaping future designs of social robotics.

As nurses, we should embrace the renewed awareness of digital technology and view it as an impetus for positive change. The pandemic has presented us with an opportunity to make fundamental and systemic changes in our preparedness for future pandemics, and we should seize it with enthusiasm and determination. Nurses have a critical role in achieving universal health coverage by 2030. To achieve this ambitious goal, we must revolutionize our relationship with digital technology [15]. Nurses are expected to embrace Ubuntu and lead the way towards a healthier, and more equitable future. We must do so within the context of our Ubuntu caring ethics, which emphasizes the interconnectedness of all individuals and the importance of treating everyone with care, respect, and engagement. By adopting the spirit of Ubuntu, nurses can better engage, empower, enable, and emancipate the patients and clients they serve, leading to better healthcare outcomes for all [22].

4. The need for digitalization

According to the strategic directions for nursing and midwifery 2021–2025 [19], nurses and midwives must be trained to acquire cross-cutting competencies in digital technology. The statement advocates for nurses to embrace digital technology. However, it acknowledges that digital transformation does not only need technical advancement but also a change of attitude and adaptation among the health workforces. Successful implementation of digital technologies requires understanding of the nursing workforce as demographic variables such as gender, age, voluntariness, use, and experience may influence their acceptance and utilization of digital tools [27]. Women are more likely than men to own a mobile phone, but they are 20% less likely to use it to access the internet. Given that more than 90% of nurses are women, the digital gender gap poses serious challenges for this sector [27]. It is time for us to act and address this issue by providing access to resources and training that empower women in the nursing community to improve their digital skills. This initiative is especially crucial in low- and middle-income countries with scarce resources, and the gender digital divide is even more pronounced. There is a need to close this gap and ensure that every woman in the nursing field can access digital tools and improve their skills.

5. Ubuntu values and digital inclusion

Digital inclusion is defined as "*equitable, meaningful, and safe access to use, lead, and design of digital technologies, services, and associated opportunities for everyone, everywhere*" [28]. It is a notion that everyone, regardless of their background, should have access to technology and the internet. According to Amugongo [29], the principles of Ubuntu that can be aligned with digital technology and AI are fairness, community

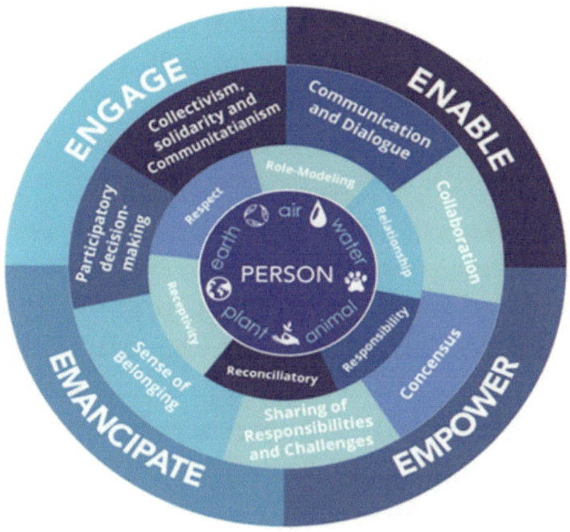

Figure 1.
Ubuntu model of nursing.

good, safeguarding, humanity, and respect. The Ubuntu principles must be infused in the design deployment and the use of digital technologies. Furthermore, we propose digital technology and digital inclusion should be aligned with Ubuntu principles that form part of the Ubuntu model of nursing (see **Figure 1**). The principles that can be applied include collectivism and solidarity, participatory decision-making, a sense of belonging, and consensus [30].

6. Ubuntu community model of nursing

Ubuntu community model of nursing proposes a framework that acknowledges that a person exists in an environment and belongs to a community. The environment is composed of earth, air, water, animal, and plant. As reflected in **Figure 1**, the community has values which include respect, role-modeling, responsibility among others. In addition, there are principles namely collectivism, solidarity, and communitarianism; collaboration; participatory decision-making; sense of belonging; sharing of responsibilities and challenges; consensus; communication and dialog. When these principles are applied in healthcare, the consumers of care feel engaged, enabled, empowered, and emancipated. Therefore, we propose that the principles of the model be applied in the integration of digital technology in health practice.

6.1 Collectivism, solidarity, and communitarianism

The principle of collectivism, solidarity and communitarianism emphasize that communities must work together and be there for each other [31]. The common good for all becomes a priority rather than individualism. Digital inclusion prioritizes equity, access, and community at its core [29]. The essence of Ubuntu is the belief that the community is more important than the individual. Ubuntu enables people to think and act collaboratively and communally. It is important to ensure that digitalization embraces the principle of communalism [32]. This principle is commensurate with the principle of utilitarianism which is used in western bioethics. Utilitarianism emphasizes that ethical decisions are made based on moral values which allow most community members to benefit [33]. In this case, if nurses embrace digital transformation and allow digital inclusion in their scope of practice, quality patient care will be provided as digitalization will ease the load on nurses through electronic records, robotics, and telehealth. These will enable them to have enough time to focus on nursing duties only and render quality patient care. Patients will also benefit from the digitalization.

6.2 Collaboration

Collaboration involves working together for a common goal. It is important that everyone, including nurses, possesses the necessary skills and knowledge to participate fully in our digital society. We need to acknowledge and appreciate the diversity of our communities, including differences in language, culture, and ability. Therefore, it is essential to design technologies and digital experiences that are accessible and inclusive for all, ensuring that everyone has a voice and a seat at the table from the design phase of the automated machines. For instance, an AI tool that was created to detect skin cancer was trained on a dataset of images primarily from fair-skinned people. As a result, the tool may fail to provide an accurate diagnosis for individuals with dark skin [29]. As caregivers, we must prioritize human interaction and care above all else. By neglecting this responsibility, we risk damaging the trust that nurses place in technology, which can lead to reluctance towards its usage [12]. Let us make sure we always put the needs of patients and nurses first and utilize technology in a way that enhances their experience and outcomes.

The use of technology in the clinical workplace is becoming more prevalent. However, this widespread use can also create reluctance towards its usage. Additionally, as more medical professionals interact with each other online, there is a growing concern about the perpetuation of gender-based violence [12]. To mitigate this risk, it is essential to have safety features such as accountability settings, and spam and harassment filters to ensure a safe and secure online environment.

6.3 Participatory decision-making

Participatory decision-making is the ability to respect other human beings, their views, and opinions. Respect in Ubuntu is not one-sided but reciprocated. There is mutual respect as both parties respect each other [30]. Ubuntu's philosophy emphasizes patient autonomy while at the same time recognizing the interconnectedness and interdependence between community members. Amugongo et al. [29] argue that the emphasis of Ubuntu on the needs of communities may compromise individual rights. Indeed, Ubuntu emphasizes communalism but at the same time guarantees every person's rights and responsibility to be able to exercise moral obligation to think on behalf of others. Thus, while designing our digital machines we will have to understand the incorporation of cultural values. Coeckelberg et al. [26] suggested that cultural robotics be incorporated to ensure that the machines resemble the cultural values of the communities we serve. Participatory decision-making constitutes respect for everyone's integrity, freedom of speech, and expression.

The Ubuntu philosophy emphasizes the ability to respect a person's integrity and freedom of choice [22]. Respect in digitalization and AI will involve incorporation of the users views from the conception and design to utilization phase [29]. In the digitalization space respect entails involving people in decision-making from the inception of the project, the design of machines, and the utilization phase. The process will enable nurses to be receptive and accept changes. They will get an opportunity to give inputs to ensure that the caring aspects are included. Van Norren [34] posits that when a machine algorithm is programmed by Westerners there is usually a gap as the inputs of Africans who are using the machines are often not incorporated. The principle of Ubuntu promotes values such as reciprocity, benevolence, and humility.

Respect also entails freedom of choice and the ability to make decisions in health care issues [23]. People need full information about the advantages and disadvantages of the procedures that are undertaken in hospitals and clinics. With the introduction of AI, there are a lot of new machines and medical tools introduced for assessment and diagnosis. The issue of informed consent becomes paramount to providing people with their inherent dignity [29]. However, the challenge of informed consent is individual informed consent versus communal informed consent. With the introduction of other procedures and AI tools that affect communities, there may be challenges concerning informed consent related to AI models that affect the whole community. For example, there is a proliferation of websites that can access people's data and publish health information and education without obtaining informed consent or following proper channels [29]. Social media can also be a challenge where photos of patients can be posted to platforms such as Facebook without the knowledge of the hospital authorities and patients themselves. Policies such as the Information and Data Protection Acts must be available to protect people from harm. Vulnerable users must be protected from risks and harm that can be inflicted by technology [35].

6.4 Sense of belonging, sharing of responsibilities and challenges

The sense of belonging is also another principle of Ubuntu which refers to sharing of opportunities, responsibilities, and challenges. In African communities, people learn to share resources and basic needs such as housing and food at very tender ages. Thus, when educational opportunities present themselves, people prefer to share information to empower each other with knowledge and skills [22]. Similarly, it will be paramount to embrace the principles of Ubuntu in digital technology to facilitate learning among nurses and other health professionals. Nurses must learn more about digital technology to acquire skills.

There is a need for fairness in the distribution of resources, knowledge, and skills to ensure equity. This notion is supported by Amugongo et al. [29], who argue that the Ubuntu philosophy promotes fairness which ensures that there is equity and justice in the distribution of resources in digital technology and AI especially in low-income countries. The course of action taken in the decision-making regarding training and designing of digital machines must be fair and just [33].

There is an inequity of digital resources between developed and low-income countries. In addition, some of the nurses lack skills in digital technology. This can be attributed to a lack of resources and technophobia. The incorporation of Ubuntu in embracing technology can assist in addressing inequity as it promotes virtues such as mutual inclusivity, supporting each other, a sense of belonging, and obligations to each other. Factors such as gender and age may also have a bearing on inequity. Women may lag in adopting technology due to financial constraints [29]. Ubuntu is a justice theory that promotes fairness [33].

6.5 Consensus

One of the principles of Ubuntu is to resolve problems by seeking consensus to ensure that all members of the community are satisfied and happy with the decisions taken [30]. The involvement of healthcare practitioners and nurses in decision-making during the designing of the models will enable them to give inputs that will incorporate caring values. The designers of digital tools and models must involve all stakeholders and users of those technologies to get more inputs and buying in. Decision-making must be based on consensus.

6.6 Communication and dialog

In the African setting, communication is essential for informing communities about messages, and activities. The communication often takes place through dialog. Ubuntu-centered communication values online communities that are interactive and characterized by respectful communication, reciprocity, and mutual trust [36]. Through the lens of Ubuntu, the introduction of technology in health practice including nursing should be a negotiated activity that respects the values of proper communication and dialog with the communities, the consumers of healthcare and other relevant stakeholders. Similarly, the online communication platforms must incorporate the values of the communities.

7. Barriers to digital transformation in nursing

Nurses often view digital technologies as a hindrance to the intimate and empathetic relationships they build with their patients and their families. They perceive these technologies as a distraction from their hands-on caring role. This resistance to adopting digital approaches to healthcare is primarily due to the belief that it contradicts traditional nursing ideals, such as compassionate care. Nurses' resistance to technology has been well documented. When digital tools such as computers were introduced, nurses resisted through avoidance, and criticism to the extent that some just refused to use them [27].

Resistance to change may be seen from all health care professionals due to lack of awareness regarding the benefits that new technology may bring to the organization. The cost of digital tools is often very high which makes access to the tools difficult. Resistance can also be from patients who are not willing to try new technology for fear of the unknown. Digitalization must be designed in a way that will benefit patients [37].

Processes that can inflict harm to clients, nurses themselves and the profession must be avoided at all costs. The use of technology can be addictive and harmful. It can lead to both physical and mental conditions such as depression and anxiety. In response, the World Health Organization has incorporated gaming disorder under the classification of disease [35]. With regards to harm to clients and the profession, there are many questions that we need to ask ourselves; do we see ubuntu on social media these days or do we see criticism, blame, shaming, defamation, abuse, hate speeches, negative comments, sexism, xenophobia, Afrophobia and so many other negative things? Additionally, nurse educators are facing challenges in incorporating ChatGPT (generative pre-trained transformer) into their teaching curriculum. Plagiarism is rife and difficult to control. Ultimately, this will negatively affect the competence of our newly qualified nurses.

8. Recommendations

There is a need for Ubuntu-based action guidelines principles for all AI stakeholders. African countries need individual, institutional, and national digital and

AI governance capabilities at continental and global levels. Digital technology and AI machines and robots must reflect the African ethos and wisdom. Facilitation of deeper discussions and scientific research regarding access, cost, electronic resource use or wastage, is necessary to ensure proper guidance on the use of digital tools. Digitalization of nurse-patient relationships will also need to be thoroughly explored. We need to change our mindset and embrace Ubuntu even in our interactions through social platforms. Nurses must be vigilant and establish ethical committees that will ensure that the digital models designed through AI incorporate cultural and ethical values.

There is a need to take steps to address the challenges that were exposed by the pandemic through investing in nursing education and enabling nurses to be empowered in digital health. Change management is critical to ensure buy-in from nurses, administrators, and patients. Training and education of staff is critical to ensure that they are equipped with knowledge that will boost their self-esteem and confidence in the use of digital technology.

In addition, ethical frameworks that govern digital technology in health care must be in place in all countries to protect individuals and communities from the risks and harm that can be caused by digital technology. Formalizing a connection and aligning synergies between the whole of nursing and digital health will lead to improved technology and health outcomes. The African philosophy of Ubuntu can be applied as a foundation of caring and the basis for the Ubuntu model of healthcare in the digital era.

9. Conclusion

Digital technology is here to stay, it is our future. Ethical challenges such as lack of privacy, safety, security, fairness, transparency, accountability, and lack of promotion of cultural and human values have arisen in nursing practice due to innovations in digital technology. Digital competencies are still not well defined for the nursing profession or formally integrated into nursing education and practice. Nursing education must incorporate digital technology to equip nurses with digital skills and knowledge. Ubuntu's ethical framework will ensure digital inclusion, equity, participatory decision-making, a sense of belonging, consensus, and mutual respect. Without proactive strategic self-reflection, planning, and action, nursing will fail to control its digital trajectory. The continuous development of nurses should also prioritize digital skills. Eventually, this will help to address and minimize the ethical challenges posed by digital technology.

Acknowledgements

This chapter was written during a writing retreat which was funded by the National Research Foundation in South Africa through the Ubuntu Community Model of Nursing Project at the University of Pretoria.

Conflict of interest

None.

Author details

Fhumulani Mulaudzi* and Rodwell Gundo
Department of Nursing Sciences, University of Pretoria, Pretoria, South Africa

*Address all correspondence to: mavis.mulaudzi@up.ac.za

References

[1] Konttila J et al. Healthcare professionals' competence in digitalization: A systematic review. Journal of Clinical Nursing. 2019;**28**(5-6):745-761

[2] Jiang Z et al. Twelve tips for teaching medical students online under COVID-19. Medical Education Online. 2021;**26**(1):1-10

[3] Pailaha AD. The impact and issues of artificial intelligence in nursing science and healthcare settings. SAGE Open Nursing. 2023;**9**:1-4

[4] Stoumpos AI, Kitsios F, Talias MA. Digital transformation in healthcare: Technology acceptance and its applications. International Journal of Environmental Research and Public Health. 2023;**20**(4):3407

[5] Mhlambi S. From rationality to relationality: Ubuntu as an ethical and human rights framework for artificial intelligence governance. Car Center for Human Rights Policy. 2020. Available from: https://carrcenter.hks.harvard.edu/publications/rationality-relationality-ubuntu-ethical-and-human-rights-framework-artificial

[6] Alotaibi YK, Frank F. The impact of health information technology on patient safety. Saudi Medical Journal. 2017;**38**(12):1173-1180

[7] Koukourikos K et al. Simulation in clinical nursing education. AIM: Journal of the Society for Medical Informatics of Bosnia & Herzegovina. 2021;**29**(1):15-20

[8] Zhu Q, Williams T, Wen R. Confucian robot ethics. In: Wittkower D, editor. Computer Ethics - Philosophical Enquiry (CEPE) Proceedings, 2019. 2019. 11 p. DOI: 10.25884/5qbh-m581. Available from: https://digitalcommons.odu.edu/cepe_proceedings/vol2019/iss1/12

[9] Henry D. Rediscovering the art of nursing to enhance nursing practice. Nursing Science Quarterly. 2018;**31**(1):47-54

[10] Samani H et al. Cultural robotics: The culture of robotics and robotics in culture. International Journal of Advanced Robotic Systems. 2013;**10**(12):1-10

[11] Haleem A et al. Telemedicine for healthcare: Capabilities, features, barriers, and applications. Sensors International. 2021;**2**(100117):1-12

[12] Troncoso EL, Breads J. Best of both worlds: Digital health and nursing together for healthier communities. International Nursing Review. 2021;**68**(4):504-511

[13] Spaulding R, Smith CE. How telehealth care exploded due to COVID: What nurse researchers need to know. Research in Nursing & Health. 2021;**44**(1):5-8

[14] World Health Organization. WHO Guideline: Recommendations on Digital Interventions for Health System Strengthening. Geneva: World Health Organization; 2019

[15] Lee J, Cho HS, Shin SR. Nursing strategies for the post-COVID-19 era. International Nursing Review. 2021;**68**:149-152

[16] Catton H, Iro E. How to reposition the nursing profession for a post-covid age. BMJ. 2021;**373**(n1105)

[17] Joy GV et al. Nurses' self-esteem, self-compassion and psychological resilience during COVID-19 pandemic. Nursing Open. 2023;**10**(7):4404-4412

[18] Aydın M, Aydın AI, Kulakaç Ö. Nurses as the leading fighters during the COVID-19 pandemic: Self-transcendence. Nursing Ethics. 2022;**29**(4):802-818

[19] World Health Organisation. The WHO Global Strategic Directions for Nursing and Midwifery (2021-2025). Geneva: World Health Organisation; 2021

[20] Assaye BT et al. Perception towards the implementation of telemedicine during COVID-19 pandemic: A cross-sectional study. BMC Health Services Research. 2023;**23**(967):1-12

[21] Mugumbate JR, Chereni A. Now, the theory of Ubuntu has its space in social work. African Journal of Social Work. 2020;**10**(1):v-xv

[22] Mulaudzi FM et al. Perceptions of retired nurses on factors preventing younger professional nurses from applying the ethos of Ubuntu in professional care. Sage Open Nursing. 2022;**8**:1-9

[23] Downing C, Hastings-Tolsma M. An integrative review of Albertina Sisulu and Ubuntu: Relevance to caring and nursing. Health SA Gesondheid. 2016:214-227

[24] Galafa B. Exploring possibilities of an undergirding Umunthu philosophy in Malawi's social studies curriculum. Ethiopian Journal of the Social Sciences and Humanities. 2019;**2**:53-78

[25] Kapuire GK et al. Framing technology design in Ubuntu: Two locales in pastoral Namibia. In: Proceedings of the Annual Meeting of the Australian Special Interest Group for Computer Human Interaction. 7 Dec 2015. pp. 212-216

[26] Coeckelbergh M. Ubuntu robot: Towards a relational conceptual framework for intercultural robotics. Science and Engineering Ethics. 2022;**28**(16):1-15

[27] Wynn M et al. Digitizing nursing: A theoretical and holistic exploration to understand the adoption and use of digital technologies by nurses. Journal of Advanced Nursing. 2023;**79**:3737-3747

[28] United Nations. Digital Inclusion. United Nations. n.d. Available from: https://www.un.org/techenvoy/sites/www.un.org.techenvoy/files/general/Definition_Digital-Inclusion.pdf

[29] Amugongo LM, Bidwell NJ, Corrigan CC. Invigorating Ubuntu ethics in AI for healthcare: Enabling equitable care. In: Proceedings of the 2023 ACM Conference on Fairness, Accountability, and Transparency. 12 Jun 2023. pp. 583-592

[30] Mulaudzi FM et al. Perceptions of retired nurses on factors preventing younger professional nurses from applying the ethos of Ubuntu in professional care. Sage Open Nursing. 2019;**8**:1-9

[31] Muhammad-Lawal AT et al. Ubuntu as an instrument to foster holistic nursing: The views of south African student nurses. Journal of Holistic Nursing. 2023;**41**(3):303-309

[32] Nicolaides A. Considering the philosophy of Ubuntu in south African healthcare ethical practices. The Journal of Medical Laboratory Science & Technology South Africa. 2023;**5**:71-76

[33] Mabvurira V. Hunhu/Ubuntu philosophy as a guide for ethical decision making in social work. African Journal of Social Work. 2020;**10**(1):73-77

[34] van Norren DE. The ethics of artificial intelligence, UNESCO and the African Ubuntu perspective. Journal of Information, Communication and Ethics in Society. 2023;**21**(1):112-128

[35] Kuss DJ et al. Tackling Digital and Gaming Addiction: A Challenge for the 21st Century. Report. University of Tasmania; 2019. Available from: https://hdl.handle.net/102.100.100/495406

[36] Steenkamp H, Rensburg R. Utilising an Ubuntu-centred communication management framework to analyse CSR messages on SNSS. Communication. 2018;**44**(3):17-40

[37] Alohali M, Carton F, O'Connor Y. Investigating the antecedents of perceived threats and user resistance to health information technology: A case study of a public hospital. Journal of Decision Systems. 2020;**29**(1):27-52

Chapter 9

Methods to Learn Clinical Pediatric Nursing for Nurse Students

Frøydis Vasset, Ingeborg Ulvund and Hildegunn Sundal

Abstract

It is useful to learn about somatically ill children when implementing project-based learning. The students interview children's nurses/parents with sick children and this enables/strengthens the students' learning. Students learned pediatric nursing after completing *the pediatric project,* which is part of the nursing program. Some students learned in an international clinical placement in a pediatric ward. Combined learning from inside and outside educational institutions is useful. How can nursing students learn pediatric nursing in nursing education in the future, with large cohorts of nurses and few internships? This chapter is composed of several studies, both quantitative studies with questionnaires from 159 nursing students and qualitative studies with individual interviews of 18 nursing students after international clinical placement in a pediatric ward and eight nurses who had an international clinical placement in a pediatric ward as nurse students. And some studies about simulation in nursing studies and studies about clinical practice in other countries.

Keywords: nursing students, project-based learning, pediatric nursing, simulation, international clinical placement

1. Introduction

Why and how should nursing students learn pediatric nursing?

EU directive (European Communities) states that pediatric nursing must be included in nurse education.

Increased global competence and intercultural society can indicate that part of practice, such as children's nursing, can also be learned in other countries/ parts of the world.

New subject areas, as technology and innovation etc., in nursing education compete for time and resources. It can lead to less time for pediatrics.

The European Communities (EU) developed the Bologna Agreement [1, 2] to safeguard common standards in higher education in Europe. The regulations in each country's nursing education regulate learning outcomes through knowledge of the normal development and special needs of children and young people.

Nursing students must have practical studies, and according to the EU, it must be 50% of the study, but there is no mention of how much of this time should be pediatric nursing. In Norway, the standards were introduced in 2003/2004 [3]. Regulation on common framework plan for health and social education regulates Norwegian bachelor's education in nursing in compliance with the Bologna Agreement.

Nursing students must have clinical experiences with patients throughout their lifetime to be in line with the European Union (EU) directive. Included is knowledge of pediatric nursing and experiences with children as patients. The bachelor program in nursing must ensure that the students acquire knowledge of pediatric nursing, according to Anon [4–6]. Further, it means that nurse students should learn pediatrics through internships in pediatric wards [7]. However, the lack of such internships makes it challenging to meet the quality requirements for providing adequate clinical care for pediatric patients [8, 9]. In addition, the level of documentation of learning clinical pediatric nursing in a bachelor's degree in nursing is inadequate [8].

To solve the problem of lack of internship, alternative work requirements have been developed. It can be useful for nursing students to learn about somatically ill children by implementing project-based learning in nursing programs, simulation, and/or international clinical placements, or all.

In summary, there is a need for nursing expertise and practice for pediatric nursing (children under 18 years), but we can also see that there is a shortage of internships in pediatrics for nursing students, especially in the specialist health service.

This chapter emphasizes different models for clinical pediatric nursing for nursing students. The theoretical part of pediatric nursing is not emphasized because it is not a special challenge. There are several good textbooks.

2. Pediatric nursing

International studies show that nursing students' learning through clinical practice was central and important in the practice of nursing in the subject [10–12], and Norwegian nursing students had clear learning benefits from clinical practical experience [13, 14]. Learning through clinical practice in a pediatric practice setting underlined the importance of learning in that type of practice [7]. American study shows that the Society of Pediatric Nursing recommended a minimum of 61 to 80 hours of pediatric clinical experience for Registered Nurses [8].

How learn nurse students pediatric nursing

- *Project-based learning at universities.*
- *Simulation.*
- *Placement for pediatric nursing.*

In case of lack of clinical practice experience is, project-based learning an alternative way for nursing students and an important contribution to achieve learning outcomes about children as somatic sick patients. Project-based learning (PjBL) is a pedagogical method in which the students manage the learning process to a greater extent himself, while the teacher functions more as a facilitator [15]. The method involves a problem analysis of the topic to be studied and preparing a solution to the problem [16], as well as it is suitable when students must learn new topics [17]. PjBL contributes to students becoming more independent in their work [17]. The method supports students' autonomy in the learning process and contributes to self-regulated learning [18, 19].

Key features of the project are the nursing students choose the composition of the group (three to five students), choose a topic and prepare a problem under supervision, which includes a delimitation of the child's age. They interview relevant healthcare personnel, pediatric nurses, or people/parents they know who have experience that can answer the problem. They write a report and submit it to the student portal. Then, they make an oral presentation (30 min) for supervisors, examiners, and fellow students. The students must have the supervisor's approval of the issue, interview guide, and information letter, which emphasizes ethical considerations regarding voluntary participation and safeguarding the confidentiality of the interviewees and that important information in the interview situation is noted in an anonymized manner [20].

The study is designed as a quantitative study with anonymized data obtained through a structured questionnaire of 159 nursing students. The questionnaire [21] has been prepared to gain insight into the learning outcome nursing students achieve about somatically ill children and their relatives and about nursing practice in that connection through the group examination project "Project Child" in the bachelor's program [20].

The nursing students experienced the 2 weeks with PjBl as useful learning outcomes about somatically ill children when completing PjBL (76,8% positive response). This even though they answered they were less motivated to perform the project (69.2 positive response). They underlined that at future meetings with somatically ill children as students, the learning outcomes were very useful (80,5 positive responses). The learning outcomes from the project were considered important for the students as a future nurses in dealing with somatically ill children (0–18 years) in hospital (70,0 positive response) [20].

In the PjBl, the students' emphasis is placed on creating themes and problem formulation themselves as important (90,6% positive response) and on interviewing people with experience in pediatric nursing as motivating and useful. Their learning outcomes of interviewing are high (92,2% positive response). The students experience learning outcomes from having written a project report in the group as important (81,1% positive response). The students are less positive that they learned from their own oral presentation (39.5 positive response), and they learned more from their fellow students' oral presentation (69.2 positive response) and giving fellow student's responses to another group's presentation and report learned they even more of (74.9 positive response). They rated searching, finding, evaluating, and including research articles in the project slightly less positively (57.9 positive response), as well as the learning outcomes of the guidance from the teacher (59.7 positive response). Having been prepared for the project through information, study plan, and teaching, slightly less than half experienced it positively (49.0 positive response) [20].

The student thinks it is important to gain practical experience with somatically ill children (0–18 years) in a hospital during the education (90,5% positive response), and they think that nursing education emphasizes somatically ill children (0–18 years) in hospital in a small degree (8,6% positive response) [20]. Sundal & Vasset's [20] study also shows that if students do not get clinical practice in the pediatric ward, interviewing and discussing pediatric nursing with a knowledgeable pediatric nurse can also provide learning.

Discussion and conclusion: PjBL, especially the students' interviews of people with experience, enables students' learning outcomes, which contributes to nursing students' learning outcomes requirements in pediatric nursing [20].

3. Pediatric learning in simulation laboratory

Simulation has been implemented as a pedagogical method in the curriculum for bachelor's degrees in several educational institutions. Simulation is especially suitable for training communication and interaction in acute situations in pediatrics. To equip nursing students for practice studies, there has been a tradition of practical training in procedures at training departments. To improve this, simulation laboratories have set up one or more simulator machines, such as SimMan and SimPad [22, 23]. Simulation-based training is one of the most important measures to improve patient safety in pediatrics and reduce the number of adverse events in hospital departments [22–24]. Simulation can be conducted in the field of practice or through school-based education [24, 25]. A study indicated that simulation in the laboratory was a useful instrument in learning pediatric nursing. They believed it was mostly used in cardiopulmonary resuscitation and could have been used more [26]. Using a SimMan that could receive a venflon can facilitate this performance of care for children. The students could learn more about how they use such dolls in hospitals. To divert children's attention, or are there other purposes? A study [27] noted that intravenous-access procedures in children are one of the most stressful because it is invasive, and using needles generates anxiety, insecurity, and fear. Playful strategies using SimMan and even the materials used for venipuncture can assist children in understanding, accepting, and coping with the procedure.

Studies underlined that students expressed the view that making mistakes was uncomfortable, even though this was just a simulation situation [22, 23, 28, 29]. This was especially related to an occurrence in a scenario in another study where a child needed a blood transfusion. Here, the informants reported that during the simulation, several teams had given the wrong blood because the patient's identity was not managed properly [22, 23]. Simulation is considered one of the most practice-oriented methods to learn practical competencies, and these findings correspond with other research in the field [30–33] that underlines simulation-based training as one of the most important measures to improve patient safety [29–31, 33, 34].

3.1 Reflection as a pedagogical method in simulation laboratory

Students construct their own learning within social frameworks. According to David Kolb's theory, learning is a process in which knowledge is formed through the transformation of experience in four stages [35]. First, students experience a given situation (in pediatrics). Next, students reflect on their experiences and what they think and mean. Based on reflective observation, students' structure and generalize or formalize the learning outcomes of their experiences. Later, this knowledge will be tested in new pediatric contexts. Then, it will be clear whether the student has learned and reflected on pediatric nursing challenges.

Philosopher Donald Schön's [36] theory of the reflective practitioner can provide an understanding of learning and performing tasks in practice, including examining the processes of thinking, talking, and interacting through a series of cases in practice. His theory addresses knowledge-in-action and reflection-in-action. According to Schön [36], teachers or managers must guide the reflection process. Knowledge-in-action and reflection-in-action. Reflection afterward a simulations section is particularly useful in the simulation work for increasing knowledge. Debriefing after the simulation work is fundamental for students' learning, according to Hammer and Vasset; Vasset, Helberget, and Almås [22, 29].

One study [22] shows that scenario-based simulation experiences in themselves are no guarantee of learning; they need to be part of a systematic process that incorporates reflection on the action. Without reflection, simulation experiences result in limited learning. Several other studies show that debriefing with an emphasis on reflection helps ensure learning in the simulation situation [22, 29].

Where learn nursing students in pediatric nursing?

- *In their own country*
- *International clinical internships (ICI)*

4. Learning outcome in national versus international clinical internships

Nursing education in European countries must be 50% of the education [1–6]. With increasing numbers of nurse students, there is often a problem when it comes to hospital practice in pediatric nursing [20].

One method of offering nursing students experience in pediatric nursing is to integrate clinical placement in a pediatric ward or in health centers in exchange studies (ICI). There are several advantages to this. From a different context, in which they study nursing, they can bring home new perspectives on pediatric nursing related to health prevention and health promotion, as well as care for sick children and their next-of-kind. The challenges regarding public health work aimed at children and young people, the prevalence of disease, and the treatment offered will include similarities and differences. Students learn through comparison between contexts. In some contexts, students will encounter diseases they would not get experience with at home, and thus, they gain a wider range of experience than if they stayed home. In addition, the students get insight into some migrants' acquired understanding of health, illness, and treatment according to children. Moreover, their cultural competence increases [36, 37].

Several bachelors's programs in nursing offer international clinical placement in both low- and high-income countries [38, 39]. Another focus in international placement is an increased focus on developing a global perspective in children's nursing.

A program for practice in the pediatric department in the ICI

- Context for the pediatric department
- Organization of the pediatric service
- Organization of students' practice
- Learning theory
- Nurse students' learning outcomes after homecoming
- Nurses' experience after attending ICI as a student retrospectively.

Learning outcomes will be discussed – using teaching—theory, and development of cultural competence and personal and professional development. In Ulvund and colleagues' [36] study, when Norwegian nurse students had internships in a hospital in Ethiopia, they compared similarities and differences, which can lead to increased cultural awareness. Parents had to pay for parts of or all treatment, such as for the painkillers and antibiotics. As a result, many children develop some complications after fractures, such as osteomyelitis, because they did not receive antibiotics. Many children also received no painkiller either after surgery or when a nurse performed a painful procedure [40].

In North Europe, the treatment and medicine are free for children. The students gained experience with and insights into more unknown medical conditions—for example, meningitis, tetanus, malaria, tuberculosis, and other infectious diseases. There are few such diseases in Norway, but they exist mostly because of increasing immigration. The students learn that children may die from diseases because their parents cannot pay for their treatment [40]. The students gain more knowledge on pediatric patients, the roles of parents and nurses, and the treatment methods and various diseases that are relevant to pediatric nursing. This placement helps them provide some level of cultural knowledge, awareness, and sensitivity because of the contrasting conditions in their home country.

5. Summary

This chapter of the book emphasizes nursing students' clinical practice in pediatric nursing. It can be implemented in various ways, such as project-based learning with interviews of professionals in pediatrics. Then, simulation learning will take place in simulation laboratory. Clinical placement in hospitals is discussed both as a part of the program in exchanges studies and as internships in hospitals nearby campus. The chapter is built on our own research on these topics. In addition, we have used some research from other researchers.

Acronyms and abbreviation

EU	European communities
Anon	the European parliament and the council of the european union
PjBL	project-based learning
SimMan	well-known patient simulators in healthcare simulation
SimPad	used to operate device used to control leardal simulations.
ICI	international clinical internships.

Author details

Frøydis Vasset*, Ingeborg Ulvund and Hildegunn Sundal
Molde University College, Norway

*Address all correspondence to: froydis.p.vasset@himolde.no

References

[1] The European Parliament and the Council of the European Union. Directive 2013/55/EU of the European Parliament and of the Council of 20 November 2013. Strasbourg, France: The European Parliament and the Council of the European Union; 2013. Available from: https://eur-lex.europa.eu/LexUriServ/LexUriServ.do?uri=OJ:L2013:354:0170:en:PDF

[2] The European Parliament and the Council of the European Union. Directive 2005/36/EC of the European Parliament and the Council of the European Council. Strasbourg, France: The European Parliament and the Council of the European Union. Available from: https://eur-lex.europa.eu/LexUriServ/LexUriServ.do?=OJ:L:2005:255:0022:0142:en:PDF

[3] Sjøberg S. Bolognaprosessen. Leksikon: European Higher Education Area (EHEA); 2023. Available from: https://snl.no/Bolognaprosessen

[4] Anon. The European Parliament and the Council of the European Union. Directive 2005/36/EC of the European Parliament and the Council of the European Council. Strasbourg, France: The European Parliament and the Council of the European Union; 2005. Available from: https://eur-lex.europa.eu/LexUriServ/LexUriServ.do?uri=OJ:L:2005:255:0022:0142:en:PDF

[5] Anon. The European Parliament and the Council of the European Union. Directive 2013/55/EU of the European Parliament and of the Council of 20 November 2013. Anon. Strasbourg, France: The European Parliament and the Council of the European Union; 2013. Available from: https://eur-lex.europa.eu/LexUriServ.do?uri=OJ:L:2013:354:0132:0170:en:PDF

[6] Anon. Ministry of Education. Regulations on National Guidelines for Nursing Education. Anon. Ministry of Education; 2019. Available from: https://lovdata.no/dokument/SF/forskrift/2019-03-15-412

[7] Carey MC, Chick A, Kent B, Latour JM. An exploration of peer-assisted learning in undergraduate nursing students in pediatric clinical settings: An ethnographic study. Nurse Education Today. 2018;**65**:212-217. DOI: 10.1016/j.nedt.2018.03.014

[8] Bowling AM, Cooper R, Kellish A, Kubin L, Smith T. No evidence to support number of clinical hours necessary for nursing competency. Journal of Pediatric Nursing. 2018;**39**:27-36. DOI: 10.1016j.pedn.2017.12.012

[9] McCarthy AM, Wyatt JS. Undergraduate pediatric nursing education: Issues, challenges, and recommendations. Journal of Professional Nursing. 2014;**30**(2):130-138. DOI: 10.1016/j.profnurs.2013.07.003

[10] Lamont S, Brunero S, Woods KP. Satisfaction with clinical placement–The perspective of nursing students from multiple universities. Collegian. 2015;**22**(1):125-133. DOI: 10.1016/j.colegn.2013.12.005

[11] Warne T, Johansson U-B, Papastavrou E, Tichelaar E, Tomietto M, Van den Bossche K, et al. An exploration of the clinical learning experience of nursing students in nine European countries. Nurse Education Today. 2010;**30**(8):809-815. DOI: 10.1016/j.nedt.2010.03.003

[12] Jonsén E, Melender H-L, Hilli Y. Finnish, and Swedish nursing students'

experiences of their first clinical practice placement—A qualitative study. Nurse Education Today. 2013;**33**(3):297-302. DOI: 10.1016/j.nedt.2012.06.012

[13] Andreasen EM, Høigaard R, Haraldstad K. Sykepleiestudentenes kliniske praksis–om klinisk læringsmiljø og studenttilfredshet. Nordisk tidsskrift for helseforskning. 2020;**16**(2):1-17. DOI: 10.7557/14.5414

[14] Vae KJU, Vae KJ, Kvalevaag HK, Löfmark A. Nursing students' perceptions of peer learning as a learning model in clinical practice and students' learning through peer learning-an evaluation study. Nordisk tidsskrift for helseforskning, (Nordic Journal of Health Research). 2017;**13**(2):1-15. DOI: 10.7557/14.4218

[15] Bell S. Project-based learning for the 21st century: Skills for the future. The Clearing House. 2010;**83**(2):39-43. DOI: 10.1080/00098650903505415

[16] Chua K. A comparative study on first-time and experienced project-based learning students in an engineering design module. European Journal of Engineering Education. 2014;**39**(5):556-572. DOI: 10.1080/03043797.2014.895704

[17] Chang C-C, Kuo C-G, Chang Y-H. An assessment tool predicts learning effectiveness for project-based learning in enhancing education of sustainability. Sustainability. 2018;**10**(10):3595. DOI: 10.3390/su10103595

[18] Stefanou C, Stolk JD, Prince M, Chen JC, Lord SM. Self-regulation, and autonomy in problem-and project-based learning environments. Active Learning in Higher Education. 2013;**14**(2):109-122. DOI: 10.1177/1469787413481132

[19] Stolk J, Harari J. Student motivations as predictors of high-level cognitions in project-based classrooms. Active Learning in Higher Education. 2014;**15**(3):231-247

[20] Sundal H, Vasset F. Prosjektbasert læring i pediatrisk sykepleie. [project-based learning in pediatric nursing]. Klinisk Sykepleje. 2022;**36**(4):240-252. DOI: 10.18261/ks.36.4.3

[21] Eberhard-Gran M. Spørreskjema Som Metode for Helsefagene. [Questionnaire as a Method for Health Subjects]. Oslo: Universitetsforlaget; 2017

[22] Vasset F, Helberget LK, Almås SH. Nursing and biomedical laboratory science (BMLS) Students' Interprofessional training in the simulation laboratory. Journal of Research in Interprofessional Practice and Education. 2018;**8**:1, v8n1a271. DOI: 10.22230/ijepl.2018

[23] Ødegården T, Struknes S, Hofmann B. Pasientsimulering – En Praktisk innføring [Patient Simulation - a Practical Introduction]. NO: Gyldendal; 2015

[24] Aase I. Interprofessional teamwork training for nursing and medical students in Norway [thesis]. Stavanger, NO: University of Stavanger; 2016

[25] Lockeman KS, Appelbaum NP, Dow AW, Orr S, Huff TA, Hogan CJ, et al. The effect of an interprofessional simulation-based education program on perceptions and stereotypes of nursing and medical students: A quasi-experimental study. Nurse Education Today. 2017;**58**:32-37

[26] Vasset F, Sundal H. Pediatric nursing for nursing students. Social Sciences and Humanities Open. 2024. (Under review)

[27] da Silva JRS, Pizzoli LML, do Prado Amorim AR, Pinheiros FT, Romanini GC, da Silva JG, et al. Using

therapeutic toys to facilitate venipuncture procedure in preschool children. Pediatric Nursing. 2016;**42**(2):61

[28] Shoemaker MJ, Voest M, Booth A, Meny L, Victor J. A virtual patient educational activity to improve interprofessional competencies: A randomized trial. Journal of Interprofessional Care. 2015;**29**(4):395-397

[29] Hammer H, Vasset F. Laboratory; nursing and pharmacy students' experiences. Journal of research in interprofessional practice and education. 2019;**9**(1):1-14. DOI: 10.22230/jripe.2019v9n1a277

[30] Aase I, Aase K, Dieckmann P, Bjørshol CA, Hansen BS. Interprofessional commu-22. Nication in simulation-based training session in healthcare: A student perspective. Journal of Nursing Education and Practice. 2016;**6**(7):91-99

[31] Willhaus J. Working toward interprofessional education with simulation. Nursing Education Perspectives. 2012;**33**(2):134

[32] Page JT, Garbee DD, Kozmenko V, Quingzhao Y, Kozmenko L, Tong Y, et al. Getting a head start: High fidelity, simulation-based operating room team training & interprofessional students. Education. 2014;**218**(1):140-149

[33] Palaganas J, Epps C, Raemer D. The history of simulation enhances interprofessional education. Journal of Interprofessional Care. 2014;**28**:1-6

[34] Kolb DA. Experiential Learning: Experience as the Source of Learning and Development. Englewood Cliffs, NJ: Prentice Hall; 1984

[35] Schön DA. Education the Reflective Practitioner. U.S: Jossey-Bass Inc; 1990

[36] Ulvund I, Dadi GB, Sundal H. Nurse benefit from international clinical placement as nurse students: A qualitative study. Nurse Education Today. 2017;**121**:105663

[37] White. Paper 16. (2016-2017). Ministry of Education and Research. A world of Opportunities-International student mobility within higher education. Available from: https://www.regjeringen.no/no.documenter/meld.st-7-20202021/id2779627/.N

[38] Bagnasco A, Rossi S, Dasso N, Cansanzi L, Timmins F, Aleo G, et al. A qualitative descriptive enquiry of nursing students' perceptions of international clinical placement experiences. Nurse education Practice. 2020;**43**:102705-102705

[39] Ulvund I, Mordal E. The impact of short-term clinical placement in a developing country on nursing students: A qualitative descriptive study. Nurse Education Today. 2017;**55**:96-100. DOI: 10.1016/j.nedt

[40] Sundal H, Ulvund H. Experiences after international clinical placement as nursing students in a pediatric ward. Nurse Education in Practice. 2023;**66**:103512

Chapter 10

Pediatric Nursing for Appropriate Healthcare Environment Based on United Nations Convention on Rights of Child

Hiroyuki Ogihara

Abstract

Children's rights and decision-making are central to pediatric nursing care for patients and their families. This descriptive questionnaire-based cross-sectional study aimed to identify school children's perceptions of the United Nations Convention on the Rights of the Child (UNCRC) and their healthcare decision-making and strengthen pediatric nursing practices in consideration of children's rights. From September to November 2015, a questionnaire was administered to 525 healthy 9–12-year-old fourth- to sixth-grade students attending a typical elementary school in Asahikawa City, Hokkaido. Data were analyzed using Pearson's chi-square test, Bonferroni's test, and φ coefficient. A logistic regression analysis was performed with forced imputation and likelihood ratio of increasing variables to examine the factors influencing UNCRC application. UNCRC was well known to 11-year-old children who had been hospitalized. Many children who needed explanations came from families of four and had been given explanations. The factor that influenced the knowledge of UNCRC was hospitalization. Nursing orientations based on school-aged children can help create an appropriate healthcare environment for pediatric patients and their families, but further validation is needed using other qualitative research methods.

Keywords: United Nations convention on the rights of the child (UNCRC), child decision-making, ethical issues, pediatric nursing, healthcare environment, school children

1. Introduction

Children's rights and decision-making are central to pediatric nursing care for patients and their families. Today, children visit hospitals and clinics to be briefed on specialized medical care that meets their needs. According to the National Hospital Ambulatory Medical Care Survey, approximately 118 million children under the age of 15 visited outpatient clinics in the United States in 2019 [1]. Furthermore, the overall age for clinic visits is declining in Japan, with the rate of these visits increasing for children aged 5–14 years [2, 3]. When children visit healthcare facilities, they encounter doctors, nurses, and other unfamiliar medical personnel and experience psychological outcomes that increase perceptions of pain, anxiety, fear, and presumed danger [4, 5]. Critically ill children are often characterized by dependency and immaturity. They have been described as becoming frightened by the lack of autonomy in their illness and are theoretically excluded from the informed consent process [6]. Emotional reactions associated with the common experience of hospitalization can also lead to post-traumatic stress disorder [7] and increase parental anxiety [8].

Recently, nurses' participation in ethical discussions has increased the involvement of pediatric patients and their understanding of the decision-making process [9], while the endowment of choices to children during invasive procedures allows for support tailored to their individual needs [10]. In this context, a professional self-efficacy pathway model of pediatric nursing quality has been proposed [11], the Distracted Ingenuity Promotion Scale (DIPS) has been developed as a nursing strategy that respects children's rights [12], and specific viable and creative methods of distraction are also being considered [13]. While the United Nations Convention on the Rights of the Child (UNCRC) emphasizes the importance of providing health and welfare information to children, children are not usually supported in healthcare settings [14–16]. Reports that children do not fully understand their care process or whom to talk to if they feel anxious after returning home reflect this conclusion [17]. These studies provide evidence that pediatric nurses must respect children's rights and improve medical explanations to facilitate decision-making of pediatric patients and their families.

2. Background

In a survey of 13,261 children between the ages of 8 and 15 years, fewer than half (46%) said they were involved "a lot" in decisions about their care and treatment [17]. Furthermore, approximately 23% of all parents did not feel that nursing staff kept them "suitably" informed about their child's care [17]. Interestingly, school-aged children were less likely to say they were involved "a lot" (43%) than adolescents (48%) [17].

School age is a developmental stage associated with trait anxiety [18], and active involvement with children has been effective in reducing pain and fear [19]. The examination of the necessary decision-making by pediatric patients and the development of established pediatric ethics research and medical protocols is gaining momentum [20, 21]. Nurses are responsible for creating an environment wherein children can be heard, understood, and respected with unprecedented dignity [22].

However, few studies reveal the extent to which nursing staff makes children feel involved and aware of their rights when receiving healthcare. For pediatric nurses to further promote practical nursing strategies toward pediatric patients and their families, child perceptions need clarification, and the gap between these and medical support needs to be eliminated. Nursing care that considers the rights of the child is expected to provide adequate support in healthcare settings, which is a psychological outcome and essential to a child-centered approach to care [10, 23]. Therefore, this study aimed to identify the perceptions of school-aged children, with a focus on the UNCRC and decision-making processes to improve pediatric nursing care that considers children's rights.

3. Study design

3.1 Operational definitions

Following Article 1 of the Convention on the Rights of the Child, adopted and enacted as an international treaty by the United Nations, a child is any human being under the age of 18 [24]. Furthermore, based on the Commentary on Informed Consent/Consent [25–27], a "child" in this study was defined as a healthy 9–12-year-old individual attending a typical elementary school.

This school-age period was the focus because it is the age at which children experience psychological outcomes, such as trait anxiety, pain, and fear [18, 28, 29], and pediatric nurses are called upon to provide support [9, 19]. The rights of the child are to be guaranteed access to medical care, education, and support for life, so that he or she can grow up with the best interests of the child at heart and develop to his or her full potential [24, 30].

"Child decision-making" is the art of respecting the interests of the child and the family considering evidence, values, and beliefs [30, 31]. These definitions are important concepts that detail the realities and challenges of school-age children's perceptions; this study is based on the basic evidence established to date [32, 33].

3.2 Design

This descriptive questionnaire-based cross-sectional study was conducted to determine school-aged children's perceptions of the UNCRC and the clinical decision-making process to strengthen pediatric nursing care in the context of children's rights.

4. Methods

4.1 Participants and setting

From September to November 2015, a questionnaire was administered to 525 healthy 9–12-year-old fourth- to sixth-grade students attending a typical elementary school in Asahikawa City, Hokkaido. The selection of target children was based on the results of the 2014 Basic School Survey, which provides basic data for school education administration [34]. In 2014, Japan's youth population (0–14 years old) was 1,666,491, while that of Asahikawa was 40,525 [35]. The sample size was calculated using G* Power 3 software with an effect size of 0.5 [36], an alpha error probability of 0.05, and a detection rate of 0.95 [37]. The calculated sample size was more than 210 children, which was justified as a reliable measurement. The inclusion criteria were as follows: (1) children between 9 and 12 years, (2) fourth- to sixth-graders attending regular elementary school, and (3) physically and mentally healthy children. The exclusion process was as follows. First, participants who had one or more unanswered items in the questionnaire were excluded. Second, children unaware that they had visited a medical facility were excluded. These procedures were important to determine accurate and step-by-step data analysis to meet the research objective of identifying school-aged children's perceptions of having seen a healthcare provider (**Figure 1**). Furthermore, to conduct this quantitative study, it was necessary to avoid statistical bias in the selection of pediatric participants.

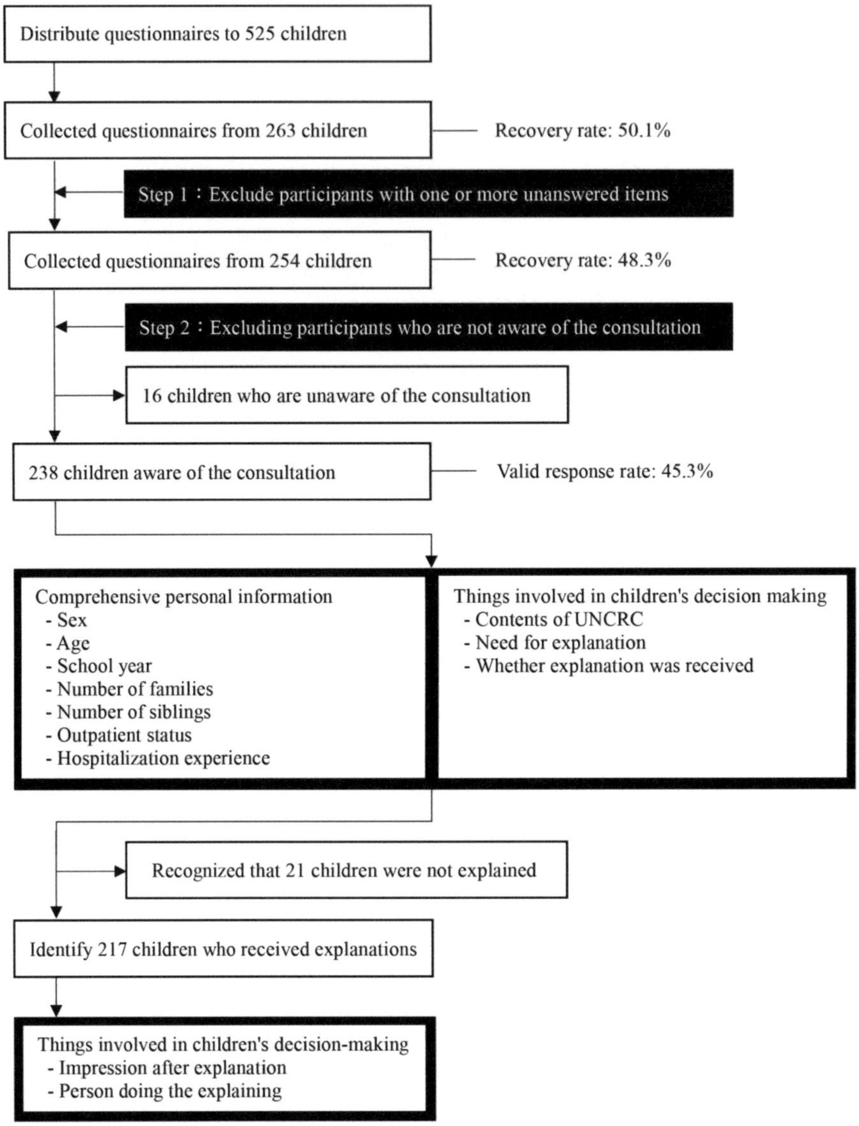

Note. UNCRC, United Nations Convention on the Rights of the Child

Figure 1.
Flowchart of participants based on the selection criteria for analysis.

A pseudorandom number was applied to the municipalities and survey participants were selected from each elementary school for random sampling. The study's research plan was explained to the Asahikawa City Board of Education, and approval and permission were received from the committee to conduct the survey. Next, each elementary school's principal was asked to participate in the survey by phone. The necessary number of questionnaires was created after receiving their approval. Precise procedures were followed to ensure that survey forms were distributed to the participants by their classroom teachers. Two study instructions—one for the participant and one for the parents—were included in the questionnaires. Standard procedures were followed to collect the questionnaires after obtaining parents' consent. Participants completed the distributed questionnaires at home, which were then submitted by the respondents and their parents after providing informed consent.

4.2 Participant characteristics

Information on 10 attributes was collected: sex, age, school grade, number of family members, number of siblings, hospital visit status, hospitalization experience, awareness of UNCRC, desire to receive explanations and experience of receiving explanations. For participants who answered that they had received explanations, two additional items were added: feelings after receiving explanations and perception of the person who gave the explanations; this resulted in a total of 12 attributes.

4.3 Rationale for focusing on the attributes of Children's rights and decision-making

This study followed the best interest standard (BIS) of ethical principles in children's healthcare and shared decision-making (SD-M) available to patients, parents, and healthcare professionals (HCPs) [38]. BIS and SD-M have received criticism for their respective concepts, especially the misunderstanding of "best" and "shared" and their independent functions [39, 40]. Hence, the shared optimization approach (SOA) was recently generated as a coherent framework combining BIS and SD-M in UNCRC publications [31]. Based on the principles of participation, provision, and protection, it is designed to address various tasks (limiting harm, showing respect, defining options, and executing plans) with discrete dimensions and steps (**Figure 2**).

From these, one can see that the SOA's overarching maxims [31] require an understanding of the child's age, elementary school grade, and comprehensive life background of the family, including that of parents and siblings. It is necessary to ensure that the attributes of this study and the SOA's "goal-oriented principles" [31] are considered appropriate to capture children's experience of hospital visits and hospitalizations, which are opportunities for them to face medical care.

The SOA "Dimensions of Implementation" [31] provides an environment where school-age children make decisions based on the UNCRC; it also simultaneously refers to a condition in which pediatric nurses are cautious in nursing practice. To fully consider the evidence, values, and beliefs that respect the interests of children and their families considering these factors, knowledge about the UNCRC, desire to receive explanations, the experience of receiving explanations, feelings after having received explanations, and perception of the person who provided these explanations cannot be excluded as attributes. The superficial validity of the questionnaire was pre-tested on children aged 9–12 years (n = 4) and checked by a university professor (n = 2) with knowledge of pediatric nursing. After the pre-test, modifications were made to avoid difficult terms, limit the number of questions, and ensure that the intent of the questions was understood.

4.4 Statistical analyses

All statistical analyses were performed using SPSS version 23.0 (IBM, Armonk, NY, USA). The descriptive statistics of the participants are expressed as numbers and percentages. For the nominal scale of each attribute, Pearson's chi-square test was

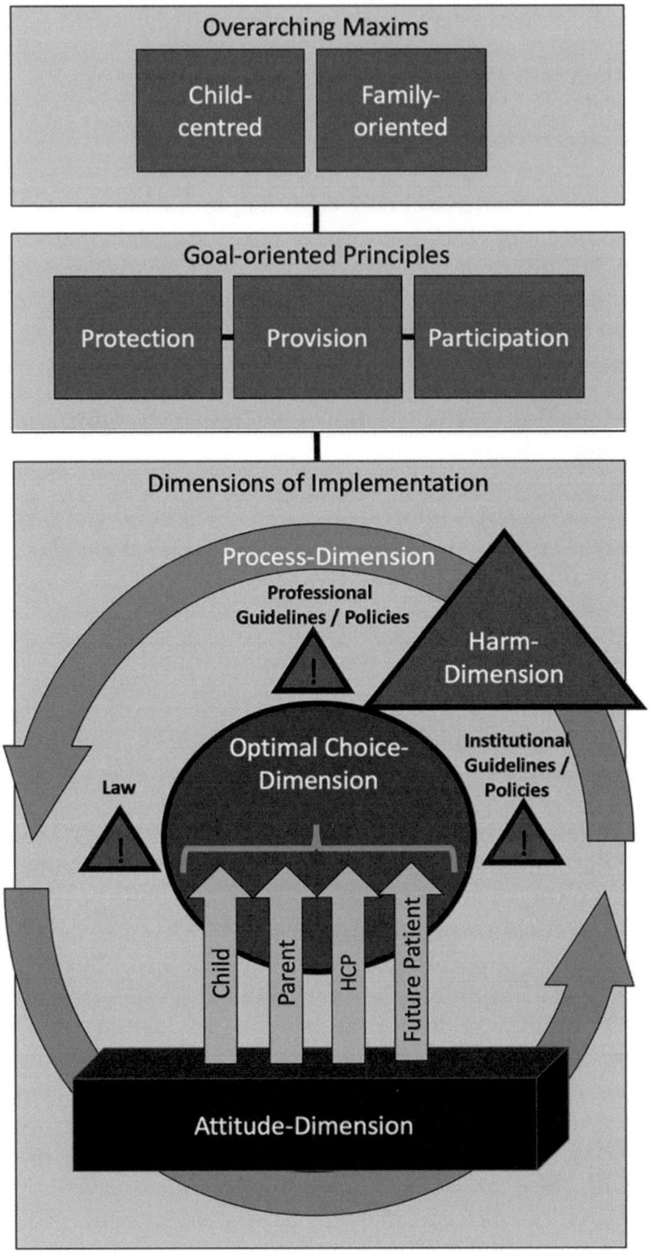

Figure 2.
Shared optimal approach for reconciling the best interest standard and shared decision-making. HCP, health care professional: Note. ***Figure 2*** *is reproduced with permission from the copyright holder as reference material for this research (Springer Link: Reproduction permitted).*

employed to analyze the pattern of occurrence and adjusted residuals for multiple groups and multiple classifications. When the sample size was small, Fisher's exact probability test and Yates's correction were used to check whether there was a statistically significant association between the two variables, and Bonferroni's test was used for multiple comparisons. The degree of association of each attribute is referred to as the φ or Cramer V coefficient. To examine the influencing factors, the dependent variable was knowledge of UNCRC, and a logistic regression analysis was performed using the forced imputation method to ensure that the independent variables were treated equally. The likelihood ratios of the method to increase the variables were also checked to confirm the significance of the entire regression equation. The evaluation indices of the regression model were calculated using the goodness of fit, significance, and positive discrimination rate.

4.5 Ethical approval

Ethical considerations such as participant anonymity, data confidentiality, and voluntary participation were explained to the study participants' parents, who then choose whether to convey this to their children. By returning completed anonymous questionnaires, participants and their parents/guardians consented to participate in this study. This study was approved by the Asahikawa Medical University Research Ethics Committee (approval no. 15075).

5. Results

5.1 Comprehensive demographic data on participants

A total of 263 participants were selected through questionnaires. Of these, 9 (3%) were excluded by step 1 of the exclusion criteria, and 16 (6%) were excluded in step 2. The participants in the study cohort were 238 children aged 9–12 years (mean ± standard deviation [SD]: 10.64 ± 0.91 years). **Table 1** shows the comprehensive demographic data of the entire participant population. Of these, 99 children (41.6%) had experienced hospitalization and 68 (28.6%) had visited the hospital as outpatients. The number of children reporting knowledge of UNCRC was 11 (4.6%), which did not correspond to 5% of the total. **Table 2** shows the comprehensive demographic data of the participants who received the explanation. All 217 (100.0%) participants who received the explanation reported that they were positive and the explanations were provided by 133 doctors (61.3%), 31 nurses (14.3%), and 53 doctors/nurses/family members (24.4%).

5.2 Comparison of attributes between groups related to Children's rights and decision-making

The sample size for this study was carefully considered when dividing the children into appropriate groups, which allowed for reasonable comparisons. UNCRC was well known to children who were 11 years old ($p < 0.05$, $\varphi = 0.206$) and had been hospitalized ($p < 0.01$, $\varphi = 0.220$) (**Table 3**).

In addition, older children, children in higher grades, and those with more family members and siblings tended to have more knowledge about the UNCRC. Among the children who knew about the UNCRC, all reported that they required and had received an explanation. Many who answered that they needed explanations were children in a family of four ($p < 0.05$, $\varphi = 0.160$) and children who had been given explanations ($p < 0.001$, $\varphi = 0.321$) (**Table 4**).

Children who answered that they did not receive an explanation tended to say that they did not need an explanation more than children who had received one, and

Variables	n	%
Sex		
Male	106	44.5
Female	132	55.5
Age		
9 years	28	11.8
10 years	73	30.7
11 years	94	39.5
12 years	43	18.1
School year		
Fourth grade	66	27.7
Fifth grade	71	29.8
Sixth grade	101	42.4
Number of family members		
2–3	43	18.1
4	129	54.2
>5	66	27.7
Number of siblings		
1	35	14.7
2	141	59.2
>3	62	26.1
Outpatient status		
During outpatient visit	68	28.6
Not during outpatient visit	170	71.4
Hospitalization experience		
Experienced	99	41.6
No experience	139	58.4
About UNCRC		
I just know	11	4.6
I do not know	227	95.4
Need for explanation		
I need it	217	91.2
I don't need it	21	8.8
Whether explanation was		
Received	217	91.2
Not received	21	8.8

Note. UNCRC, United Nations Convention on the Rights of the Child.

Table 1.
Comprehensive demographic data of all participants (n = 238).

Variables	n	%
Impression after explanation		
It was good	217	100.0
It was not good	0	0.0
The person who explained		
Doctor	133	61.3
Nurse	31	14.3
Doctors, nurses, and families	53	24.4

Table 2.
Comprehensive demographic data of the participants who received the explanation (n = 217).

children who received an explanation were more likely to want to receive one from a doctor ($p < 0.05$, $\varphi = 0.201$) (**Table 5**). On the other hand, all the children who answered that no explanation was necessary felt that no explanation was required from the doctor. None of the children indicated that they did not need an explanation from the nurse or doctor/nurse/family.

5.3 Factors affecting the knowledge of the UNCRC

Factors affecting the knowledge of UNCRC were evaluated using binomial logistic regression analysis. The regression equation obtained by the forced imputation method was guaranteed to be significant by the Cox and Snell R-square (0.093), Nagelkerke R-square (0.282), and omnibus test of model coefficients ($p < 0.05$). The results of the model χ-square test revealed that the factor influencing UNCRC was hospitalization experience (B = 2.708, 95% confidence interval [CI]: 1.698, 132.404, $p < 0.05$) (**Table 6**). The odds ratio (OR) for having been hospitalized was 14.996, indicating that children who had been hospitalized were about 15 times more likely to know about the UNCRC than those who had not been hospitalized. The goodness of fit of this regression equation was high with the Hosmer–Lemeshow test ($p = 0.442$), and the discriminant accuracy rate was 94.9%. In addition, when these binomial logistic regression analyses adopted the method of variable increase by the likelihood ratio, independent variables other than hospitalization experience were excluded. The results of the final procedure were the omnibus test of the model coefficients ($p < 0.001$), model χ-square test (B = 2.757, 95% CI: 1.978, 125.396, $p < 0.01$), and OR of the hospitalization experience of 15.750. Thus, the results of the independent variables affecting knowledge of the dependent variable UNCRC are warranted.

6. Discussion

School-aged children's perceptions of the UNCRC and decision-making indicate the need for nurses to consider children's rights in pediatric nursing. The results of this study support the important concept of nurses implementing the best interest criteria to support a child-centered, family-oriented process [12, 30, 31]. The UNCRC and decision-making as perceived by school-aged children experiencing psychological

Variables	About UNCRC: ■ I just know (%)	■ I do not know (%)	*p*	ϕ / *V*
Sex			ns	-
Male (n=106)	2.9	41.6		
Female (n=132)	1.7	53.8		
Age			<0.05*	0.206
9 years (n=28)	0.0	11.8		
10 years (n=73)	0.0	30.7		
11 years (n=94)	3.8	35.7		
12 years (n=43)	0.8	17.2		
School year			ns	-
Fourth grade (n=66)	0.0	27.7		
Fifth grade (n=71)	2.5	27.3		
Sixth grade (n=101)	2.1	40.3		
Number of family members			ns	-
2–3 (n=43)	0.0	18.1		
4 (n=129)	2.9	51.3		
>5 (n=66)	1.7	26.1		
Number of siblings			ns	-
1 (n=35)	0.0	14.7		
2 (n=141)	3.8	55.5		
>3 (n=62)	0.7	25.2		
Outpatient status			ns	-
During outpatient visit (n=68)	2.1	26.5		
Not during outpatient visit (n=170)	2.5	68.9		
Hospitalization experience			<0.01 †	0.220
Experienced (n=99)	4.2	37.4		
No experience (n=139)	0.4	58.0		
Need for explanation			ns	-
I need an explanation (n=217)	4.2	87.0		
No explanation needed (n=21)	0.4	8.8		
Whether explanation was received			ns	-
Received (n=217)	4.6	86.6		
Not received (n=21)	0.0	8.8		

Note. UNCRC, United Nations Convention on the Rights of the Child; *p*, *p*-value; ns: not significant; φ: coefficient of association; *V*: Cramer's V.

* Pearson's chi-squared test, † Fisher's exact test

Table 3.
Attribute relationships with children who do not know about UNCRC (n = 238).

outcomes, such as trait anxiety, pain, and fear, were proved to be closely related to the healthcare environment [16, 18, 28]. Based on these findings and resulting from the clarification of perceptions of school-aged children, the responsibility of nurses in creating a respectful environment for children may be fulfilled at the behavioral level. This section provides a detailed rationale for school-aged children's perceptions of the UNCRC and their decision-making process, so that pediatric nurses can provide appropriate care to all children and their families.

Variables	About the need for explanation: I need (%)	I do not need it (%)	*p*	ϕ / *V*
Sex			ns	-
Male (n=106)	41.2	3.4		
Female (n=132)	50.0	5.5		
Age			ns	-
9 years (n=28)	10.1	1.7		
10 years (n=73)	27.7	2.9		
11 years (n=94)	37.0	2.5		
12 years (n=43)	16.4	1.7		
School year			ns	-
Fourth grade (n=66)	24.4	3.4		
Fifth grade (n=71)	28.2	1.7		
Sixth grade (n=101)	38.7	3.8		
Number of family members			<0.05*	0.160
2–3 (n=43)	15.5	2.5		
4 (n=129)	51.7	2.5		
>5 (n=66)	23.9	3.8		
Number of siblings			ns	-
1 (n=35)	13.4	1.3		
2 (n=141)	55.5	3.8		
>3 (n=62)	22.3	3.8		
Outpatient status			ns	-
During outpatient visit (n=68)	26.5	2.1		
Not during outpatient visit (n=170)	64.7	6.7		
Hospitalization experience			ns	-
Experienced (n=99)	37.8	3.8		
No experience (n=139)	53.4	5.0		
Whether explanation was received			<0.001*	0.321
Received (n=217)	85.7	5.5		
Not received (n=21)	5.7	3.4		

Note. p, p-value; ns: not significant; φ: coefficient of association; *V*: Cramer's V.

* Pearson's chi-squared test

Table 4.
Attribute relationships with children who needed explanations (n = 238).

6.1 Ethical issues faced by school-aged children

According to Piaget's theory of cognitive development, school-aged children are in the concrete operational stage when they begin to solve problems logically, but can only solve those problems that apply to a specific event or problem [41]. According to Erikson's theory of personality, school-aged children strive to prove their ability to be rewarded in society and require a supportive environment to improve their ability to achieve these goals [42]. Thus, school-age development was scientifically proven, children's rights and freedoms were respected, and laws and guidelines were formed. For example, Article 17 of the UNCRC states that "children have the right to access information that is important to their health and well-being" [33]. Furthermore,

Variables	Explainer: Doctor	Nurse	Doctors, nurses, and families (%)	p	ϕ / V
Sex				ns	-
Male (n=95)	28.6	4.1	11.1		
Female (n=122)	32.7	10.1	13.4		
Age				ns	-
9 years (n=25)	6.0	2.8	2.8		
10 years (n=69)	19.8	2.8	9.2		
11 years (n=84)	24.0	6.0	8.8		
12 years (n=39)	11.5	2.8	3.7		
School year				ns	-
Fourth grade (n=62)	15.2	4.6	8.8		
Fifth grade (n=66)	20.3	3.2	6.9		
Sixth grade (n=89)	25.8	6.5	8.8		
Number of family members				ns	-
2–3 (n=38)	11.1	1.4	5.1		
4 (n=122)	32.7	9.2	14.3		
>5 (n=57)	17.5	3.7	5.1		
Number of siblings				ns	-
1 (n=32)	9.7	0.9	4.1		
2 (n=131)	35.5	9.7	15.2		
>3 (n=54)	16.1	3.7	5.1		
Outpatient status				ns	-
During outpatient visit (n=65)	18.9	3.7	7.4		
Not during outpatient visit (n=152)	42.4	10.6	17.1		
Hospitalization experience				ns	-
Experienced (n=90)	25.3	5.5	10.6		
No experience (n=127)	35.9	8.8	13.8		
About UNCRC				ns	-
I just know (n=11)	3.2	0.9	0.9		
I do not know (n=206)	58.1	13.4	23.5		
Need for explanation				<0.05*	0.201
I need (n=204)	55.3	14.3	24.4		
I do not need it (n=13)	6.0	0.0	0.0		

Note. UNCRC, United Nations Convention on the Rights of the Child; p, p-value; ns: not significant; φ: coefficient of association; V: Cramer's V.

* Pearson's chi-squared test

Table 5.
Attribute relationship between the explainer and children (N = 217).

Predictive variables	B	SE	Wald	df	*p*	Exp (B)	95% CI for Exp (B)	
							Lower	Upper
Sex	0.578	0.718	0.647	1	0.421	1.782	0.436	7.287
Age	−1.042	0.792	1.730	1	0.188	0.353	0.075	1.667
School year	0.455	0.938	0.235	1	0.628	1.576	0.251	9.907
Number of family members	−1.523	0.813	3.508	1	0.061	0.218	0.044	1.073
Number of siblings	0.795	0.776	1.049	1	0.306	2.214	0.484	10.135
Outpatient status	−0.120	0.725	0.027	1	0.869	0.887	0.214	3.675
Hospitalization experience	2.708	1.111	5.937	1	0.015	14.996	1.698	132.404
Need for explanation	−0.900	1.284	0.492	1	0.483	0.407	0.033	5.034
The person who explained	−0.043	0.423	0.010	1	0.919	0.958	0.418	2.194

Note: UNCRC, United Nations Convention on the Rights of the Child; B, partial regression coefficient; SE, standard error; df, degree of freedom; p, p-value; CI, confidence interval.

Table 6.
Factors affecting knowledge of UNCRC (n = 217).

Article 5 of the European Association for Children in Hospitals states that "children and parents have the right to be informed participants in all decisions related to their health care" [43]. However, the perception of school-age involvement in decisions regarding care and treatment is low [17], which exacerbates children's fears and anxieties [44].

These are salient ethical issues for school-aged children and their families who are about to receive medical care. Therefore, pediatric nurses must strengthen the environment in which they contribute to the resolution of ethical issues and the decision-making process and become advocates for the dignity of the child [22, 45]. The results of this study provide information that can help pediatric nurses focus on and improve UNCRC and decision-making processes in the context of these ethical issues.

6.2 Awareness of children's rights and decision-making

In this study, it was necessary to understand UNCRC and decision-making in school-aged children to enhance pediatric nursing care that considers children's rights. First, it has been suggested that the older the age, the greater the knowledge school-aged children have about the UNCRC, and that their understanding may increase with the developmental stage. This can be viewed positively from the perspectives of the cognitive developmental theory [41] and ego theory [42] as children trying to become aware of the UNCRC. This study also found that the demand for explanations may depend on the number of family members and that children's decision-making processes require family involvement. This can also be interpreted as an attribute that is supported as a construct in SOA [31].

In contrast, more than 90% of school-aged children who had previously been briefed in hospitals and clinics stated that they wanted to continue, but more than 95% were unaware of the UNCRC. This result parallels children's lack of support in the healthcare environment [16] and the lack of participation in decisions regarding their care and treatment [17]. In other words, the inability of children to self-determine their personal needs is expected to increase their fear [44, 46] and induce parental anxiety [8]. Furthermore, 13 of the 217 children who received the explanation and 8 of the 21 children who did not receive the explanation said that they did not need an explanation. Children should be allowed to receive explanations and be able to make decisions about whether they want to receive another explanation [33, 43]. However, it was found that about half of the children who did not receive an explanation were in a serious condition for which they did not want any further explanation. To increase the participation and understanding of pediatric patients in the decision-making process and instill trust in team members, it is important to focus on nursing ethics [9]. Therefore, increasing opportunities for school-aged children to learn about UNCRC and decision-making before they go to the hospital or clinic needs to be addressed.

6.3 Benefits to children and families of explanations of individual healthcare

In practice, it is necessary to focus on HCPs to consider ethical principles in children's healthcare as well as evidence of respect for the interests of children and families, values, and beliefs [31, 38, 47]. The results of this study showed that school-aged children often sought clarification from physicians. This is a time when school-aged children develop the concept of illness [48], and based on this, they have proven to be proactive and willing to engage in treatment [42]. This is also consistent with previous research on physicians building moral trust in school-aged children [49, 50].

However, on examining the relationship between HCPs and the need for explanations, the results indicated that school-aged children who did not want explanations concentrated on physicians. This could be related to the fact that they were not involved in decision-making regarding care and treatment [17]. They may also have previously undergone invasive medical procedures without being given the option to receive explanations, which may have been distressing to experience [7]. Furthermore, the lack of explanation to parents for painful emotional experiences in school-aged children may be one of the causes of increased parental anxiety [8, 16]. Conversely, there were no school children who did not want explanations from nurses alone or doctors, nurses, and their families. These results also support the need for the promotion of SOAs to consider HCPs comprehensively based on the UNCRC [31].

Therefore, it can be said that pediatric nursing is currently required to foster the creation of an environment where children and their families can receive appropriate explanations at the right developmental age of the child. Specifically, the use of DIPS is recommended [12], as it can be implemented by pediatric nurses, including nursing ethics, in addition to the SOA [31]. These tools, and the study results, which have focused on HCPs and explanatory needs, demonstrate the need to ensure benefits to children and families in UNCRC-aware nursing management.

6.4 The UNCRC and inpatient experience

The UNCRC has stated that Sisom, an eHealth service, has created a communication space in medical settings allowing for the voices of school-aged children to be heard [51]. HCPs' actions have influenced children's active participation in decision-making processes, including medical care, indicating the need to increase awareness among health professionals [23]. While school-aged children experience psychological consequences that increase their perceptions of pain, anxiety, fear, and perceived threat when receiving medical care, they are also more likely to be exposed to the UNCRC as a result [4, 5]. Our study results demonstrate that hospitalization of school-aged children is an opportunity to learn about the UNCRC.

However, pediatric nurses should pay special attention to whether children can learn about UNCRC without hospitalization. In other words, since a child's autonomy is known to be under threat from disease [6], they should be aware of the UNCRC before they see a doctor, so that they can exercise their rights. For example, if a pediatric nurse explains the UNCRC before and after a pediatric patient's visit or treatment, it can facilitate decision-making for these patients and their families [23]. Pediatric nurses can also create a respectful environment for children by providing a forum for discussing the UNCRC not only in the medical field but also through elementary schools and institutions. Thus, enhancing school-aged children's awareness and pediatric nursing practice regarding UNCRC and decision-making will contribute to the best interests of children and their families [22].

6.5 Strengths and limitations

6.5.1 Strengths

Pediatric nursing research on UNCRC and decision-making interventions, especially from the perspective of children, remains challenging. This study carefully examined decision support that respects children's rights from the perspective of school-aged children and provided insights useful for pediatric nurses in their clinical practice.

6.5.2 Limitations

This study has two major limitations. First, to gain the understanding and support of the survey participants, only school-aged children living in some parts of Japan were included in the study, and older data were used. This limits the generalizability of the findings. Second, the analysis of school-aged children's perceptions considered only quantitative data on attributes extracted from previous research rather than open-ended textual data. Further validation of our findings will require sufficient sample size, stability checks, new data including participants from different ethnic groups, and further research using induction.

7. Conclusion

Nursing orientations derived from the perceptions of school-aged children can help create an appropriate healthcare environment to support pediatric patients and their families. This concept, based on the UNCRC, adds to the rights of the child that must be respected by all pediatric nurses and underlines the efforts required by medical staff to share healthcare information with families to determine the best approach for pediatric patients. Awareness of the child's age is an indicator for pediatric nurses to optimize their planning and practice in pediatric and family nursing. However, considerations regarding awareness of school-aged children need to be further validated using other qualitative research methods.

Acknowledgements

The author would like to thank all school-aged children and parents who participated in this study. The author would also like to thank Editage (www.editage.com) for English language editing.

Funding and role of the funding source

This study was funded by Asahikawa Medical University's Innovative Research in Life Science.

Conflict of interest

The author declares that there is no potential or existing conflict of interest relevant to this article.

Ethics statement

This study complies with the principles enunciated in the Declaration of Helsinki, which is the ethical principles for medical research involving human participants.

Author details

Hiroyuki Ogihara[1,2]

1 Faculty of Nursing, Ashikaga University, Ashikaga, Tochigi, Japan

2 Graduate School of Science and Technology, Gunma University, Kiryu, Gunma, Japan

*Address all correspondence to: ogihara.hiroyuki@g.ashikaga.ac.jp

References

[1] Santo L, Kang K. National Hospital Ambulatory Medical Care Survey: 2019 National Summary Tables. USA: National Ambulatory Medical Care Survey; 2023. DOI: 10.15620/cdc:123251

[2] Ministry of Health, Labour and Welfare. List of Health, Labor and Welfare Statistics, Outline of Patient Survey (in Japanese). 2017. Available from: https://www.mhlw.go.jp/toukei/saikin/hw/kanja/17/dl/01.pdf [Accessed: November 01, 2023]

[3] Ministry of Health, Labour and Welfare. List of Health, Labor and Welfare Statistics, Outline of Patient Survey (in Japanese). 2019. Available from: https://www.mhlw.go.jp/toukei/saikin/hw/kanja/20/dl/suikeikanjya.pdf [Accessed: November 01, 2023]

[4] De Mula-Fuentes B, Quintana M, Rimbau J, Martínez-Mejías A, Úriz MS, Rivera-Pérez C, et al. Anxiety, hospital fears and conduct and behavioral alterations during pediatric hospitalization. Actas Españolas de Psiquiatría. 2018;**46**(2):42-50. DOI: 10.15620/cdc:123251

[5] Jurko A, Minarik M, Jurko T, Tonhajzerova I. White coat hypertension in pediatrics. Italian Journal of Pediatrics. 2016;**42**(4):1-5. DOI: 10.1186/s13052-016-0213-3

[6] Alderson P. Consent to children's surgery and intensive medical treatment. Journal of Law and Society. 1990;**17**(4):52-65. DOI: 10.2307/1409954

[7] Triantafyllou C, Matziou V. Aggravating factors and assessment tools for posttraumatic stress disorder in children after hospitalization. Psychiatriki. 2019;**30**(3):264-270. DOI: 10.22365/jpsych.2019.303.256

[8] Oommen S, Shetty A. Does parental anxiety affect children's perception of pain during intravenous cannulation? Nursing Children and Young People. 2020;**32**(3):21-24. DOI: 10.7748/ncyp.2019.e1187

[9] Bartholdson C, Sandeberg MA, Molewijk B, Pergert P. Does participation in ethics discussions have an impact on ethics decision-making? A cross-sectional study among healthcare professionals in paediatric oncology. European Journal of Oncology Nursing. 2021;**52**(101950):1-9. DOI: 10.1016/j.ejon.2021.101950

[10] Maslak K, Favara-Scacco C, Barchitta M, Agodi A, Astuto M, Scalisi R, et al. General anesthesia, conscious sedation, or nothing: Decision-making by children during painful procedures. Pediatric Blood and Cancer. 2019;**66**(5):e27600, 1-8. DOI: 10.1002/pbc.27600

[11] Yoo SY, Cho H. Exploring the influences of nurses' partnership with parents, attitude to families' importance in nursing care, and professional self-efficacy on quality of pediatric nursing care: A path model. International Journal of Environmental Research and Public Health. 2020;**17**(15):5452, 1-13. DOI: 10.3390/ijerph17155452

[12] Ogihara H. Development and validation of the distracting ingenuity promotion scale for paediatric nurses to support the psychological outcomes of paediatric patients and their families: A survey-based cross-sectional cohort study. Nursing Open. 2022;**9**(3):1653-1666. DOI: 10.1002/nop2.1190

[13] Ogihara H, Funato Y, Oku H. Proposal for a distraction technique using two-screen projection for stress relief

in children with medical complexity. IEEE Access. 2023;**11**:105749-105760. DOI: 10.1109/ACCESS.2023.3316226

[14] Coyne I, Hallström I, Söderbäck M. Reframing the focus from a family-centred to a child-centred care approach for children's healthcare. Journal of Child Health Care: For Professionals Working with Children in the Hospital and Community. 2016;**20**(4):494-502. DOI: 10.1177/1367493516642744

[15] Eklund R, Kreicbergs U, Alvariza A, Lövgren M. Children's views are not taken into account in accordance with article 12 of the United Nations convention on the rights of the child in the family talk intervention when a parent is cared for in palliative care. Omega. 2020;**85**(1):126-154. DOI: 10.1177/0030222820941283

[16] Przybylska MA, Burke N, Harris C, Kazmierczyk M, Kenton E, Yu O, et al. Delivery of the UN convention on the rights of the child in an acute paediatric setting: An audit of information available and service gap analysis. BMJ Paediatrics Open. 2019;**3**(1):e000445, 1-8. DOI: 10.1136/bmjpo-2019-000445

[17] Care Quality Commission. Children and Young People's Survey: Statistical release2020. p. 2021. Available from: https://www.cqc.org.uk/publications/surveys/children-young-peoples-survey-2020 [Accessed: November 01, 2023]

[18] Jovanovic T, Nylocks KM, Gamwell KL, Smith A, Davis TA, Norrholm SD, et al. Development of fear acquisition and extinction in children: Effects of age and anxiety. Neurobiology of Learning and Memory. 2014;**113**:135-142. DOI: 10.1016/j.nlm.2013.10.016

[19] Lee VY, Caillaud C, Fong J, Edwards KM. Improving vaccine-related pain, distress or fear in healthy children and adolescents–a systematic search of patient-focused interventions. Human Vaccines and Immunotherapeutics. 2018;**14**(11):2737-2747. DOI: 10.1080/21645515.2018.1480238

[20] Quist N. Pediatric decision making: Ross, Rawls, and getting children and families right. Journal of Clinical Ethics. 2019;**30**(3):240-246. DOI: 10.1086/JCE2019303240

[21] Nicholl A, Evelegh K, Deering KE, Russell K, Lawrence D, Lyons-Wall P, et al. Using a respectful approach to child-centred healthcare (ReACH) in a paediatric clinical trial: A feasibility study. PLoS One. 2020;**15**(11):e0241764, 1-32. DOI: 10.1371/journal.pone.0241764

[22] Petronio-Coia BJ, Schwartz-Barcott D. A description of approachable nurses: An exploratory study, the voice of the hospitalized child. Journal of Pediatric Nursing. 2020;**54**:18-23. DOI: 10.1016/j.pedn.2020.05.011

[23] Quaye AA, Coyne I, Söderbäck M, Hallström IK. Children's active participation in decision-making processes during hospitalisation: An observational study. Journal of Clinical Nursing. 2019;**28**(23-24):4525-4537. DOI: 10.1111/jocn.15042

[24] MacPherson S. The convention on the rights of the child. Social Policy & Administration. 1989;**23**(1):99-101. DOI: 10.1111/j.1467-9515.1989.tb00500.x

[25] Hein IM, De Vries MC, Troost PW, Meynen G, Van Goudoever JB, Lindauer RJL. Informed consent instead of assent is appropriate in children from the age of twelve: Policy implications of new findings on children's competence to consent to clinical research. BMC Medical Ethics. 2015;**16**:1-7. DOI: 10.1186/s12910-015-0067-z

[26] Hein IM, Troost PW, Broersma A, De Vries MC, Daams JG, Lindauer RJL. Why is it hard to make progress in assessing children's decision-making competence? BMC Medical Ethics. 2015;**16**:1-6. DOI: 10.1186/1472-6939-16-1

[27] Katz AL, Webb SA, Macauley RC, Mercurio MR, Moon MR, Okun AL, et al. Informed consent in decision-making in pediatric practice. Pediatrics. 2016;**138**(2):1-16. DOI: 10.1542/peds.2016-1485

[28] Öztürk Şahin ÖÖ, Topan A. Investigation of the fear of 7-18-year-old hospitalized children for illness and hospital. Journal of Religion and Health. 2019;**58**(3):1011-1023. DOI: 10.1007/s10943-018-0688-x

[29] Rennick JE, Rashotte J. Psychological outcomes in children following pediatric intensive care unit hospitalization: A systematic review of the research. Journal of Child Health Care: For Professionals Working with Children in the Hospital and Community. 2009;**13**(2):128-149. DOI: 10.1177/1367493509102472

[30] UNICEF. Representing Children: Then and Now. Unicef. 2019. Available from: https://www.unicef.org/stories/representing-children-then-and-now [Accessed: November 02, 2023]

[31] Streuli JC, Anderson J, Alef-Defoe S, Bergsträsser E, Jucker J, Meyer S, et al. Combining the best interest standard with shared decision-making in pediatrics—Introducing the shared optimum approach based on a qualitative study. European Journal of Pediatrics. 2021;**180**(3):759-766. DOI: 10.1007/s00431-020-03756-8

[32] Jaroslawska AJ, McCormack T, Burns P, Caruso EM. Outcomes versus intentions in fairness-related decision making: School-aged children's decisions are just like those of adults. Journal of Experimental Child Psychology. 2020;**189**(104704):1-53. DOI: 10.1016/j.jecp.2019.104704

[33] UN Committee on the Rights of the Child (CRC). General Comment No. 12 (2009): The Right of the Child to be Heard. CRC/C/GC/12. 2009. Available from: https://www.refworld.org/docid/4ae562c52.html [Accessed: November 02, 2023]

[34] Asahikawa City Hall. 2014 School Basic Survey Results (in Japanese). 2015. Available from: https://www.city.asahikawa.hokkaido.jp/700/701/705/p007266.html [Accessed: November 02, 2023]

[35] Ministry of Internal Affairs and Communications. Population, Vital Statistics and Number of Households Based on the Basic Resident Register (in Japanese). 2014. Available from: https://www.soumu.go.jp/menu_news/s-news/01gyosei02_02000062.html [Accessed: November 02, 2023]

[36] Cohen J. Statistical Power Analysis for the Behavioral Sciences. 2nd ed. UK: Routledge; 1988. Available from: https://www.utstat.toronto.edu/~brunner/oldclass/378f16/readings/CohenPower.pdf [Accessed: November 02, 2023]

[37] Cohen J. A power primer. Psychological Bulletin. 1992;**112**(1):155-159. DOI: 10.1037/0033-2909.112.1.155

[38] Bester JC. The best interest standard and children: Clarifying a concept and responding to its critics. Journal of Medical Ethics. 2019;**45**(2):117-124. DOI: 10.1136/medethics-2018-105036

[39] Ross LF, Swota AH. The best interest standard: Same name but different roles in pediatric bioethics and child rights frameworks. Perspectives in Biology

and Medicine. 2017;**60**(2):186-197. DOI: 10.1353/pbm.2017.0027

[40] Salter EK. Deciding for a child: A comprehensive analysis of the best interest standard. Theoretical Medicine and Bioethics. 2012;**33**(3):179-198. DOI: 10.1007/s11017-012-9219-z

[41] Ginsburg H, Opper S. Piaget's Theory of Intellectual Development. 2nd ed. USA: Prentice Hall; 1979

[42] Erikson EH. Identity and the Life Cycle. USA: W. W. Norton & Company; 1994

[43] European association for children in hospital (EACH). The EACH Charter with Annotations. 2016. Available from: https://www.childrenshealthscotland.org/wp-content/uploads/2017/06/Charter_AUG2016_oSz.pdf [Accessed: November 02, 2023]

[44] Coyne I. Children's experiences of hospitalization. Journal of Child Health Care: For Professionals Working with Children in the Hospital and Community. 2006;**10**(4):326-336. DOI: 10.1177/1367493506067884

[45] Bagnasco A, Cadorin L, Barisone M, Bressan V, Iemmi M, Prandi M, et al. Ethical dimensions of paediatric nursing: A rapid evidence assessment. Nursing Ethics. 2018;**25**(1):111-122. DOI: 10.1177/0969733016631161

[46] Broström L, Johansson M. Involving children in non-therapeutic research: On the development argument. Medicine, Health Care, and Philosophy. 2014;**17**(1):53-60. DOI: 10.1007/s11019-013-9486-0

[47] Birchley G. Deciding together? Best interests and shared decision-making in paediatric intensive care. Health Care Analysis. 2014;**22**(3):203-222. DOI: 10.1007/s10728-013-0267-y

[48] Bibace R, Walsh ME. Development of children's concepts of illness. Pediatrics. 1980;**66**(6):912-917. DOI: 10.1542/peds.66.6.912

[49] Díaz-Pérez A, Navarro Quiroz E, Aparicio Marenco DE. Moral structuring of children during the process of obtaining informed consent in clinical and research settings. BMC Medical Ethics. 2020;**21**:1-10. DOI: 10.1186/s12910-020-00540-z

[50] Luchtenberg ML, Maeckelberghe ELM, Locock L, Verhagen AAE. Understanding the child-doctor relationship in research participation: A qualitative study. BMC Pediatrics. 2020;**20**:1-10. DOI: 10.1186/s12887-020-02243-1

[51] Carlsson IM, Arvidsson S, Svedberg P, Nygren JM, Viklund Å, Birkeland AL, et al. Creating a communication space in the healthcare context: Children's perspective of using the ehealth service, Sisom. Journal of Child Health Care: For Professionals Working with Children in the Hospital and Community. 2021;**25**(1):31-43. DOI: 10.1177/1367493520904804

Chapter 11

Perspective Chapter: Nurse-Led Education for Patients with Chronic Inflammatory Arthritis

Stefka Stoilova

Abstract

As an integral part of disease monitoring and management of patients with chronic inflammatory arthritis, patient education is highly recommended to help patients optimize their health and well-being rather than be limited to the disease. Rheumatology nurses have been shown to play a major role in patient education, thus enabling them to increase their knowledge about their health condition as well as change their health behavior. Since patients with chronic inflammatory arthritis have different educational needs, patient education can be provided in a variety of ways tailored to the specific and unique needs of each patient. The extent to which nurses in various regions of the world are involved in patient education depends on both their professional background and the organization of the relevant health system.

Keywords: nurse-led education, patients, chronic inflammatory arthritis, educational needs, disease management

1. Introduction

The need for patient education is widely recognized [1]. It is an important aspect of nursing care that would allow patients to manage their disease and improve their health outcomes [2], thus maintaining a better quality of life (QoL) [3].

To improve the health of patients with chronic diseases, such as chronic inflammatory arthritis (CIA), patient education provided by healthcare professionals plays a tremendous role [4]. CIA has an adverse effect on the physical and psychological functioning of individuals; this negative impact increases the severity of the disease [5], worsens the prognosis, and is often associated with a significant socioeconomic burden. CIA has a lasting impact on the daily activities and quality of life of over 100,000 people in Bulgaria [6].

The fast development of medicine and technology in recent decades has highlighted the need for a well-trained, highly skilled nursing workforce capable of adapting to new changes and challenges. The introduction of biologic disease-modifying antirheumatic drugs (bDMARDs) in recent years has led to a dramatic improvement in the treatment of CIA. The application of this new class of medications in rheumatology is associated with continued learning and knowledge advancement in this field attained by healthcare providers as well as by patients and their families.

 IntechOpen

bDMARDs are effective in the treatment of CIA, including rheumatoid arthritis (RA), spondyloarthritis (SpA), and psoriatic arthritis (PsA); they make it possible to achieve control of disease activity and manage functional impairment in order to improve disease prognosis [7]. In the context of rheumatology, nurses, together with physicians and other healthcare professionals, participate in the treatment of CIA [8], with nurses playing a major role in the patient education [9]. Patient education is highly recommended for better management of chronic diseases such as CIA, as it would help patients master specific skills necessary to manage the disease [7].

The chronic course of the disease suggests that patients with CIA are constantly in need of education throughout their entire illness—an education that is tailored to their individual needs for learning and information [10]. Nurses contribute to patient education by teaching patients to self-inject medications [11, 12]; their support may also be helpful for the maintenance of a healthier lifestyle by encouraging patients to increase their physical activity [13] or quit smoking [14]. In addition, patient education enables nurses to provide patients with the information and emotional support they need [12].

There is a large body of evidence suggesting that patient education programs, based on long-term interactions with nurses, provide knowledge to patients during the entire course of their illness and may also positively change their lifestyle [13, 15].

2. Characteristics of patient education

1. Focus

2. Problem-oriented

3. Compliance with regulated principles and recommendations

4. Dynamism and relevance

5. Applicability

6. Measurability

7. Formation of attitudes and behaviors as part of coping with the disease process

As defined by the European League Against Rheumatism (EULAR), patient education "is a planned interactive learning process designed to support and enable people to manage their life with CIA and optimize their health and well-being, rather than be limited to the disease" [16], and it has become the core principle in rheumatology. This overarching principle applies to other chronic diseases as well [17, 18].

Through provision of education, health professionals convey information to patients and their caregivers in order to improve patients' health and encourage them to make decisions in relation to the care provided to them. During the process of education, patients can put in practice their knowledge, skills, values, and attitudes associated with specific or general medical topics related to the adoption of a healthier lifestyle and appropriate use of medicines [19].

Perception of patient education as an integral part of CIA treatment ensures that patients will be able to perform self-management activities and will adhere to their treatment. Patient education aims at improving patients' self-efficacy as a prerequisite for self-management [5].

A number of authors consider patient education as an integral part of disease management in people with CIA [16, 20–26]. It is, however, emphasized that educational needs may differ from one individual to another and may change over the course of the disease. It is recommended that patient education should begin immediately after the patient has been diagnosed or as early as possible; it also should be individually tailored and should address different aspects of the disease [3]. It has also been shown that patients need knowledge in order to exercise appropriate behavior and practices to manage their symptoms and complaints associated with their disease. Patients therefore seek information about their illness and its treatment, including pharmacological and non-pharmacological treatment options; they search for information about managing the psychological and emotional impacts of the illness and information about nutrition, exercise, pain control, and how to lead a stress-free life. Studies have also shown that patients' educational needs depend on the characteristics of their diagnosis, sex, age, and duration of illness [10].

Being an essential part of nursing practice, patient education lies at the heart of all self-management interventions adapted to the type and severity of disease, individual social circumstances, and available resources [27]. Efforts to conduct effective education should be the task of both health professionals and the patients themselves.

2.1 The role of the nurse in patient education

In 2012, the European League Against Rheumatism (EULAR) released its recommendations on the role of nurses in the management of CIA, which includes rheumatoid arthritis (RA), ankylosing spondylitis (AS), and psoriatic arthritis (PsA). According to a 2018 update of these recommendations, patients should have access to a nurse for needs-based education and self-management support to improve knowledge about CIA and its management throughout the entire course of their disease. The recommendations focus on rheumatology nursing care and aim at educating patients based on their needs and satisfaction with care; these recommendations also aim at ensuring timely access to care, facilitating disease management, increasing care efficiency, providing psychosocial support, and promoting self-management [9].

The implementation of EULAR recommendations is based on the specialized training of rheumatology nurses. It has been noted, however, that the implementation of the recommendations varies in different regions of the world and they are least followed in Southern, Eastern, and Central Europe [8].

The EULAR recommendations state that non-pharmacological treatment should include patient education; they also highlight that providing information to patients is an important part of the treatment and emphasize the opportunity for implementation of educational programs as additional interventions in the treatment of early arthritis and ankylosing spondylitis (AS) [28, 29].

There are three overarching principles and eight recommendations included in the updated EULAR recommendations.

The principles define the nurse as an integral member of the healthcare team who provides evidence-based care and encourages shared decision-making when counseling a patient.

2.1.1 Overarching principles

1. Rheumatology nurses are part of a healthcare team

Being part of a multidisciplinary team, rheumatology nurses play an integrated role in patient care; they work in collaboration with the patient (and their family) and the rheumatologist or are involved in the process as part of a larger healthcare team [30].

2. Rheumatology nurses provide evidence-based care

Evidence-based nursing care provided by rheumatology nurses includes: (i) research evidence; (ii) clinical nursing experience; (iii) patients' experiences, preferences, and values; and (iv) the local context [31, 32].

3. Rheumatology nursing is based on shared decision-making with the patient

Collaborative decision-making between the healthcare provider and the patient is crucial for providing quality health care [33, 34], with a commitment to understanding patient's values and preferences.

2.1.2 Updated recommendations

- *Recommendation 1 states that patients should have access to a nurse for needs-based education to improve knowledge of CIA and its management throughout the course of their disease.*

The positive contribution of patient education refers to a number of educational activities, such as therapeutic and health education and health promotion, with the principal aim of improving patients' knowledge and skills related to disease control so that they can manage their lives themselves [16].

- *According to Recommendation 2, patients should have access to nurse consultations in order to enhance satisfaction with care.*

In terms of ensuring quality of care, patients' satisfaction with nursing care is given top priority and is considered of utmost importance. Maintaining a long-term patient–nurse relationship makes patients more confident and comfortable in managing their treatment, which emphasizes nurses' holistic and professional approach to care [35].

- *Recommendation 3 states: Patients should have the opportunity of timely access to a nurse for needs-based support; this includes telehealth.*

The opportunity for patients to use new forms of communication, such as telehealth, provides them with access to a competent healthcare team and a sense of personalized care and support [36].

- *Recommendation 4 states: Nurses should participate in comprehensive disease management to control disease activity, reduce symptoms and improve patient-preferred outcomes; this leads to cost-effective care.*

The role of nurses as part of the healthcare team is to provide patient education and control and management of the disease, which may help lower the healthcare costs [24].

- *Recommendation 5: Nurses should address psychosocial issues to reduce patients' symptoms of anxiety and depression.*

Dealing with symptoms of anxiety and depression requires nurses to identify them and support patients with psychosocial issues by means of referring them to special treatment or counselling [37].

- *Recommendation 6: Nurses should support self-management skills to increase patients' self-efficacy.*

Self-management involves the patient's ability to understand the disease and gain adequate knowledge and skills to manage the physical and psychosocial effects of the disease and to make lifestyle changes [38]. By mastering self-management skills, patients can achieve and maintain an independent lifestyle and become more confident and empowered to manage their illness.

The remaining two recommendations apply to education and access to advanced training in rheumatology for nurses so that they can maintain and improve their knowledge and skills and be encouraged to take on extended roles in compliance with national regulations.

In addition, rheumatology nurses play a major role in patient education with regard to infection prevention in screening for comorbidities and increasing the prescription of vaccines by the rheumatologist or general practitioner (GP). Therefore, rheumatology nurses help increase patients' safety skills related to the administration of bDMARDs [7].

2.2 Goals of patient education

The main goal of patient education is to provide comprehensive care to patients with CIA.

Setting appropriate goals and objectives is crucial for the proper conduct of the educational process. Nurses need to have a good knowledge and understanding of educational goals, content, and materials. According to Wingard R., the effectiveness of patient education depends on the proper formulation of specific, measurable, and achievable goals [39]. By using appropriate tools to assess patient needs, nurses set goals and educational strategies aimed at providing appropriate patient care [40].

1. Understanding the impact of nurse-led education and its effect on the patient

2. Through education and training, nurses help patients take control of their health and thus improve their health status. Patient education should provide adequate information aimed at increasing the understanding of disease and provoking behavior directed toward protection and improvement of health [40]. Studies have shown that patients receive much of the information related to their health mainly from the nurse [41]. In this way, nurses have the opportunity to better assess patients' educational needs and prepare them for learning [42]. Analyzing the nurse–patient interaction including promoting autonomy and empowerment, with the ability to adapt to the new life situation

3. An important aspect of caring for people with inflammatory arthritis (IA) is empowering them to acquire a good understanding of their disease and build abilities to deal effectively with the physical and psychological challenges of the disease. Nurses are in closest contact with patients; they spend much more time with them than any other member of the healthcare team, which helps them build trusting relationships with each other. Patient's autonomy to make decisions is influenced by the nurse–patient relationship, which also has an effect on the quality and satisfaction of care received. Patient education, as a leading component of nursing care, has a positive impact on the patient's life and can bring about lasting changes in their life [19]. Supporting patients in their self-management skills, including changes in lifestyle, physical activity, nutrition, and fighting bad habits such as smoking and alcohol consumption

4. Collaboration with patients in promoting healthy behavior includes avoiding harmful substances (e.g., alcohol and tobacco), maintaining physical activity, and developing healthy eating habits [43]; it also turns out to be the foundation on which nurses can empower patients and support their self-efficacy. Patient self-management support focuses on self-care, self-efficacy, and empowerment. The support provided by nurses can strengthen patients' willpower as this can be done by acquiring the right knowledge and problem-solving skills. Interventions should be individually targeted and tailored to patient's specific needs; they should also take into account various social and economic factors. Evaluation of the nurse's role as part of a multidisciplinary team

As members of a multidisciplinary team, nurses are involved in the education, management, psychosocial support, and promotion of self-care in patients with CIA.

a. Patient education and counseling

b. To be effective patient educators, nurses must have special training in rheumatology and be familiar with the theoretical basis of patient education, which ensures the use of personalized tools for each individual patient in order to achieve optimal outcomes [44]. Involvement of all members of the healthcare team can contribute to the ongoing patient education, with each team member having some educational component to provide to the patient. Nurse-led education offers adequate resources including knowledge to improve skills needed to be involved in disease management. Formation of motivation to learn and cope with health problems

c. Knowledge and education are essential to motivate people to make changes in their lives. A better educated patient tends to take greater care of themselves by developing skills aimed at understanding and managing their own health throughout their entire life [45]. The drive to improve their own knowledge and skills encourages patients to be active participants in the management of their health. Receiving adequate information increases patients' confidence and satisfaction; it also represents an important incentive to encourage patients to participate actively in their healthcare process [46]. Formation in the patient of willingness and need for a higher level of knowledge and self-efficacy

   Patient education aims at providing relevant clinical information in order to increase the understanding of the disease and health promoting behavior [40].

With the right support, patients can learn how to use the resources provided in health programs.

5. Maintaining the quality of life of patients with CIA

Many educational programs have demonstrated improvement in patients' understanding of their health status as well as in their knowledge, which has resulted in slowing or halting disease progression and maintaining quality of life [47]. Patient activation leads to an improvement of self-management; it is also associated with disease prevention, increased interest toward seeking health information and results in better quality of life, greater satisfaction with care, improved adherence to treatment, better knowledge, enhanced health status, and lower use of health services [48]. Studies confirm that nurse-led patient education provides opportunities and perspectives for a better life [49] as a prerequisite for maintaining a good quality of life.

2.3 Learning objectives

1. Acquiring knowledge, skills, and habits related to disease management by patients with CIA

Knowledge and skills allow patients to be involved in the management and treatment of the disease. Patients' knowledge as part of a complex intervention influences patients' beliefs and behaviors and is related to medical treatment [50]. Nurses can help patients acquire skills necessary to achieve health goals related to disease management.

a. Providing information and education to increase knowledge about the disease

b. Patients with inflammatory arthritis have high information demands; they seek up-to-date and individualized information [51]. Keeping patients informed about their health condition promotes the activation of self-management.

c. Improvement in care quality and patient safety

   Patient education has been shown to improve patients' quality of life, increase their understanding of their treatment program, and encourage self-management [40], with the potential to involve them in the management of their disease.

2. Conducting and achieving positive changes in patients' self-care behaviors and health status

Involvement in disease control and management as well as providing information, awareness, and support prove to be a solid foundation for increasing patients' sense of empowerment [52]. Patient education helps increase patients' knowledge about their own health condition and provides an opportunity for them to change their health behaviors [50].

a. Building trusting relationships with patients

Nurses inspire a sense of safety, trust, hope, and confidence in patients. Patients prefer discussing issues with nurses rather than with doctors, which is why patient–nurse relations predominate over patient–doctor relations [52].

3. Adapting the treatment regimen to the disease activity

In the management of CIA, it is recommended to adapt treatment regimen to the disease activity. It involves adequate treatment and provision of appropriate educational support [53], thus encouraging patients to self-care.

4. Providing psycho-emotional support to patients

The first step in satisfying patients' psychological needs is identifying psychological distress, which means recognizing the necessity for specialized training in this field. Nurses and other members of the healthcare team should be trained to provide adequate psychological support to patients with IA [54].

5. Use of resources appropriate for the patient

Patients may have different preferences for resources or may suffer specific limitations (visual or hearing impairment or limited motor skills) to which resources need to be tailored.

6. Assessment of patient's needs, concerns, their willingness to learn, and their preferences

Patients should be offered only the amount of information they can handle at a time. There is a need to develop a care and support plan for the entire course of the disease that includes readiness for education and treatment preferences.

7. Assessment of patient's abilities and provision of individualized treatment

Individual patient education cannot be substituted for any other resource.

8. Checking the patient's understanding after patient education and analysis of possible obstacles to learning

Maintenance of knowledge and skills acquired in educational programs is important. Key elements to effective patient education include use of an open communication style, compliance with standards, and dealing with barriers to learning [55]. Continuous measurement of learning outcomes is necessary to improve patients' health literacy. The feedback received from patients is a commonly used way to measure learning outcomes. The effectiveness of patient education may be affected by multiple factors, such as patient's learning ability, literacy level, cultural environment, lack of resources and educational tools, lack of sufficient time, and so forth [56].

3. Patient education (PE): EULAR recommendations

In 2015, EULAR developed eight recommendations for education of patients with inflammatory arthritis; these are guidelines on the provision of PE and training of healthcare professionals to perform PE across Europe.

PE includes all educational activities provided to patients such as therapeutic training, health education, and health promotion. Patients are considered to be active participants in the management of their own disease.

PE achieves not only transfer of knowledge and control of disease; it also empowers patients to manage their disease, adapt to their condition, and maintain a better quality of life.

It has been shown that provision of PE varies across European countries. In some countries, PE is used only to provide knowledge, thus aiming at patient adherence to treatment. The extent to which different healthcare professionals (HP) are involved in PE according to their competence, availability, and education, as well as the organization of the relevant health system, is also essential. The implementation of the EULAR recommendations for education of patients with inflammatory arthritis would allow standardization and improvement of education for people with IA across Europe [16].

Based on evidence and expert opinion, two overarching principles and eight recommendations have been developed.

3.1 Overarching principles

1. PE is a planned interactive learning process designed to support and enable people to manage their life with IA and optimize their health and well-being.

2. Communication and shared decision-making between people with IA and their healthcare professionals are essential for effective PE.

EULAR recommendations for patient education (PE) for people with inflammatory arthritis (IA)

- Recommendation 1: PE as an integral part of standard care

PE should be provided for people with IA as an integral part of standard care in order to enhance patient involvement in disease management. PE improves adherence to treatment and helps recognize side effects of medications.

- Recommendation 2: PE throughout the course of the disease

All people with IA should have access to PE throughout the entire course of their disease, including at the time of diagnosis, in case of change in the pharmacological treatment or when required by the patient's physical or psychological condition.

- Recommendation 3: personalized and needs-based physical training

The content and delivery of PE should be individually tailored and needs-based for people with IA.

- Recommendation 4: Modes of delivery of PE

PE for people with IA should include individual and/or group sessions, which can be provided through face-to-face or online interactions and supplemented by phone calls and written or multimedia material.

- Recommendation 5: theoretical framework and evidence for PE

PE programs for IA patients should have a theoretical framework and be evidence-based. Interventions can be: educational programs, self-management programs (SMPs), cognitive behavioral therapy (CBT), or stress management.

- Recommendation 6: PE results

The effectiveness of PE for people with IA should be evaluated, and the outcomes must reflect the objectives of the PE program.

- Recommendation 7: competence in providing PE

PE should be carried out by competent healthcare specialists—for the most part, they should be HP and/or trained patients.

- Recommendation 8: competence to teach PE

Providers of PE for people with IA should have access to and undertake specific training in order to obtain and maintain knowledge and skills.

Patient education, as defined in the recommendations, can facilitate patients to make informed choices in order to manage their disease [57].

4. Patient education practice guidelines for healthcare professionals

The guidelines address the following important questions:

1. What are the PE guidelines?

A patient education guide to evidence-based practice for healthcare professionals

2. Who should use the guidelines?

Any healthcare professional who provides patient education

3. Where should the guidelines be used?

In any setting where patients learn how to achieve healthcare goals

4. When should the guidelines be used?

Any time patient instructions are being given such as disease information, test preparation/results, treatment, accessing care, appointments, and resources

5. Why should the guidelines be used?

Provides care for consumers in achieving optimal levels of health.

6. How do you use the guidelines?

By following the steps in each section of the guidelines (assessment, planning, implementation, and evaluation)

The Patient Education Practice Guidelines for Healthcare Professionals was developed by the Health Care Education Association (HCEA). The guidelines are based on the four components of the patient education process.

The education process includes assessment, planning, implementation, and evaluation (APIE) [58].

The first step involves *assessment* of patients' learning needs, their learning style, and readiness to learn. The assessment includes what patients know, what they want and need to know, what they are competent to learn, and what is the best way to teach. Understanding patient needs and related factors is linked to the patient-centered nursing approach.

The second step is to develop a *plan*. A successful patient education program depends on a well-designed plan comprising the goals and objectives of the educational process.

The third step in the process is the *implementation* of an individual learning plan that includes interactive learning.

Lastly, an *evaluation* that shows whether or not the goals of care have been achieved [40].

5. Forms of education

Patient education is offered to patients in groups or individually. Group education facilitates patients' learning from each other, while individual education offers easier responsiveness to patients' personal needs. In rheumatology, individual patient education is often carried out by nurses and covers a wide variety of different aspects of medical treatment. Individual consultations with an expert nurse have shown to have a positive impact on patients' ability to control and manage their disease [59]. The following training tools can be used: brochures or other printed materials, podcasts, videos, presentations, posters, or diagrams or discussion with the patient to create individual tools for the patient's needs. It is important to obtain patient feedback in order to gain information on the materials provided to the patient.

6. Conclusion

The role of nurses in CIA management varies considerably across countries and regions due to a variety of factors such as educational level, training, and experience.

EULAR recommendations support the involvement of nurses in the overall management of the disease and promotion of self-management to achieve a greater sense of self-efficacy and patient empowerment.

To improve the process of health care provided by nurses, it is appropriate to ensure continuous training in order to maintain and upgrade basic and advanced knowledge and skills in compliance with the recommendation of the EULAR for the improvement of their competencies, thus ensuring better quality of health care provided.

The guidelines provided above are applicable to the work of nurses practicing in the field of rheumatology, kinesitherapy, balneotherapy, and so on.

Author details

Stefka Stoilova
UMHAT "Sveti Georgi" - Plovdiv, Rheumatology Clinic, Bulgaria

*Address all correspondence to: ef_i@abv.bg

References

[1] Behar-horenstein LS et al. Improving patient care through patient-family education programs. Hospital Topics. 2005;**83**(1):21-27. DOI: 10.3200/HTPS.83.1.21-27

[2] Thompson DL, May EJ, Leach M, Smith CP, Fereday J. The invisible nature of learning: Patient education in nursing. Collegian. 2021;**28**(3):341-345. DOI: 10.1016/j.colegn.2020.08.002

[3] Raunsbæk Knudsen L, Lomborg K, Ndosi M, Hauge E-M, De Thurah A. The effectiveness of e-learning in patient education delivered to patients with rheumatoid arthritis: The WebRA study—protocol for a pragmatic randomised controlled trial. BMC Rheumatology. 2021;**5**(1):57. DOI: 10.1186/s41927-021-00226-y

[4] Ma L et al. Assessment of the practicability of implementing the EULAR recommendations for the role of nurses in the management of chronic inflammatory arthritis in China. European Journal of Inflammation. 2020;**18**:205873922093522. DOI: 10.1177/2058739220935225

[5] Ndosi M et al. Effects of needs-based patient education on self-efficacy and health outcomes in people with rheumatoid arthritis: A multicentre, single blind, randomised controlled trial. Annals of the Rheumatic Diseases. 2016;**75**(6):1126-1132. DOI: 10.1136/annrheumdis-2014-207171

[6] Organization of Patients with Rheumatological Diseases. Socioeconomic burden of RD and MSDs and the role of biological treatment in its reduction [Online]. 15 October 2015. Available from: https://www.revmatologia.org/images/pages/%D0%A2%D0%95%D0%96%D0%95%D0%A1%D0%A2%20%D0%9D%D0%90%20%D0%A0%D0%97%20%D0%98%20%D0%9C%D0%A1%D0%97%20%5BCompatibility%20Mode%5D.pdf

[7] Beauvais C et al. Efficacy of a nurse-led patient education intervention in promoting safety skills of patients with inflammatory arthritis treated with biologics: A multicentre randomised clinical trial. RMD Open. 2022;**8**(1):e001828. DOI: 10.1136/rmdopen-2021-001828

[8] Vivienne L, Michael S. Nurses' roles in the management of chronic inflammatory arthritis: A systematic review. Rheumatology International. 2018;**38**(11):2027-2036. DOI: 10.1007/s00296-018-4135-9

[9] Bech B et al. 2018 update of the EULAR recommendations for the role of the nurse in the management of chronic inflammatory arthritis. Annals of the Rheumatic Diseases. 2020;**79**(1):61-68. DOI: 10.1136/annrheumdis-2019-215458

[10] Grønning K, Lim S, Bratås O. A longitudinal study of educational needs among patients with inflammatory arthritis. Musculoskeletal Care. 2022;**20**(1):151-157. DOI: 10.1002/msc.1575

[11] Fitzgerald P, Hale C. Moving the injectable methotrexate service closer to home: A practice development initiative. Musculoskeletal Care. 2014;**12**(3):182-189. DOI: 10.1002/msc.1070

[12] Fall E, Chakroun N, Dalle N, Izaute M. Is patient education helpful in providing care for patients with rheumatoid arthritis? A qualitative study involving French nurses. Nursing

& Health Sciences. 2013;**15**(3):346-352. DOI: 10.1111/nhs.12042

[13] Knittle K et al. Targeting motivation and self-regulation to increase physical activity among patients with rheumatoid arthritis: A randomised controlled trial. Clinical Rheumatology. 2015;**34**(2):231-238. DOI: 10.1007/s10067-013-2425-x

[14] Naranjo A et al. Results of a specific smoking cessation program for patients with arthritis in a rheumatology clinic. Rheumatology International. 2014;**34**(1):93-99. DOI: 10.1007/s00296-013-2851-8

[15] Arvidsson S, Bergman S, Arvidsson B, Fridlund B, Tingström P. Effects of a self-care promoting problem-based learning programme in people with rheumatic diseases: A randomized controlled study. Journal of Advanced Nursing. 2013;**69**(7):1500-1514. DOI: 10.1111/jan.12008

[16] Zangi HA et al. EULAR recommendations for patient education for people with inflammatory arthritis. Annals of the Rheumatic Diseases. 2015;**74**(6):954-962. DOI: 10.1136/annrheumdis-2014-206807

[17] Prothero L, Barley E, Galloway J, Georgopoulou S, Sturt J. The evidence base for psychological interventions for rheumatoid arthritis: A systematic review of reviews. International Journal of Nursing Studies. 2018;**82**:20-29. DOI: 10.1016/j.ijnurstu.2018.03.008

[18] Isidori V et al. Digital technologies and the role of health care professionals: Scoping review exploring nurses' skills in the digital era and in the light of the COVID-19 pandemic. JMIR Nursing. 2022;**5**(1):e37631. DOI: 10.2196/37631

[19] Fereidouni Z, Sabet Sarvestani R, Hariri G, Kuhpaye SA, Amirkhani M, Kalyani MN. Moving into action: The master key to patient education. Journal of Nursing Research. 2019;**27**(1):e6. DOI: 10.1097/jnr.0000000000000280

[20] Combe B et al. 2016 update of the EULAR recommendations for the management of early arthritis. Annals of the Rheumatic Diseases. 2017;**76**(6):948-959. DOI: 10.1136/annrheumdis-2016-210602

[21] Deighton C, O'Mahony R, Tosh J, Turner C, Rudolf M, Guideline Development Group. Management of rheumatoid arthritis: Summary of NICE guidance. BMJ. 2009;**338**:b702. DOI: 10.1136/bmj.b702

[22] Dejaco C et al. 2015 recommendations for the management of polymyalgia rheumatica: A European League Against Rheumatism/American College of Rheumatology Collaborative Initiative. Arthritis & Rheumatology. 2015;**67**(10):2569-2580. DOI: 10.1002/art.39333

[23] Richette P et al. 2016 updated EULAR evidence-based recommendations for the management of gout. Annals of the Rheumatic Diseases. 2017;**76**(1):29-42. DOI: 10.1136/annrheumdis-2016-209707

[24] Smolen JS et al. Treating rheumatoid arthritis to target: 2014 update of the recommendations of an international task force. Annals of the Rheumatic Diseases. 2016;**75**(1):3-15. DOI: 10.1136/annrheumdis-2015-207524

[25] van der Heijde D et al. 2016 update of the ASAS-EULAR management recommendations for axial spondyloarthritis. Annals of the Rheumatic Diseases. 2017;**76**(6):978-991. DOI: 10.1136/annrheumdis-2016-210770

[26] Grønning K, Lim S, Bratås O. Health status and self-management in patients

with inflammatory arthritis—A five-year follow-up study after nurse-led patient education. Nursing Open. 2020;7(1):326-333. DOI: 10.1002/nop2.394

[27] Nikiphorou E et al. 2021 EULAR recommendations for the implementation of self-management strategies in patients with inflammatory arthritis. Annals of the Rheumatic Diseases. 2021;**80**(10):1278-1285. DOI: 10.1136/annrheumdis-2021-220249

[28] Combe B et al. EULAR recommendations for the management of early arthritis: Report of a task force of the European Standing Committee for International Clinical Studies Including Therapeutics (ESCISIT). Annals of the Rheumatic Diseases. 2006;**66**(1):34-45. DOI: 10.1136/ard.2005.044354

[29] Zochling J. ASAS/EULAR recommendations for the management of ankylosing spondylitis. Annals of the Rheumatic Diseases. 2006;**65**(4):442-452. DOI: 10.1136/ard.2005.041137

[30] Kilpatrick K, Lavoie-Tremblay M, Ritchie JA, Lamothe L. Advanced practice nursing, health care teams, and perceptions of team effectiveness. Health Care Manag (Frederick). 2011;**30**(3):215-226. DOI: 10.1097/HCM.0b013e318225e03a

[31] Sackett DL, Rosenberg WMC, Gray JAM, Haynes RB, Richardson WS. Evidence based medicine: What it is and what it isn't. BMJ. 1996;**312**(7023):71-72. DOI: 10.1136/bmj.312.7023.71

[32] Rycroft-Malone J, Seers K, Titchen A, Harvey G, Kitson A, McCormack B. What counts as evidence in evidence-based practice? Journal of Advanced Nursing. 2004;**47**(1):81-90. DOI: 10.1111/j.1365-2648.2004.03068.x

[33] Makoul G, Clayman ML. An integrative model of shared decision making in medical encounters. Patient Education and Counseling. 2006;**60**(3):301-312. DOI: 10.1016/j.pec.2005.06.010

[34] Dy SM, Purnell TS. Key concepts relevant to quality of complex and shared decision-making in health care: A literature review. Social Science & Medicine. 2012;**74**(4):582-587. DOI: 10.1016/j.socscimed.2011.11.015

[35] Vinall-Collier K, Madill A, Firth J. A multi-centre study of interactional style in nurse specialist- and physician-led Rheumatology clinics in the UK. International Journal of Nursing Studies. 2016;**59**:41-50. DOI: 10.1016/j.ijnurstu.2016.02.009

[36] Primdahl J, Wagner L, Hørslev-Petersen K. Being an outpatient with rheumatoid arthritis – a focus group study on patients' self-efficacy and experiences from participation in a short course and one of three different outpatient settings: Being an outpatient with RA. Scandinavian Journal of Caring Sciences. 2011;**25**(2):394-403. DOI: 10.1111/j.1471-6712.2010.00854.x

[37] Mawson M, Hardy S. Using a psychological approach in rheumatoid arthritis. Practice Nursing. 2017;**28**(10): 431-436. DOI: 10.12968/pnur.2017.28.10.431

[38] Glasgow RE, Davis CL, Funnell MM, Beck A. Implementing practical interventions to support chronic illness self-management. The Joint Commission Journal on Quality and Safety. 2003;**29**(11):563-574. DOI: 10.1016/S1549-3741(03)29067-5

[39] Wingard R. Patient education and the nursing process: Meeting the patient's needs. Nephrology Nursing Journal: Journal of the American Nephrology Nurses' Association. 2005;**32**(2):211-215

[40] Seyedin H, Goharinezhad S, Vatankhah S, Azmal M. Patient education process in teaching hospitals of Tehran University of Medical Sciences. Medical Journal of the Islamic Republic of Iran. 2015;**29**:220

[41] Oermann MH, Harris CH, Dammeyer JA. Teaching by the nurse: How important is it to patients? Applied Nursing Research. 2001;**14**(1):11-17. DOI: 10.1053/apnr.2001.9236

[42] Farahani MA, Mohammadi E, Ahmadi F, Mohammadi N. Factors influencing the patient education: A qualitative research. Iranian Journal of Nursing and Midwifery Research. 2013;**18**(2):133-139

[43] Espinosa-Salas S, Gonzalez-Arias M. Behavior Modification for Lifestyle Improvement. Treasure Island, FL: StatPearls Publishing; 2023. Available from: https://www.ncbi.nlm.nih.gov/books/NBK592418/

[44] Syx RL. The practice of patient education: The theoretical perspective. Orthopaedic Nursing. 2008;**27**(1):50-54. DOI: 10.1097/01.NOR.0000310614.31168.6b

[45] Marcus C. Strategies for improving the quality of verbal patient and family education: A review of the literature and creation of the EDUCATE model. Health Psychology and Behavioral Medicine. 2014;**2**(1):482-495. DOI: 10.1080/21642850.2014.900450

[46] Karaca A, Durna Z. Patient satisfaction with the quality of nursing care. Nursing Open. 2019;**6**(2):535-545. DOI: 10.1002/nop2.237

[47] Gurjar NR. Effect of educational program on knowledge and self-care behavior among arthritis patients: Pre-experimental research design. International Journal of Orthopaedic and Trauma Nursing. 2023:101038. DOI: 10.1016/j.ijotn.2023.101038

[48] Bahrom NH, Ramli AS, Isa MR, Baharudin N, Badlishah-Sham SF, Mohamed-Yassin MS, et al. Validity and reliability of the Patient Activation Measure® (PAM®)-13 Malay version among patients with Metabolic Syndrome in primary care. Malaysian Family Physician: The Official Journal of the Academy of Family Physicians of Malaysia. 2020;**15**(3):22-34

[49] Grønning K, Bratås O, Steinsbekk A. Patients' perceptions of having a good life one year after arthritis patient education: A qualitative study nested within a randomized controlled trial. Nursing Medical Journal of Nursing. 2017;**7**(1):1. DOI: 10.14710/nmjn.v7i1.15123

[50] Grønning K, Midttun L, Steinsbekk A. Patients' confidence in coping with arthritis after nurse-led education; a qualitative study. BMC Nursing. 2016;**15**(1):28. DOI: 10.1186/s12912-016-0150-x

[51] Connelly K et al. Patients' perceived health information needs in inflammatory arthritis: A systematic review. Seminars in Arthritis and Rheumatism. 2019;**48**(5):900-910. DOI: 10.1016/j.semarthrit.2018.07.014

[52] Uthman I et al. Nurse-led care for the management of rheumatoid arthritis: A review of the global literature and proposed strategies for implementation in Africa and the Middle East. Rheumatology International. 2021;**41**(3):529-542. DOI: 10.1007/s00296-020-04682-6

[53] Nadrian H, Morowatisharifabad MA, Bahmanpour K. Development of a Rheumatoid Arthritis Education

Program using the PRECEDE_PROCEED Model. Health Promotion Perspectives. 20 Dec 2011;**1**(2):118-129. DOI: 10.5681/HPP.2011.013. PMID: 24688908; PMCID: PMC3963622

[54] Dures E et al. A survey of psychological support provision for people with inflammatory arthritis in secondary care in England. Musculoskeletal Care. 2014;**12**(3):173-181. DOI: 10.1002/msc.1071

[55] Aghakhani N, Nia HS, Ranjbar H, Rahbar N, Beheshti Z. Nurses' attitude to patient education barriers in educational hospitals of Urmia University of Medical Sciences. Iranian Journal of Nursing and Midwifery Research. 2012;**17**(1):12-15

[56] Wu Z et al. The effects of patient education on psychological status and clinical outcomes in rheumatoid arthritis: A systematic review and meta-analysis. Frontiers in Psychiatry. 2022;**13**:848427. DOI: 10.3389/fpsyt.2022.848427

[57] Jones B et al. Disseminating and assessing implementation of the EULAR recommendations for patient education in inflammatory arthritis: A mixed-methods study with patients' perspectives. RMD Open. 2022;**8**(1):e002256. DOI: 10.1136/rmdopen-2022-002256

[58] Health Care Education Association. Patient education practice guidelines for health care professionals. 2021. Available from: https://www.hcea-info.org/assets/hcea%20guidelines_BW%201-25-2021.pdf

[59] Grønning K, Rannestad T, Skomsvoll JF, Rygg LØ, Steinsbekk A. Long-term effects of a nurse-led group and individual patient education programme for patients with chronic inflammatory polyarthritis – a randomised controlled trial. Journal of Clinical Nursing. 2014;**23**(7-8):1005-1017. DOI: 10.1111/jocn.12353

Chapter 12

Nursing Process for an Orthopedic Patient

Princess Busisiwe Siphiwe Mbatha

Abstract

A nursing care plan is a tool that the nursing team uses to communicate with each other regarding the treatment of the patient. It also promotes continuity of care as one of the patient's rights in the Patient Rights Charter in South Africa. The purpose of this chapter is to look at the needs of an orthopedic patient and to create a nursing care plan. Once the problems of the patient have been identified, the expected outcome will be formulated and nursing interventions will be implemented. This will provide a framework on how the treatment plan of the patient should be structured. There are many academic books with standardized nursing care plans for surgical nursing. In orthopedic wards, even if two patients are admitted for the same orthopedic condition, their nursing care plan will not be the same. Their treatment should be individualized. There are many factors that will affect the nursing care plan of an individual patient such as age, if the patient has any comorbidities and the patient's attitude towards rehabilitation and treatment.

Keywords: nursing care plan, fractures, orthopedics, SMART mnemonic, outcomes, nursing intervention

1. Introduction

Nursing care plan is a written document that has information regarding the condition of the patient, nursing diagnoses, expected outcomes, as well as the nursing interventions [1–3]. There are five steps of nursing process that need to be followed before a nursing care plan is formulated, namely assessment, nursing diagnosis, outcomes, implementation and evaluation [4]. After emergency management and treatment of an orthopedic patient with fractures, the nursing management and treatment of the patient will be based on the individual problem or injury that is presented by the patient. As the Orthopedics Unit is a specialty unit, an individualized nursing care should be formulated instead of a standardized nursing care.

2. Assessment

Assessment is the first step in delivering nursing care. A nurse must collect and analyze data in a systematic manner. A health assessment is a term used to describe a process whereby a nurse identifies the needs of a patient by doing a comprehensive physical examination of the patient and obtaining the health history of the patient [5].

A brief history is essential in order to assess the mechanism of injury and to raise suspicion of other, less apparent injuries such as a pathological fracture where the skeletal system is weakened by a disease. If the violence has been minimal and hardly sufficient to have caused a fracture, then this may arouse a suspicion that the fractured bone has been weakened by a disease or previous damage, for example, a pathological fracture. The mechanism of injury and the mode of application are frequently important to determine additional injury. Taking the occupation of the patient into account is frequently helpful in planning rehabilitation and recuperative efforts once the fracture has been managed. Activity level before injury directs the type of treatment given for a specific injury. Deformity and swelling must be carefully evaluated physically so that complications can be avoided. It is vitally important that the neurovascular status of the extremity be carefully evaluated to avoid long-term or permanent damage to limbs. The neurovascular integrity of the extremity, or lack thereof; should be documented. Integrity of the skin should be monitored as well. Care must be taken to ensure that there is no breakdown of the skin in the area of the fracture site.

There are four types of health assessments that are done in the health care setting, which are further discussed in the following sections:

2.1 Initial assessment or head-to-toe assessment

Initial assessment is done by a nurse who is admitting the patient. This nurse must obtain biographical information about the patient and also details of past medical history, surgical history as well as social history [6]. The reason for this is to make a correct diagnosis when diagnosing an orthopedic patient because most orthopedics conditions are specific to certain demographics; for example, rickets (vitamin D deficiency), sickle cell disease, and slipped capital femoral epiphysis are all pediatric conditions which means they are age specific and multiple myeloma affects people who are much older. Race and ethnicity also play a role in certain musculoskeletal conditions. Asian women, as well as women who are menopausing, are more likely to be diagnosed with osteoporosis. Finding out whether a patient smokes or not will affect the patient's diagnosis because smoking delays fracture healing [6] and affects the patient's response to analgesics.

2.2 Focused assessment

Focused assessment is a close examination of a disease. In nursing, the focused assessment is involved in relieving pain and stabilizing the condition of the patient, especially when the medical diagnosis is fully understood. Focused assessment also helps the nurse to identify a problem in a patient in order to formulate a specific plan related to the main problem that she is focusing on. A patient who is diagnosed with a tibia fracture might complain of shortness of breath and chest pains. The nurse will then focus on monitoring the vital signs of the patient, checking neurovascular compromise, and monitoring that patient for fat embolism syndrome [6].

DOI: http://dx.doi.org/10.5772/intechopen.1005323

2.3 Emergency assessment

During admission, a patient may have low hemoglobin, that is a hemoglobin of less than 8 g/dl. That patient may need a blood transfusion that will be prescribed by an orthopedic surgeon and administered by a professional nurse. This forms part of emergency assessment. Also, a patient with low peripheral saturation, which is SATS of below 94% on room air or an unresponsive orthopedic patient, will also need emergency attention. Patients might need emergency resuscitation for a number of reasons. It might be pulmonary embolus or fat embolus (life-threatening conditions). Different health care workers, for example, orthopedic surgeons, nephrologists, cardiologists and nurse professionals, will perform different emergency assessments until the patient is stabilized [6].

2.4 On-going or time-lapsed assessment

Nurses take care of the patients for a longer period based on the initial diagnosis or problem that patients presented with on admission. In this assessment, the patient is constantly evaluated monitoring his or her progress and response to treatment. Patient progress or lack thereof will be noted on the patient's file through a document called nursing progress chart. A care plan will be formulated using the needs and problems that the patient will be presenting during their hospital stay. This can last for months.

The nurse personnel will need to continuously gather and interpret information from the patient in order to meet the needs of the patient and act accordingly [6].

3. Diagnosis

The nurse will use her knowledge, skills and experience to diagnose a patient [1]. The diagnoses may also reflect the causes of the illness that the patient would be presenting with at an orthopedic ward. A patient, for example; might complain of falling and sustaining a fracture of a neck or femur. If the patient has a history of prostate cancer, the nurse will make an initial diagnosis of a pathological fracture (when a bone has been weakened by a disease), and the plan of treatment will differ from someone presenting with a fracture after falling without any prior medical history.

4. Planning

Planning is a process whereby the goals and outcomes are formulated to impact patient care. These goals should bring a positive outcome in the life and well-being of the patient. A care plan should be unique to an individual patient. No two care plans should look the same even if the patients present with a similar condition.

Outcome statements should contain five components that are easily remembered using the SMART mnemonic (**Table 1**) [7].

5. Implementation

Implementation means actually doing what, as a nurse, you have outlined and set out to do in your nursing care plan [8]. This is a nursing intervention stage. This is

Specific	Outcome statement should state precisely what it is to be accomplished. They must not be ambiguous.
Measurable/ meaningful	Measurable outcomes have numeric parameters for judging whether the outcome was met, for example, administer, identify, verbalize and have absence of.
Attainable/action-oriented	Outcome statement should be written so that there is a clear action to be taken by the patient. They must also be possible to achieve.
Results-oriented/ realistic	Realistic outcomes consider the patient's physical and mental condition, their cultural and spiritual values, beliefs and preferences. They should be within reach. They should be achievable with available resources for the patient, nursing staff and the health care setting.
Timely	Outcomes statements should include the time frame for evaluation, for example, within 24 hours, by discharge, and throughout hospitalization. There should be a starting date and end date for outcomes.

Table 1.
SMART mnemonic.

where a nurse administers analgesics, elevates the affected limb, collaborates with a physical therapist to mobilize the patient from bed to chair, etc.

6. Evaluation

This is the final stage of the nursing process [8]. If a nurse has provided an intervention to the patient, they must come back and evaluate if it did bring a positive outcome to the patient. For example, did elevating the affected limb reduce swelling? The nursing care plan may be changed depending on the evaluated condition of the patient.

7. Fractures

7.1 Definition

A fracture is a break in the continuity of the cortical and/or cancellous bone.

7.2 Causes

1. Physical trauma e.g. motor vehicle accident, falling from height

2. Overuse e.g. sport injuries

3. Health condition e.g. metastatic bone disease

7.3 Types of fractures

1. Closed fracture

2. Open fracture

3. Greenstick fracture

4. Hairline fracture

5. Avulsion

6. Compression fracture

Some fractures are classified by their pattern, for example, oblique fracture, transverse fracture and longitudinal fracture, and others are diagnosed by their pattern of not breaking the bone in a straight line such as greenstick fractures, segmental fractures, spiral fractures and comminuted fractures [9].

7.4 Signs and symptoms of fractures

A sign is an objective, observable phenomenon that can be identified by another person, in this case, a nurse. A symptom is an effect noticed and experienced only by the person who has the condition, and this is where, as a nurse, you will get your subjective data. Subjective data is largely reported by the patient.

7.4.1 Altered comfort

Patient will complain of pain on the fractured site. Depending on the time of presentation at the clinic, the level of pain will range from moderate to severe. The patients' response to pain is not the same. There are many factors that affect the patient's response to pain such as language barrier and analgesic that a patient has taken, for example, Grand Pa headache powder (which is not recommended by any South African government hospital due to its side effects on the gastrointestinal tract), cultural belief or anxiety and expectations of patient regarding pain.

7.4.2 Inability to use the limb

Postinjury, the patient may or may not be able to move the limb or put weight on the limb.

7.4.3 Diminished sensation

Numbness or tingling sensation can be experienced by the patient in the affected area. This could be due to a nerve injury.

7.4.4 Altered normal limb alignment

Postinjury, the bone may position incorrectly, causing poor alignment. Bones may be angulated (bent), rotated (twisted), translated or displaced, which may be described as a position shift or limb length discrepancy (LLD or difference in length of the bone).

7.4.5 Edema

A fracture will cause swelling. There is an increased flow of blood to a fractured area, which causes more fluid to pass through the affected area. The soft tissues will subsequently be inflamed.

7.4.6 Increased warmth

Not all fractures will lead to infection, but if increased warmth is noted on the affected limb, this may be a sign of infection, especially on compound fractures.

7.4.7 Crepitus

This is a grating sound that can occur when two bone ends or fragments move or rub against each other.

7.4.8 Ecchymosis

Bruising will be caused by leaking blood vessels underneath the skin of the affected limb. The color may be brown, black or blue [9].

8. Complications of fractures

1. Fat embolism
2. Vascular injuries
3. Nerve damage
4. Pulmonary embolism
5. Thromboembolism
6. Compartment syndrome
7. Infection
8. Shock
9. Reaction to internal fixation devices
10. Limb length discrepancy
11. Osteonecrosis
12. Reflex sympathetic dystrophy
13. Non-union, mal-union and delayed union
14. Amputation [9].

9. Nursing priorities for patients with fractures

1. Patient should be pain-free.

2. Fracture should be immobilized with a splint or traction.

3. Prevent and control infection in case of an open fracture.

4. Provision of adequate nutrition especially high protein diet for wound and bone healing.

5. Allay fear and anxiety.

6. Give health education on exercising and prevention of falls and refracture.

10. General principles of nursing care

1. Body parts must be in alignment.

2. Prevent foot drop.

3. Logrolling body is moved as one unit using two or more individuals, aligning with pillows, blankets, etc.

4. Circulatory/neurovascular checks "The 6P's."

    - Pulselessness

    - Pallor

    - Pain

    - Paresthesia

    - Paralysis

    - Poikilothermia

11. Discharge goals

1. Patient should be able to administer medication, that is, analgesics as well as anticoagulants, on their own

2. Patient should be able to perform activities of daily living

3. Patient should be able to take the prescribed diet

4. Patient should be able to come for wound review and/or follow-up X-rays

12. Nursing diagnosis

The nursing diagnoses should include pain management, risk of infection and mobility problems. These nursing diagnoses provide a guide for developing and implementing individual nursing interventions that aim to optim ize patient care (**Table 2**).

12.1 Acute pain

Acute pain related to:
- Trauma
- Muscle spasms
- Movement of bone fragments
- Soft tissue damage
- Inflammation and swelling

As evidenced by:
- Guarding behavior
- Verbalization or reports of pain
- Antalgic positioning to avoid pain
- Facial grimacing
- Restlessness

Table 2.
Common nursing diagnoses associated with fractures.

12.2 Impaired physical mobility

Impaired physical mobility can be temporary (fractured tibia/fibula), permanent (spinal cord injury) or worsening (multiple myeloma) (**Table 3**).

Impaired physical mobility may be caused by, that is, "related to":
- Loss of integrity of the bone
- Neuromuscular impairment
- Pain
- Reluctance to initiate movement
- Prescribed restrictions or immobilizers etc.

Looking back at the signs and symptoms of fractures is where a nurse will obtain the "as evidenced by":
- Verbalization of pain and discomfort with mobilizing
- Refusal to mobilize
- Limited range of motion
- Uncoordinated movements
- Contractures of limbs

Table 3.
Common nursing diagnoses associated with fractures.

13. Other common nursing diagnoses for fractures

1. Anxiety
2. Impaired skin integrity
3. Risk for infection
4. Risk for compartment syndrome

5. Risk for hypovolemic shock/risk for deficient fluid volume
6. Self-care deficit
7. Ineffective coping
8. Ineffective peripheral tissue perfusion
9. Risk for injury
10. Risk for additional trauma
11. Risk for disuse syndrome
12. Knowledge deficit

14. Desired/expected outcomes

1. Expected outcomes for acute pain in a patient with a fracture
2. The patient will show an increased comfort level
3. The patient will verbalize non-pharmacological strategies to relieve pain
4. Patient will reach a tolerable pain level maximum 2 on a scale of 1–10 within 48 hours after receiving pain medication
5. Patient will verbalize relief of pain
6. Patient will display a relaxed manner, able to participate in activities and sleep and rest appropriately

15. Nursing interventions

15.1 Nursing intervention categories

15.1.1 Independent

These are nursing tasks that requires only one nurse who independently provides the treatment intervention without assistance from other staff members. An example is of this is a nurse administering medication to a patient [10].

15.1.2 Dependent

These are nursing tasks that require a direct order or permission from a doctor such as prescribing medication, Plaster of Paris, and urinary catheter as well as providing negative pressure wound therapy [10].

15.1.3 Interdependent or collaborative

These tasks require the medical team to care for a patient and depend on orders from physicians and Orthopedics trained nursing practitioners. For example, in a patient with a neck or femur fracture whereby a doctor will prescribe medication, the nurse will administer it and apply skin weight traction, and a physical therapist helps with rehabilitation of the patient [10].

15.2 Types of nursing interventions

15.2.1 Health promotion

Nurses can provide health education to quit smoking as it delays fracture healing and to eat a healthy diet and exercise healing to promote wound healing. Patient can also be advised to reduce alcohol intake and to avoid mixing prescribed medication together with traditional medicine from *inyanga* or *isangoma* [10].

15.2.2 Disease prevention

Disease prevention aims at reducing the risk of developing specific illnesses and diseases. If you work on a computer, take breaks to avoid conditions like carpal tunnel syndrome [10].

15.2.3 Treatment

Treatment aims to manage and treat existing health problems. The most common treatment nurses provide is pain control. Nurses administer analgesics and anti-hypertensives, reposition patients four hourly, provide ice packs for edematous limbs and joints, and elevate injured extremities [10].

15.2.4 Rehabilitation

Assisting the patient to mobilize from bed to chair after surgery such as ORIF (open reduction and internal fixation) of the tibia or fibula is part of rehabilitation for the patient (**Table 4**) [10].

16. Rationale

In most cases, nurses are not required to write rationale in the nursing care plan. The rationales for interventions mentioned above have been highlighted in italics. Rationale is statement that explains why a certain intervention was done. A nurse must use her critical thinking skills to explain the rationale; for example, elevate the lower limb of a patient with a cushion to reduce swelling. Rationales are specific to the individual patients. It happens that sometimes a patient will not exhibit any swelling before an operation, but the swelling will be noticed operatively, so the nursing care plan of that patient will change, and the reason for elevation will be stated under rationale. Also, repositioning the patient four hours a day can be used as an example. The rationale would be to promote circulation, prevent pressure injuries, which are one of the complications of fractures, and to prevent respiratory problems such as pneumonia (**Table 5**).

Acute pain • Smile at the patient *to make the environment as comfortable as possible.* • Explain procedure to the patient to allay any anxiety. • Provide calm, quiet environment. *Promotes effects of analgesics and to decrease any form of stimuli.* • Monitor pain intensity every 2 hours. Utilize appropriate method of assessment (e.g., numeric pain scales (0–10), behavior assessment). *Pain is subjective in nature, and only the patient can fully describe it.* • Evaluate and document reports of pain or discomfort, noting location and characteristics, including intensity. • Consider non-pharmacological treatment (RICE therapy), for example, ice packs *to reduce swelling.* • Produce immobilization of affected limb by bedrest, back slab, POP and traction. *This relieves pain and prevents further tissue injury.* • Elevate affected extremity above heart level. *This promotes venous return, decreases swelling and reduces pain.* • Avoid the use of plastic linen savers and pillows under the limb in cast. *It increases pain by enhancing heat in the drying cement.* • Elevate bed linen and keep it away from patient's toes using a bed cradle. *This helps with keeping the limb warm without causing more pain to the patient with the heaviness of bed linen.* • Reposition the limb. Maintain alignment with pillows or a folded blanket. *This helps stimulate blood circulation.* • Administer pain medication as prescribed. *Response to pain and pain medication differs from patient to patient.* • Monitor vital signs at least every 4 hours while awake. *Detects early changes.*
Impaired physical mobility • Assess degree of immobility produced by the fracture. *Patient may be restricted by self-perception disproportionate to the physical limitations.* • Educate the patient regarding proper use of assistive devices. *Maintains muscle tone and prevents complications of immobility.* • Provide progressive mobilization as tolerated. Schedule increased mobilization on a daily basis. Medicate for pain as needed, especially before activity. *Pain interferes with ability to ambulate by inhibiting muscle movement.* • Perform ROM exercises (passive, active, and functional) of affected and unaffected extremities every 2 hours. *Increases circulation, maintains muscle tone and prevents joint contractures.* • Implement measures to prevent falls, such as keeping bed in low position, wearing appropriately fitting shoes or non-skid slippers. *Basic safety measures.* • A patient on traction to stabilize the fracture should be placed on a supine position. *It reduces the risk of flexion contracture on the hip.* • Maintain adequate nutrition with the assistance of a dietician. *Provides nutrients for energy and prevents protein loss due to immobility.* • Observe for complications of immobility (e.g., constipation, muscle atrophy, pressure injuries and orthostatic hypotension). *Allows early detection and prevention of complications.* • Assist and encourage the patient with self-care activities such as bathing. *Improves muscle strength and circulation.* • Encourage diversional and recreational activities such as reading newspapers, watching TV, personal possessions (smartphones with social media such as Facebook, X, Instagram and TikTok), and family visits. *Provides opportunity to focus patient's attention elsewhere and enhance patient's sense of self control.* • Include the patient and family or significant other in carrying out plan of care. *Allows time for practice under supervision. Increases likelihood of effective management of therapeutic regimen.* • Assist with mobility with crutches, wheelchair, walking frame and initiate physical therapy and/or occupational therapy as soon as possible. *Reduces complications of bedrest.*

Table 4.
Nursing interventions [11].

17. Health education

Preserving skeletal health may involve:
Avoiding falls

Evaluation
Acute pain • Patient verbalizes relief of pain. • Patient follows prescribed pharmacological regimen. • Patient displays relaxed manner, is able to participate in activities and sleeps appropriately. • Demonstrates use of relaxation exercises. Impaired physical mobility • Patient's mobility will be improved • Pain and discomfort decreased • Independence restored • Physical mobility will be stabilized • Patient satisfaction

Table 5.
Evaluation of acute pain and impaired physical mobility.

Taking calcium supplements
Getting enough vitamin D
Avoiding carbonated beverages (phosphates deplete bone)
Getting regular exercise.

18. Examples of nursing care plan in an orthopedics setting

18.1 Clinical nursing document progress report-nursing care plan: A patient with multiple myeloma

No*	Need list		
1	Comfort	5	
2	Mobility	6	
3		7	
4		8	

When admitting a patient ensure the Nursing Care Plan is done … … The needs and/or the problems that are identified above are clearly described in the diagnosis and prioritized Clear expected outcomes are written Nursing interventions are clear The patient's reactions to interventions are evaluated and documented on the CMJAH1114/6	Use the same need names/numbers initially allocated on the needs list Delete solved needs by crossing out their numbers alongside Do not re-use deleted numbers, unless a solved need is re-activated Nursing Care Plan should be done on admission, when patients condition changes and as the needs arise.

Nursing diagnosis	Expected outcome	Nursing intervention
Self-care deficit evidenced by patient being fully dependent on nursing staff	Patient will improve participation in activities of daily living by the end of this week	Encourage patient to perform as much self-care as condition allows Assist patient with tasks that a patient cannot perform Assist patient in becoming independent and functioning

No*	Need list		
	Impaired physical mobility related to pain evidenced by patient being unable to walk unaided	Patient will increase physical mobility and demonstrate safe use of assistive devices a day after starting physical therapy	Mobilize the joint above and joint below the wound gently Promote daily physical therapy program by collaborating with physical therapist Do passive exercises
	Risk for infection related to impaired immune system functioning	Patient will obtain negative results from cultured specimen Patient will exhibit absence of fever and chills throughout admission	Implement measures to reduce the risk of infection such as maintaining hand-washing techniques when handling the patient Adhere to universal precautions Maintain adequate fluid intake Avoid invasive procedures such as catheterization
	Risk for bleeding related to excessive losses through normal routes	Patient will take measures to prevent bleeding and will recognize signs of bleeding Patient will not experience bleeding as evidenced by normal pressure, normal hemoglobin levels and desired coagulation profile during hospitalization	Monitor patient's vital signs Look for signs of orthostatic hypotension Check stools and urine for occult blood Assess skin and mucous membrane for signs of petechiae, bruising hematoma formation or oozing of blood Monitor hematocrit and hemoglobin Educate patient about precautionary measures to prevent tissue trauma or disruption of normal clotting mechanisms Use soft brittle toothbrush and non-abrasive toothpaste; avoid use of toothpicks and dental floss Avoid rectal suppositories, rectal thermometers, enemas and tampons Limit straining with bowel movements, forceful nose-blowing Monitor for skin necrosis
DATE: 2023/03/19 **TIME:** 13 h 05 **NAME:** P.B.S Mbatha **SIGNATURE: RANK:** Professional Nurse Specialty(Orthopaedics)			

Name of Patient: .... **Hospital/Reg no:** ....
Ward: .... **Doctor:** .... **Page:** 01
Diagnosis: Multiple Myeloma

18.2 Clinical nursing document progress report-nursing care plan: A patient with right subtrochanteric fracture and right fibula fracture

No*	Need list		
1	Comfort	5	
2	Mobility	6	
3		7	
4		8	

When admitting a patient ensure the nursing care plan is done … … The needs and/or the problems that are identified above are clearly described in the diagnosis and prioritized Clear expected outcomes are written Nursing interventions are clear The patient's reactions to interventions are evaluated and documented on the CMJAH1114/6		Use the same need names/numbers initially allocated on the needs list Delete solved needs by crossing out their numbers alongside Do not re-use deleted numbers, unless a solved need is re-activated Nursing Care Plan should be done on admission, when patients condition changes and as the needs arise.
Nursing diagnosis	Expected outcome	Nursing intervention
Risk for infection evidenced by elevated temperature	Patient will show absence of infection during admission Patient will report absence of drainage from the wound pre- and post-operatively Patient will report normal temperature and exhibit no swelling during admission	Use strict aseptic technique when changing the dressings Provide thorough skin care Administer antipyretic as prescribed by collaborating with Medical team Monitor patient's response to antipyretic
Altered comfort related to inflammation and swelling evidenced by blisters on the fracture site	Reports no discomfort with movement 30 minutes post administration of analgesic Patient will verbalize his pain as less than 7/10 during therapy by the end of this week	Elevate the affected area to reduce swelling and discomfort Collaborate with medical team to administer analgesic Monitor neurovascular status four hourly

DATE: 2024/01/02 **TIME:** 13 h 05 **NAME:** P.B.S Mbatha **SIGNATURE: RANK:** Professional Nurse Specialty-Orthopedics

Name of Patient: .... **Hospital/Reg no:** ....
Ward: .... **Doctor:** .... **Page:** 01
Diagnosis: Right subtrochanteric fracture and right fibula fracture

18.3 Clinical nursing document progress report-nursing care plan: A patient with right neck of fracture and open fracture left tibia postexternal fixation

No*	Need list		
1	Comfort	5	Skin integrity
2	Mobility	6	Rest and Sleep
3	Nutrition	7	Psychosocial needs
4	Elimination	8	Safety

When admitting a patient ensure the nursing care plan is done… … The needs and/or the problems that are identified above are clearly described in the diagnosis and prioritized Clear expected outcomes are written Nursing interventions are clear The patient's reactions to interventions are evaluated and documented on the CMJAH1114/6		Use the same need names/numbers initially allocated on the needs list Delete solved needs by crossing out their numbers alongside Do not re-use deleted numbers, unless a solved need is re-activated Nursing Care Plan should be done on admission, when patients condition changes and as the needs arise.

Nursing diagnosis	Expected outcome	Nursing intervention
Risk for movement of bone fragments and additional trauma related to loss of skeletal integrity	Patient will maintain stabilization and alignment of fractures while on traction	Maintain bedrest or limb rest as indicated. Provide support for joints above and below fracture site, especially when moving and turning Support fracture site with pillows or folded blankets. Maintain neutral position of affected part with sandbags, splints, trochanter roll or footboard Evaluate splinted extremity for edema resolution. Maintain position and integrity of traction Assess integrity of external fixation device Position client so that appropriate pull is maintained on the long axis of the bone Review follow-up or control x-rays. Initiate and maintain bone rehabilitation that is, early ambulation
Acute pain related to muscle spasms evidenced by protective behavior	Patient will verbalize relief of pain 30 minutes postadministration of analgesics Patient will display a relaxed manner, will be able to participate in activities, and sleep and rest appropriately by the end of the week	Maintain immobilization of affected part by means of bedrest, cast, splint and traction. Elevate and support injured extremity. Evaluate and document reports of pain or discomfort, noting location and characteristics, including intensity (scale of 0–10), relieving and aggravating factors Encourage patient to discuss problems related to injury. Explain procedures before beginning them.

No*	Need list		
			Administer medication before care activities. Let the patient know it is important to request medication before pain becomes severe. Perform and supervise passive or active ROM exercises.
	Knowledge deficit related to new diagnosis	The patient will verbalize an understanding of the disease process within a day of receiving Health Education	Identify the patient's best methods for learning. Initiate teaching when patient is most amenable to receiving information Provide relevant information only. Provide an environment conducive to learning. Explain each procedure as it is being done, and give the rationale for procedure and the patient's role. Provide the patient with enough opportunity to ask questions, for example Teach about the importance of taking antibiotics as prescribed Educate about signs and symptoms of neurovascular compromise Educate about principles of infection control and wound care
	Anxiety threat or change in role status and health status	Patient will demonstrate absence of physiological signs and symptoms of anxiety after explanation by nursing personnel	Give the patient an opportunity to verbalize perception of situation that is causing anxiety. Explain all procedures and rationales for the procedure in clear, concise, simple terms.
	Risk for all problems associated with bed rest: pressure ulcers, pneumonia, constipation, urinary stasis, DVT	Patient will not experience any orthopedic complications throughout admission	Do four hourly neurovascular checks Maintain body alignment Instruct patient on what to report, for example, pain that is disproportionate to injury Check weights and pulleys Provide adequate time and privacy during elimination Encourage patient to eat all prescribed diet
DATE: TIME: NAME: P.B.S Mbatha **SIGNATURE:** RANK: Professional Nurse Specialty-Orthopedics			

Name of Patient: Hospital/Reg no: Ward: Doctor: Page: 01

Diagnosis: Right neck of femur fracture and open fracture left tibia postexternal fixation.

18.4 Clinical nursing document progress report-nursing care plan: A patient with a spinal cord injury

No*	Need list		
1	Comfort	5	Elimination
2	Mobility	6	Skin Integrity
3	Hygiene	7	Psychosocial
4	Nutrition	8	Rest

When admitting a patient ensure the nursing care plan is done … … The needs and/or the problems that are identified above are clearly described in the diagnosis and prioritized Clear expected outcomes are written Nursing interventions are clear The patient's reactions to interventions are evaluated and documented on the CMJAH1114/6	Use the same need names/numbers initially allocated on the needs list Delete solved needs by crossing out their numbers alongside Do not re-use deleted numbers, unless a solved need is re-activated Nursing Care Plan should be done on admission, when patients condition changes and as the needs arise.

Nursing diagnosis	Expected outcome	Nursing intervention
Disturbed sensory perception related to psychological stress evidenced by motor incoordination	Patient will recognize sensory impairments and identify behaviors to compensate for deficits by the end of the week	Assess and document sensory function or deficit, progressing from area of deficit to neurologically intact area Protect from bodily harm Assist patient to recognize and compensate for alterations in sensation Explain procedures before and during care, identifying the body part involved Provide tactile stimulation, touching patient in intact sensory areas Position patient to see surroundings and activities Provide uninterrupted sleep and rest periods Note presence of exaggerated emotional responses
Altered comfort related to physical injury evidenced by burning pain below level of injury	Will report relief or control of pain 30 minutes postadministration of analgesics	Assess for presence of pain. Help patient to identify and quantify pain Evaluate increased irritability, muscle tension, restlessness, unexplained vital sign changes Assist in identifying precipitating factors Provide comfort measures, for example, warm or cold packs Encourage use of relaxation techniques Administer medication as indicated by collaborating with a Medical team
Risk for grief related to loss of feelings of inadequacy	Patient will begin to process through recognized stages of grief, focusing on 1 day at a time	Identify signs of grieving Note lack of communication or emotional response, absence of questions Provide simple, accurate information to patient

No*	Need list		
		and identifying ways to appropriately cope with grief	Do not give false reassurance while providing emotional support Encourage expression of feelings Encourage expression of sadness, grief, guilt and fear assist patient in verbalizing feelings about situation, avoiding judgment about what is expressed Note comments indicating that the patient is expecting to walk shortly and is bargaining with God Focus on present needs, for example, ROM, exercises and skin care Identify the use of manipulative behavior and reactions to caregivers Encourage the patient to take control when possible Accept expressions of anger and hopelessness Set limits on unacceptable behavior when necessary, for example, abusive language Note loss of interest in living, sleep disturbance and suicidal thoughts Arrange visit by individual similarly affected as appropriate Consult with or refer to psychiatric/ mental health nurse, social worker, psychologist and psychiatrist
	Ineffective breathing pattern evidenced by use of accessory muscles to breathe	Patient will maintain adequate ventilation and demonstrate appropriate behavior to support respiratory effort Patient will demonstrate an effective breathing pattern as evidenced by normal breath sounds and normal arterial blood gases	Assess respiratory function by asking the patient to do deep breathing exercises Note the presence and absence of spontaneous effort and quality of respirations Auscultate breath sounds Note strength and effectiveness of cough Observe skin color for cyanosis Assess for abdominal distension and muscle spasm Maintain patent airway by keeping the head in neutral position Suction as necessary Administer oxygen therapy Assist with the use of respiratory adjuncts and aggressive chest percussions in collaboration with physiotherapist
	Risk for Impaired Skin Integrity related to altered metabolic state	Patient will participate to level of ability to prevent skin breakdown by the end of this week	Inspect all skin areas, noting capillary blanching and refill, redness, swelling Encourage continuation of regular exercise program Avoid and limit injection of medication below the level of injury Massage and lubricate skin with lotion, for example, Zinc and castor oil ointment Reposition frequently Wash and dry skin, especially in high-moisture areas

No*	Need list		
			Keep linen dry and free of wrinkles and crumbs
	Risk for Autonomic Dysreflexia related to Spinal cord injury at T7 or above	Patient will cooperate with the care plan to prevent development of dysreflexia and will also be able to recognize triggers of dysreflexia by the end of the week	Identify and monitor precipitating risk factors Observe signs and symptoms of syndrome such as changes in vital signs and paroxysmal hypertension, tachycardia and bradycardia Stay with patient during episode Monitor BP frequently Elevate head of the bed Eliminate causative stimulus as such as bladder distention Inform patient of warning signs and how to avoid them Perform ROM (active or passive) every 4 hours Keep the patient warm Monitor intake and output Provide appropriate skin care
	Impaired urinary elimination related to disruption in bladder innervation evidenced by bladder distension, incontinence and overflow	Patient will verbalize understanding of condition and maintain balanced intake and output with clear odor-free urine by the end of today	Assess voiding pattern Compare fluid intake with urine output Palpate for bladder distension and observe for overflow Encourage 2 liters of fluid intake daily Begin bladder retraining as per ward protocol when appropriate Observe for cloudy or bloody urine and foul odor Cleanse perineal area and keep dry Refer for further evaluation of the bladder Keep the bladder deflated by means of indwelling catheter initially. Begin intermittent catheterization program when appropriate Measure residual urine
	Constipation related to disturbance of innervation to bowel and rectum evidenced by loss of ability to evacuate bowel voluntarily	Patient will re-establish satisfactory bowel elimination pattern in 24 hours	Auscultate bowel sounds, noting location and characteristics Observe abdominal distension if bowel sounds are decreased or absent Note reports of nausea, the onset of vomiting Record frequency, characteristics and amount of stool Check for the presence of impaction Establish regular daily bowel program Encourage a well-balanced diet that includes bulk and roughage and increased fluid intake Assist and encourage exercise and activity within individual ability Observe incontinence and help patient relate incontinence change in diet or routine

No*	Need list		
			Restrict intake of caffeine Provide skin care Collaborate with dietician and nutritional team
	Situational low self-esteem related to situational crisis evidenced by fear of rejection and negative feelings about the body	Patient will verbalize acceptance of self in situation	Acknowledge difficulty in determining degree of functional incapacity and a chance of functional improvement Listen to patient's comments and responses to situation Assess dynamics of patient Encourage family to treat patient as normally as possible Provide accurate information Discuss the meaning of loss or change with patient Accept patient, show concern for individual as a person Give positive reinforcements Include patient in care, allow patient to make decisions and participate in self-care activities as possible Be alert to sexually oriented jokes, flirting or aggressive behavior Be aware of own feelings and reaction to patient's sexual anxiety Refer for counseling
	Risk for trauma evidenced by instability of spinal column	Patient will maintain proper alignment of the spine without further damage to spinal cord	Maintain bed rest and immobilization devices such as sandbags, traction, halo, hard and soft cervical collar and braces Check external stabilization device, for example, skeletal traction apparatus Elevate head of the bed as indicated Check weights for ordered traction Reposition at intervals using for turning and support
	Impaired physical mobility related to neuromuscular impairment evidenced by inability to purposefully move	Patient will increase the strength of unaffected body parts by the end of the week	Continually assess motor function by requesting patient to perform certain actions such as shrugging shoulders, spreading fingers, squeezing and releasing examiner's hands Provide means to summon help (Bell system) Perform and assist with full ROM exercises on all extremities and joint, using slow, smooth movements Maintain ankles at 90 degrees with footboard Elevate lower extremities at intervals when in chair Assess for edema of feet and ankles Plan activities to provide uninterrupted rest periods Monitor BP before and after activity Change position slowly Prepare for weight-bearing activities like the use of tilt table for upright position

No*	Need list	
		Encourage use of relaxation techniques Inspect skin daily and provide skin care. Assist and encourage pulmonary hygiene like deep breathing, coughing and suctioning Assess for swelling, redness and muscle tension in the calf Investigate sudden onset of dyspnea and cyanosis and other signs of respiratory distress Collaborate with physiotherapist and occupational therapist Administer muscle relaxants and anti-spasticity agents as indicated.

Name of Patient:.........Hospital/Reg no:.........Ward:....Doctor:................Page: 01
Diagnosis: Spinal Cord Injury

19. Conclusion

All nursing programs teach the basics of nursing care plan. This promotes effective communication within the nursing team and improves patient care. Nursing care plan needs practice. It is not something that one can learn once and be perfect on formulating it. It should be concise but realistic, correlate with the patient's condition, and vary from time to time depending on the condition of the patient. As part of patient's records, continuity of care is maintained with a nursing care plan.

Acknowledgements

The author would like to express her gratitude to all the orthopedic surgeons at the Charlotte Maxeke Johannesburg Academic Hospital for their support to the orthopedics nursing team.

Conflict of interest

The author declares no conflict of interest.

Author details

Princess Busisiwe Siphiwe Mbatha
Charlotte Maxeke Johannesburg Academic Hospital, Johannesburg, South Africa

*Address all correspondence to: mbathaphiwe@gmail.com

References

[1] Nurselabs. Nursing Care Plans [Internet]. 2023. Available from: http://www.nurselabs.com/nursing-care-plans/#google_vignette [Accessed: February 19, 2023]

[2] South African Department of Justice. Patient Right Charter [Internet]. 2023. Available from: http://www.justice.gov.za/vc/docs/policy/patient%rights%20charter.pdf [Accessed: November 16, 2023]

[3] Study.com. Nursing Care Plan| Diagnoses, Intervention and Examples [Internet]. 2023. Available from: https://www.study.com/academy/lesson/critical-care-nursing-careplans.html [Accessed: November 23, 2023]

[4] Toney-Butler TJ, Thayer JM. Nursing Process. StatPearls Publishing; 2024. Available from: https://www.ncbi.nlm.nih.gov/books/NBK499937/.#_ NBK 499937_ai_

[5] The University of Tulsa. What is health assessment? [Internet]. 2024. Available from: https://www.online.utuls.edu/blog/what-is-a-health-assessment/ [Accessed: January 28, 2024]

[6] indeed. Career development. The 4 Types of Nursing Assessment[Internet]. 2023. Available from: https://www.indeed.com/career-advice/career-ddevelopment/types-of-nursing-assessments [Accessed: November 28, 2023]

[7] University of St. Augustine for Health Sciences. How to write a Care Plan: A Guide for Nurses. [Internet]. 2021. Available from: https://www.usa.edu/blog/how-to-write-a-care-plan/ [Accessed: December 2, 2023]

[8] Toney-Butler TJ, Thayer JM. Nursing Process. StatPearls Publishing. 2023. Available from: https://www.ncbi.nlm.nih.gov/books/NBK591807/ [Accessed: December 2, 2023]

[9] Maher AB, Salmond SW, Pellino T. Orthopaedic Nursing. 3rd ed. Philadelphia: W.B. Saunders Company: W.B; 2002. 940 p. DOI: 0721693024/9780721693026

[10] Walden University. What are nursing interventions? Definition, types, and examples [Internet]. 2023. Available from: https://www.usa.edu/blog/how-to-write-a-care-plan/ [Accessed: December 2, 2023]

[11] Doenges ME. Nursing Care Plans. Guidelines for Individualizing Client Care Across the Life Span. 8th ed. Philadelphia: F.A Davis Company; 2010. 940 p. DOI: 0-8036-2210-4/978036-2010-4

Chapter 13

Competence of Healthcare Employees in Pressure Ulcer Prevention and Care

Melita Peršolja and Rosanda Drufovka

Abstract

A pressure ulcer, from its inception, represents a multifaceted challenge, encompassing health, social, and financial dimensions, thereby deteriorating the patient's overall quality of life. The mitigation of pressure ulcers commences with a methodical evaluation of the dermal condition of individuals deemed at considerable risk. This proactive approach includes vigilant skin care, the utilization of appropriately designed support surfaces, and the regular repositioning of affected patients. This investigation's main aim is to assess the proficiency of healthcare personnel in pressure ulcer prevention and treatment within the inpatient context. This empirical study featured the participation of 115 healthcare practitioners employed at Nova Gorica General Hospital. The research instrument employed in this inquiry was an adapted questionnaire derived from the work of Pieper Zulkowski, which incorporated 83 items encompassing preventive strategies, wound characteristics, and wound stage categorization. The amassed data were subjected to statistical analysis using IBM SPSS version 29. The internal consistency reliability, as measured by Cronbach's alpha, for the comprehensive questionnaire was proven at 0.913. However, it is unmistakably evident that a pressing need for continuous and systematic educational interventions concerning pressure ulcer management remains essential and indispensable for healthcare professionals.

Keywords: decubitus, nursing care, nursing interventions, prevention, pressure ulcers

1. Introduction

Pressure ulcer is a localized injury of the skin or underlying tissue, most commonly occurring over bony prominences, caused by pressure or a combination of pressure and shear forces [1]. From the moment a pressure ulcer develops, it becomes a health, social, and financial problem that diminishes the patient's quality of life. The development of pressure ulcers is influenced by the interaction of numerous risk factors [2]. External factors for the formation of pressure ulcers include unrelieved pressure, shear force, friction, and repeated pressure [3]. Internal factors contributing to pressure ulcer development include malnutrition, immobility, impaired sensation of pressure or pain, urinary and fecal incontinence, consciousness disorders, increased body weight, age, chronic diseases, elevated body temperature, and certain medications [4]. Sites, where pressure ulcers commonly develop, include the hips, sacrum, elbows, ankles, heels, occiput, shoulders, scapulae, fingers, knees, and ears [1]. Pressure ulcers that occur in atypical locations, such as behind the ears, the nose and nostrils, cheeks, forehead, penis, urethral meatus, and lower lip, raise particular concern [5]. The most vulnerable patients for pressure ulcer development are those with limited ability to change positions, spending a significant amount of time in bed or in a chair [6], such as critically ill and injured patients in the intensive care unit, patients with spinal cord injuries, overweight patients, undernourished patients, and patients in the operating room [7].

Preventing pressure ulcers involves skin assessment, nutritional status evaluation, regular repositioning, and the use of preventive cushions. Skin is protected from excretions and excessive moisture, and lotions and skincare creams are used. During pressure ulcer prevention, it is crucial not to massage the skin or rub it in at risk-prone areas [3]. Daily skin inspections are conducted and findings are documented. Care is taken to prevent skin damage from medical devices and equipment such as nasogastric tubes, urinary catheters, oxygen catheters, etc.

The development of a pressure ulcer is a progressive process. If preventive measures to reduce contributing factors are not taken in the presence of a pressure ulcer, it can progress to a more severe stage [8]. Regular assessment of the risk of pressure ulcer development should be carried out as frequently as the patient's condition requires. The Waterlow assessment scale is most commonly used for assessing the risk of pressure ulcer development. Other scales, such as Norton's, Braden's, and others, are also known [9]. Before classifying a pressure ulcer, it is essential to assess the patient and the type of wound. Confirming the presence of pressure and/or shear force as causative factors is crucial in diagnosing pressure ulcers. The nursing staff must have adequate anatomical knowledge to correctly assess the stage of a pressure ulcer as treatment and preventive measures depend on this [10].

Despite efforts, pressure ulcers remain one of the most significant challenges in healthcare. The occurrence of pressure ulcers (the prevalence rate of pressure ulcers in Europe is ranging from 4.6% to 27.2%) represents a deviation that requires serious attention to determine the causes, timing, and key contributing factors to reduce the incidence [11, 12]. A fundamental aspect of providing quality healthcare to prevent pressure ulcer development is the planning and execution of high-quality healthcare. In Slovenia, we follow and adhere to international guidelines for pressure ulcer prevention, harmonized by the European Pressure Ulcer Advisory Panel (EPUAP) and the National Pressure Ulcer Advisory Panel (NPUAP). Healthcare personnel receive basic theoretical knowledge on pressure ulcer prevention during formal education. The continuity of professional education and training must be ensured as it elevates knowledge levels and improves the quality of care [13]. Healthcare staff must possess the necessary skills for accurate wound assessment. To ensure high-quality and effective healthcare for patients with pressure ulcers, continuous education, the study of new guidelines, and collaboration with other healthcare professionals are essential [14] as basic theoretical knowledge on pressure ulcer prevention during formal education alone is insufficient for high-quality patient care [15]. Assessing the knowledge of healthcare staff allows for identifying training needs, priorities, and supports the development of new strategies to enhance the quality of prevention and care for pressure ulcers [16].

2. Methods and materials

This research's purpose was to examine and present the competence of healthcare professionals in pressure ulcer prevention and care for hospitalized patients. The research aims were to determine the extent to which hospital healthcare employees are knowledgeable about the development, classification, other characteristics of pressure ulcers, their knowledge of preventive measures, tools, prevention, and modern pressure ulcer care.

Based on the research aims, the following research questions were formulated:

1. What is the proportion of healthcare personnel who have the requisite qualifications to competently manage pressure ulcers in the context of hospitalized patients?

2. To what degree do the attributes of the respondents correlate with their competency levels?

3. To what extent do healthcare personnel comprehend the attributes of pressure ulcers?

4. To what degree are healthcare employees acquainted with pressure ulcer prevention measures?

5. To what extent are healthcare employees well-versed in the diverse materials and tools for pressure ulcer prevention and care?

6. To what extent are healthcare employees familiar with current approaches to pressure ulcer care?

3. Instrument

Data for the research were obtained using the original PZ-PUKT questionnaire by authors Pieper and Zulkowski [17]. The authors provided us with the questionnaire *via* email. The research instrument was translated from English to Slovene, and for the purpose of verifying comprehensibility, it was distributed among 20 nurses. The results of the pilot study were considered in preparing the final version of the questionnaire, which consists of 83 questions, with 72 of them assessing the knowledge about pressure ulcers.

The research instrument is divided into two parts. The first part comprises demographic data, including gender, age, education, years of experience, specialized knowledge, and education. The second part consists of three sets of questions related to pressure ulcers: the stages and characteristics of pressure ulcer development (21 questions), wound care (20 questions), and pressure ulcer prevention (31 questions). Respondents had three options for each statement: "True," "False," and "I do not know." Completing the questionnaire required 20 to 30 minutes.

We calculated the internal reliability of the questionnaire (Cronbach's alpha coefficient), which was found to be 0.913 (n = 72). Piper and Zulkowski [17] reported a preliminary internal reliability of the original questionnaire as 0.800 (n = 72).

4. Population and sample

The research was conducted from January 2023 to February 2023, on selected departments at the General Hospital Dr. Franca Derganca in Nova Gorica, where healthcare personnel regularly meet patients with pressure ulcers. At the beginning of the research, there were 393 healthcare employees in the hospital, distributed across various departments: internal medicine department 36, orthopedics 10, gynecology 9, rehabilitation and youth disability department 34, surgery 18, intensive care unit for internal medicine, and surgical specialties 36 employees.

The research sample included 120 randomly selected healthcare employees from these departments who received a paper questionnaire during the research period. Of the 120 distributed questionnaires, 115 (95.8%) were returned properly filled out, and 5 were incomplete and had to be discarded.

Most respondents were female (n = 94), while there were 21 males. Nearly half (47.8%) of the respondents had a high school education, while 43.6% had higher professional, college, or university education. A total of 6.1% of respondents held a master's degree in nursing, and 2.6% had vocational education. The average age of the respondents was 39.28 years (min. 21, max. 63, Sd = 10.9). Slightly over half of the respondents had 15 or more years of experience in healthcare.

The majority (93.0%, n = 107) of the respondents did not have specialized knowledge in wound care. A vast majority, 98.3% (n = 113), also did not possess a license for wound care. One-third of the respondents had never attended any wound care education, and more than a third of them had received education more than 4 years ago. Only 14.4% (n = 16) of the respondents had attended wound care education within the past year or less (**Table 1**).

We see also that slightly less than one-third (n = 30) of the respondents have been reading literature on wound care in the past year, while 13.5% (n = 15) have never read anything on this topic. Internet literature on pressure ulcers had been read by 33.3% (n = 37) of the respondents within the past year.

5. Ethical aspect

We obtained permission to conduct the research from the hospital director, the nursing service, and the commission for medical ethics of the hospital under investigation. The healthcare employees voluntarily participated in the research. They were

Time	**Value**	
	N	%
Never	34	30.6
Over 4 years ago	38	34.2
2–3 years ago	15	13.5
More than one, but less than 2 years ago	8	7.2
Within the past year or less	16	14.4

Legend: n = number, % = percent.

Table 1.
Time of attendance at wound care education (n = 111).

informed about the research's purpose and the possibility to decline participation and were ensured about confidentiality and the protection of personal data. The paper questionnaire was enclosed in an envelope, which the participants filled out and sealed. The research was conducted following the Code of Ethics in Healthcare and Nursing in Slovenia (Official Gazette of the Republic of Slovenia, Principle VII, [18]).

6. Data analysis

The questionnaire responses were entered into an electronic database. Microsoft Excel 2019 was used for presenting the results in tables. Statistical analysis and data processing were performed using IBM SPSS 29.0.

In the analysis, responses were scored as either 0 (incorrect answer or "I do not know") or 1 (correct answer). At the end, the sum of points from the entire questionnaire was categorized into five levels: below 59% correct answers as low (insufficient) competence, 60–69% as moderate (acceptable) competence, 70–79% as good competence, 80–89% as particularly good competence, and 90% or more as excellent competence.

Characteristics were presented with frequency (n) and percentages (%), maximum (max), minimum (min), mean (M), and standard deviation (Sd). The normality of variable distributions was assessed using Skewness and Kurtosis tests. The association between variables was examined through linear correlation analysis, and the strength of the relationship was expressed using the Pearson coefficient. Associations, following the guidelines from Field (2009), were described with values: 0.00—no association; 0.01–0.19—negligible association; 0.20–0.39—low/weak association; 0.40–0.69—moderate/moderate association; 0.70–0.89—high/strong association; 0.90–0.99—very high/very strong association; 1.00—perfect (functional) association. An analysis of variance (ANOVA) and t-test for independent samples were also conducted to examine the significance of the results. The significance level was considered 0.05.

7. Results

7.1 Competence in professional handling

Respondents scored a minimum of 16 and a maximum of 72 points on the test, which means that the percentage of correct answers ranged from a minimum of 22% to a maximum of 100%. On average, the respondents scored 45.14 out of 72 (62.6 9%, SD = 9.26). We assessed the knowledge of the respondents on a five-point scale, where a minimum of 60% correct answers (43/72) was needed to pass the test. The average result of the entire group of respondents can be classified as "acceptable."

We found that about 40% of the respondents were unsuccessful (**Table 2**). Nine respondents (7.8%) proved very good or excellent knowledge, while 59 (51.3%) showed acceptable and good knowledge. The skewness coefficient (0.134) and kurtosis (0.447) show a normal distribution of the results.

7.2 Accuracy of responses based on respondent characteristics

The average number of correct answers increases with age and experience. However, the differences based on both parameters are too small to be statistically significant. We found that the differences in the average number of correct answers

Score	Value	
	n	%
Insufficient (0–59%)	47	40.9
Acceptable (60–69%)	31	27.0
Good (70–79%)	28	24.3
Very good (80–89%)	3	2.6
Excellent (90% or more)	6	5.2

Legend: n = number, % = percent.

Table 2.
Results of respondents' points on the test.

		Sample		Test score		
Attribute		n	%	M	F	p
Age, years	20–30	27	24.3	43.96	1.17	0.323
	31–40	33	29.7	43.60		
	41–50	31	27.9	47.51		
	More than 50	20	18.0	45.71		
Years of work	< 1	5	4.3	43.0	1179	0.324
	1–5	27	23.5	43.26		
	5–10	17	14.8	42.76		
	10–15	12	10.4	44.25		
	15–20	18	15.7	45.94		
	20 and more	36	31.3	47.86		
Education	College	59	50.4	44.03		
	University	34	29.6	43.55	3.75	0.013
	High school	16	13.9	51.81		
	Master	7	6.1	47.86		

Legend: n = number, % = percent, F = ANOVA value, p = statistical significance.

Table 3.
Test score related to demographic attributes (n = 115).

are statistically significant based on the level of education. The lowest average score is associated with university education, while the highest is associated with higher professional education (**Table 3** and **Figure 1**).

The differences in test scores between the genders are not significant (t (113) = −0.883; p = 0.379), with men averaging 43.52 (Sd = 8.35) points and women averaging 45.5 (Sd = 9.46) points.

We also investigated the relationship between the number of correct answers and various methods of knowledge acquisition (**Table 4**). The analysis showed a weak but statistically significant correlation between a successful test outcome and various learning methods such as reading professional literature, searching for content online, and education in wound care. However, we did not find significant correlations with obtaining a license and specialized knowledge in the field.

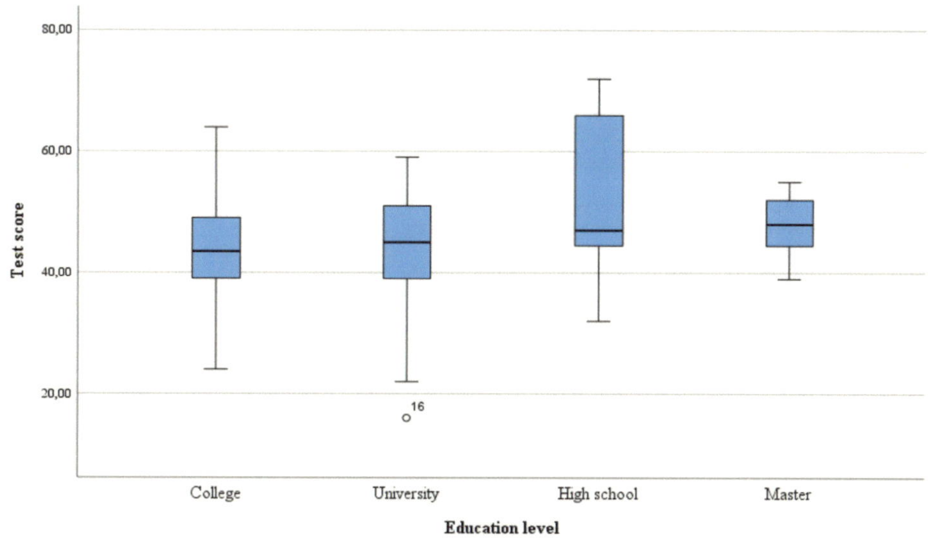

Figure 1.
Test result related to education level (n = 115).

Education methods	Test score	
	r	p
Reading nursing care literature	0.298	0.01
Searching internet	0.268	0.004
Education workshops and seminars	0.265	0.004
License	−0.125	0.182
Specialized knowledge	−0.011	0.909

Legend: r—Pearsons correlation coefficient, p—statistical significance.

Table 4.
Correlation between education methods and test score (n = 115).

7.3 Knowledge of pressure ulcer characteristics

The majority of respondents correctly knew that scars resulting from pressure ulcers are more likely to develop new ulcers than undamaged skin. They also understood that pressure ulcers of stage 3 may appear shallow if they are on the ear, ankle, or heel. Over half of the respondents were aware that moist necrosis is yellow or creamy devitalized tissue on the wound bed and that stage 1 pressure ulcers are characterized by intact skin with unbleachable redness over a bony prominence. A high proportion of respondents correctly noted that pressure ulcers can develop around the ears in individuals using oxygen. Additionally, most respondents knew that if a wound had necrotic tissue with visible or palpable bone, it would be classified as a stage 4 ulcer. The appearance of a blister on the heel was recognized as a cause for concern, and the majority knew that stage 3 pressure ulcers might appear shallow when found on the ear, ankle, or heel. Most respondents were also aware that deep tissue injury can progress to another stage of ulcer.

Statement	Answer n (%)		
	Do not know	Wrong	Correct
Wet necrosis is devitalized tissue, yellow or creamy in color, on the wound bed. (P)	7 (6.1)	32 (27.8)	76 (66.1)
A stage 3 pressure ulcer is an injury to the skin that involves the epidermis and/or dermis. (N)	12 (10.4)	58 (50.4)	45 (39.1)
A scab is a healthy tissue. (N)	11 (9.6)	39 (33.6)	65 (56.6)
A pressure ulcer of an undetermined stage, once necrotic tissue is removed, is classified as a stage 2 pressure ulcer. (N)	43 (37.4)	44 (37.4)	45 (37.4)
Healing in chronic wounds is often slowed in the proliferative phase of healing. (N)	23 (23,0)	70 (60.9)	22 (19.1)
To heal a heel wound, a dry, adherent crust should be removed. (N)	12 (10.4)	38 (33.0)	65 (56.5)
In large and deep pressure ulcers, the number of dressings used should be counted and documented so that all dressings are removed during the next change. (P)	10 (8.7)	18 (15.7)	87 (75.7)
A stage 1 pressure ulcer is intact skin with non-blanchable redness over a bony prominence. (P)	11 (9.6)	26 (22.6)	78 (67.8)
When the wound bed is entirely covered with wet necrosis, the ulcer's stage cannot be determined. (P)	30 (26.1)	57 (49.6)	28 (24.3)
A dressing should keep the wound bed moist and the surrounding area dry. (P)	15 (13.0)	9 (7.8)	91 (79.1)
Hydrocolloid and film dressings should be removed quickly to reduce pain. (N)	11 (9.6)	13 (11.3)	91 (56.5)
Skin tears are classified as stage 2 pressure ulcers. (N)	35 (30.6)	26 (22.6)	54 (47.0)
Stage 3 pressure ulcers may appear shallow when located on the ear, ankle, or heel. (P)	16 (13.9)	13 (11.3)	86 (74.8)
Hydrocolloid dressings should be used on infected stage 2 pressure ulcers. (N)	37 (32.2)	34 (29.6)	44 (38.3)
Pressure ulcers should not be cleaned with drinking water. (N)	11 (9.6)	51 (44.3)	53 (46.1)
Alginates can be used for stage 3 and 4 pressure ulcers with moderate exudate. (P)	28 (24.3)	7 (6.1)	80 (69.6)
Film dressings absorb a significant amount of exudate. (N)	14 (12.2)	36 (31.3)	65 (56.5)
Skin protection cream should be applied around the wound to protect the surrounding tissue from moisture. (P)	10 (8.7)	14 (31.3)	91 (56.5)
Non-blanchable redness anywhere on the body is a stage 1 pressure ulcer. (N)	9 (7.80)	66 (57.4)	40 (34.8)
A stage 2 pressure ulcer is a complete loss of skin thickness. (N)	27 (23.5)	33 (28.7)	55 (47.8)
A stage 2 pressure ulcer can have wet necrosis at the base. (N)	22 (19.1)	58 (50.4)	35 (30.40)
If necrotic tissue is present on the wound, and bone is visible or directly palpable, we classify the ulcer as stage 4. (P)	11 (9.6)	6 (5.2)	98 (85.2)
A pressure ulcer of an undetermined stage, once necrotic tissue is removed, is classified as a stage 2 pressure ulcer. (N)	43 (37.4)	28 (24.3)	44 (28.3)
Blanching refers to the whiteness that occurs when pressure is applied to a reddened area. (P)	26 (22.6)	16 (13.9)	73 (63.5)

Statement	Answer n (%)		
	Do not know	Wrong	Correct
A blister on the heel is not a cause for concern. (N)	5 (4.3)	18 (15.7)	92 (80.0)
Early changes related to pressure ulcer development are often overlooked in individuals with dark skin. (P)	33 (28.7)	12 (10.4)	70 (60.9)
In a stage 3 pressure ulcer, bones, tendons, or muscles may be exposed. (N)	13 (11.3)	50 (43.5)	52 (45.2)
The difference between moisture-related skin damage and pressure ulcers can be challenging. (P)	31 (27.0)	17 (14.8)	67 (58.3)
To heal a heel wound, dry, adherent crust should be removed. (N)	20 (17.4)	51 (44.3)	44 (38.3)
A pressure ulcer on mucous membranes due to medical equipment use is stage 3. (N)	46 (40.0)	30 (26.1)	39 (33.9)
Pressure ulcers can develop around the ears in individuals using a nasal cannula for oxygen. (P)	1 (0.9)	11 (9.6)	103 (89.6)
A stage 1 pressure ulcer is intact skin with non-blanchable redness over a bony prominence. (N)	11 (9.6)	26 (22.6)	78 (67.8)
When the wound bed is entirely covered with wet necrosis, its stage cannot be determined. (P)	30 (26.1)	57 (49.6)	28 (24.3)
Stage 3 pressure ulcers may appear shallow when located on the ear, ankle, or heel. (P)	16 (13.9)	13 (11.3)	86 (74.8)
Pressure ulcers should not be cleaned with drinking water. (N)	11 (9.6)	51 (44.3)	53 (46.1)
Alginates can be used for stage 3 and 4 pressure ulcers with moderate exudate. (P)	28 (24.3)	7 (6.1)	80 (69.6)
Deep tissue injury will not progress to another stage of pressure ulcer. (P)	18 (15.7)	17 (14.8)	80 (69.6)
Stage 4 pressure ulcers always lead to tissue breakdown beneath the skin. (N)	13 (11.1)	73 (67.8)	24 (20.9)

Legend: n = number, % = percent, P = positive, the statement is correct, N = negative, the statement is wrong.

Table 5.
Knowledge of pressure ulcers characteristics (n = 115).

However, there were gaps in knowledge regarding the stages of pressure ulcer formation. Only one-third believed that an unstageable pressure ulcer, after necrotic tissue removal, should be classified as a stage 2 pressure ulcer. A similar percentage correctly answered that when the wound bed is entirely covered with moist necrosis, the stage cannot be determined. More than half did not know that skin tears are classified as stage 2 pressure ulcers, nor did they realize that stage 3 pressure ulcers involve damage to the epidermis and/or dermis (**Table 3**). Most respondents were unaware that unbleachable redness occurring anywhere on the body is not a stage 1 pressure ulcer, and the majority did not know that, when a heel wound heals, a dry, adherent scab should not be removed. Most also incorrectly answered that a pressure ulcer on a mucous membrane due to medical equipment is a stage 3 ulcer. Furthermore, most respondents did not know that stage 4 pressure ulcers do not always involve tissue breakdown beneath the skin (**Table 5**).

Statement	Answer n (%)		
	Do not know	Wrong	Correct
Sitting for individuals at risk of pressure ulcers should be brief and on an appropriate chair/wheelchair with a pressure redistribution cushion. (P)	0 (0.0)	9 (7.8)	106 (92.2)
Individuals with pressure ulcers at high risk should be turned on an individualized schedule regardless of their mobility level unless contraindicated. (P)	4 (3.5)	6 (5.2)	105 (93.3)
New pressure ulcers can be expected sooner on the site of a scar resulting from a pressure ulcer than on undamaged skin. (P)	10 (8.7)	9 (7.8)	96 (83.5)
Dragging a patient across a bed increases friction. (P)	0 (0.0)	14 (12.4)	101 (87.7)
Elevated body temperature is a risk factor for pressure ulcers. (P)	4 (3.5)	21 (18.3)	90 (78.3)
Diabetes mellitus does not increase a person's risk of pressure ulcers. (N)	3 (2.6)	20 (17.4)	92 (80.0)
Individuals with pressure ulcers and incontinence should use high-absorbency incontinence products. (P)	8 (7.0)	9 (5.2)	101 (87.8)
Anti-decubitus cushions regulate tissue load and skin microclimate. (P)	2 (1.7)	6 (5.2)	107 (93.0)
Individuals at high risk of pressure ulcers should typically supplement their regular diet with nutritional supplements. (P)	16 (13.9)	12 (10.4)	87 (75.7)
When the heel is elevated, the leg's weight should be evenly distributed longitudinally to prevent pressure ulcer formation. (P)	10 (8.7)	10 (8.7)	95 (82.6)
Ring-shaped cushions help prevent pressure ulcers. (N)	11 (9.6)	85 (73.9)	19 (16.5)
New pressure ulcers can be expected sooner on the site of a scar resulting from a pressure ulcer than on undamaged skin. (P)	10 (8.7)	7 (6.1)	98 (85.2)
A nutritional assessment should be performed in individuals at risk of pressure ulcers. (P)	11 (9.6)	10 (8.7)	94 (81.7)
Critically ill patients may require slow, gradual turning due to hemodynamic instability. (P)	17 (14.8)	15 (13.0)	83 (72.2)
In immobile patients whose feet do not reach the floor, a footstool should not be used. (N)	32 (27.8)	15 (13.0)	68 (59.1)
Massaging bony prominences is essential for quality skin care. (N)	12 (10.4)	52 (45.2)	51 (44.3)
Improper positioning in a wheelchair can be a cause of pressure ulcers. (P)	4 (3.5)	7 (6.1)	104 (90.4)
In individuals with incontinence, the skin should be cleaned after elimination and at routine intervals. (P)	3 (2.6)	3 (2.6)	109 (94.8)
Patients with spinal cord injuries need knowledge about pressure ulcer prevention and self-care. (P)	3 (2.6)	2 (1.7)	110 (95.7)
A pressure ulcer on the mucous membrane resulting from medical equipment use is of stage 3. (N)	46 (40.0)	30 (26.1)	39 (33.9)
Immobile individuals who can be taught should shift their weight while sitting in a chair every 30 minutes. (P)	11 (9.6)	79 (68.7)	25 (21.7)
The selection of an anti-decubitus cushion considers the risk level for pressure ulcer development in a specific person. (N)	5 (4.3)	92 (80.0)	18 (15.7)

Statement	Answer n (%)		
	Do not know	Wrong	Correct
A patient using an anti-decubitus cushion is not at risk for shear force injuries. (N)	3 (2.6)	18 (15.7)	94 (81.7)
Patients with spinal cord injuries do not need an assessment of their sitting ability. (N)	15 (13.0)	19 (16.5)	81 (70.4)
To prevent pressure ulcers, the bed's headrest should be elevated at an angle greater than 45 degrees. (N)	16 (13.9)	17 (14.8)	82 (71.3)
The urinary catheter tube should be placed under the leg. (N)	9 (7.8)	14 (12.2)	92 (80.0)
Properly sized equipment can help prevent pressure ulcers in bariatric patients. (P)	37 (32.2)	3 (2.6)	75 (65.2)
Nurses should avoid turning the patient onto a reddened area. (P)	6 (5.2)	19 (16.5)	90 (78.3)
A person with a spinal cord injury has a lifelong responsibility for pressure ulcer care. (P)	6 (5.2)	7 (6.1)	102 (88.7)

Legend: n = number, % = percent, P = positive, the statement is correct, N = negative, the statement is wrong.

Table 6.
Knowledge of pressure ulcer prevention measures (n = 115).

7.4 Knowledge of pressure ulcer prevention measures

Table 6 presents responses to the research question regarding knowledge of preventive measures for pressure ulcer prevention.

Most respondents knew that patients with spinal cord injuries need knowledge about pressure ulcer prevention and self-care. They were also aware that individuals with incontinence should clean their skin after each elimination and at routine intervals. Respondents also knew that alternating pressure mattresses regulate both tissue pressure and skin microclimate. Most correct answers were obtained for statements such as the need to use high-absorbency incontinence products for individuals with pressure ulcers and incontinence, the likelihood of new ulcers at the scar site, and the increased risk of pressure ulcers in individuals with diabetes.

The response to the statement that ring cushions help prevent pressure ulcers surprised us. Most respondents incorrectly answered this, and just over half of the respondents provided a wrong answer to the statement that massaging bony prominences is necessary for quality skin care. Similarly, more than half of the respondents gave an incorrect answer to the statement that individuals with limited mobility who are capable should be instructed to shift their weight while sitting every 30 minutes (**Table 6**).

7.5 Knowledge of materials/equipment for care and prevention of pressure ulcers

The vast majority of respondents correctly answered that a nurse must ensure the proper operation of specialized beds and document this. Most also gave the correct response that pain-relieving agents help manage acute pain in pressure ulcers. Respondents were aware that patients using alternating pressure mattresses are less exposed to the risk of shear forces and that the head of the bed should not be elevated more than 30 degrees in pressure ulcer prevention. They also knew that overweight patients require appropriately sized equipment that can help prevent pressure ulcers (**Table 7**).

Statement	Answer n (%)		
	Do not know	Wrong	Correct
Foam dressings can increase pain in the wound. (N)	17 (14.80)	18 (17.40)	80 (67.80)
Hydrogel dressings should not be used on pressure ulcers with granulation tissue. (N)	28 (24.3)	30 (26.1)	57 (49.6)
Individuals with pressure ulcers and incontinence should use high-absorbency incontinence products. (P)	8 (7.0)	6 (5.2)	101 (87.8)
An anti-decubitus cushion regulates tissue load and skin microclimate. (P)	2 (1.7)	6 (5.2)	107 (93.0)
Ring-shaped cushions help prevent pressure ulcers. (N)	11(9.6)	85 (73.9)	19 (16.5)
The nurse's responsibility is to ensure that the specialized bed functions correctly and record its usage. (P)	10 (8.7)	7 (6.1)	98 (85.2)
Critically ill patients may require slow, gradual turning as they are hemodynamically unstable. (P)	17 (14.8)	15 (13.0)	83 (72.2)
In immobile patients whose feet do not reach the floor, a footstool should not be used. (N)	32 (27.8)	15 (13.0)	68 (59.1)
Local opioids can help manage acute pain in pressure ulcers. (P)	18 (15.7)	30 (26.1)	67 (58.3)
Biofilm on a wound is associated with reduced wound exudate. (N)	35 (30.4)	28 (33.0)	42 (36.5)
Massaging bony prominences is essential for quality skin care. (N)	12 (10.4)	52 (45.2)	51 (44.3)
In individuals with incontinence, the skin should be cleaned after elimination and at routine intervals. (P)	3 (2.6)	3 (2.3)	109 (94.8)
Immobile individuals who can be taught should shift their weight while sitting in a chair every 30 minutes. (P)	11 (9.6)	79 (68.7)	25 (21.7)
The selection of an anti-decubitus cushion considers the risk level for pressure ulcer development in a specific person. (N)	5 (4.3)	92 (80.0)	18 (15.7)
A patient using an anti-decubitus cushion is not at risk for shear force injuries. (N)	3 (2.6)	18 (15.7)	94 (81.7)
To prevent pressure ulcers, the bed's headrest must be elevated at an angle greater than 45 degrees. (N)	16 (13.9)	17 (14.8)	82 (71.3)
The urinary catheter tube should be positioned under the leg. (N)	9 (7.8)	14 (12.2)	92 (80.0)
Properly sized equipment can help prevent pressure ulcers in bariatric patients. (P)	37 (32.2)	3 (2.6)	75 (65.2)
Nurses should avoid turning the patient onto a reddened area. (P)	6 (5.2)	19 (16.5)	90 (78.2)
A person with a spinal cord injury has a lifelong risk of pressure ulcers. (P)	6 (5.2)	7 (6.1)	102 (88.7)

Legend: n = number, % = percent, P = positive, the statement is correct, N = negative, the statement is wrong.

Table 7.
Knowledge of materials/equipment for care and prevention of pressure ulcers (n = 115).

The majority of incorrect answers were provided in response to the statement that the level of risk for pressure ulcer development in a specific individual should be considered when using an alternating pressure mattress. Additionally, one-third of the respondents did not know that foam dressings do not increase pain at the wound site. Nearly the same percentage of respondents did not realize that a footrest should not be used for immobile patients whose feet do not reach the ground.

Statement		Answer n (%)	
	Do not know	Wrong	Correct
Alkaline soaps are used for wound cleaning. (P)	28 (24.30)	34 (6.10)	53 (46.10)
Hydrogel dressings should not be used on pressure ulcers with granulation tissue. (N)	28 (26.1)	30 (26.1)	57 (49.6)
Pain intensity should be assessed in individuals with pressure ulcers. (P)	7 (6.1)	10 (8.7)	98 (85.2)
Sterile dressings can be used to protect the skin. (N)	6 (5.2)	47 (40.9)	62 (53.9)
A nutritional assessment should be performed in individuals at risk of pressure ulcers. (P)	11 (9.6)	10 (8.7)	94 (81.7)
Biofilms can develop on any type of wound. (P)	28 (24.3)	28 (24.3)	59 (51.3)
Critically ill patients may require slow, gradual turning due to hemodynamic instability. (P)	17 (14.8)	15 (13.0)	83 (72.2)
Local opioids can help manage acute pain in pressure ulcers. (P)	18 (15.7)	30 (26.1)	67 (58.3)
Biofilm on a wound is associated with reduced wound exudate. (N)	35 (30.4)	28 (33.0)	42 (36.5)
Healing in chronic wounds is often slowed in the proliferative phase of healing. (N)	23 (20.0)	70 (60.9)	22 (19.1)
To heal a heel wound, a dry, adherent crust should be removed. (N)	12 (10.4)	38 (33.0)	65 (56.5)
In large and deep pressure ulcers, the number of dressings used should be counted and documented so that all dressings are removed during the next change. (P)	10 (8.7)	18 (15.7)	87 (75.7)
Dressings should keep the wound bed moist and the surrounding area dry. (P)	15 (13.0)	9 (7.8)	91 (79.1)
Hydrocolloid and film dressings should be removed quickly to reduce pain. (N)	6 (5.2)	19 (16.5)	90 (78.3)
Hydrocolloid dressings should be used on infected stage 2 pressure ulcers. (N)	37 (32.2)	34 (29.6)	44 (38.3)
Pressure ulcers should not be cleaned with drinking water. (N)	11 (9.6)	51 (44.3)	53 (46.1)
Alginates can be used for stage 3 and 4 pressure ulcers with moderate exudate. (P)	28 (24.3)	7 (6.1)	80 (69.9)

Legend: n = number, % = percent, P = positive, the statement is correct, N = negative, the statement is wrong.

Table 8.
Knowledge of modern approaches in pressure ulcer care (n = 115).

7.6 Knowledge of modern approaches in pressure ulcer care

The majority of respondents are aware that pressure ulcers are not sterile wounds. They also know that dressings should keep the wound bed moist while keeping the surrounding area dry. They understand that it is necessary to assess the pain intensity in individuals with pressure ulcers and that a nutritional assessment is needed for such patients. Respondents are also aware that hydrocolloid and film dressings should not be removed quickly, and they know that the goal of palliative care is not wound healing.

However, more than half of the respondents incorrectly believe that wound healing often slows down in the proliferative phase of chronic wounds. They are also unaware that hydrogel dressings can be used for pressure ulcers with granulation tissue, that biofilm on a wound is not associated with reduced wound exudate, and that pressure ulcers can be cleansed with drinking water (**Table 8**).

8. Discussion and conclusions

In this research, we assessed the knowledge of healthcare professionals in hospital nursing through a questionnaire. Overall, the knowledge of the participants regarding the prevention and care of pressure ulcers in hospitalized patients is considered acceptable.

We found that over half of the respondents scored above 60% of correct answers, thus successfully passing the test. Similar results have been reported in other studies employing the same questionnaire. For instance, in the study conducted by Foolbrook et al. [14], a total of 65% correct answers were achieved, while Miller et al. [19] reported a score of 72%. Researchers believe that this percentage represents satisfactory knowledge, considering the comprehensive nature of the questionnaire used.

In our study, we identified a correlation between the length of work experience and the knowledge of healthcare professionals. In contrast, a study conducted in Ireland by Eskes et al. [20] argues that long-term experience alone is not a guarantee of knowledge; rather, it requires support from healthcare policymakers, educational organizations, and employees themselves through knowledge exchange in clinical settings. Like our study, Barakat-Johnson et al. [21], Tirgari et al. [22], and Li et al. [23] suggest that respondents with several years of experience own more knowledge. Furthermore, Parisod et al. [24] report that respondents with extensive work experience not only showed better knowledge but also displayed a more positive attitude toward pressure ulcer prevention and self-evaluation, which can be used to identify individuals in the work environment who require additional training. On the opposite, Miller et al. [19] found that younger nurses with less work experience had more knowledge about wound stages.

In our research, we also saw a correlation between the level of education and the knowledge of the respondents regarding pressure ulcers. Similar conclusions have been drawn by Ebi et al. [25] and De Mayer et al. [26], who linked the level of education with knowledge about pressure ulcers. Ilesanmi et al. [27] in their study in Nigeria and Nuru et al. [28] in Ethiopia found that the knowledge of healthcare staff with higher education, additional training, and more years of work experience is better. Similarly, Fulbrook et al. [14] and Al-Shidi [29] observed that more experienced and highly educated nurses had more knowledge about pressure ulcers than others. But here we find an important finding—the lowest score on the test was from university-educated nurses. It could be the consequence of the educational system as in Slovenia we do not have a university level study for nursing, so the nurses are forced to study other sciences such as economics, management, or others. McCluskey and McCarthy [30] emphasize the importance of informal knowledge sources, which include experiential learning and intuition in pressure ulcer care. Fulbrook et al. [14] found that over half of the respondents had sought education and information about pressure ulcers online. Sengul and Karadag [31] also noted a higher level of knowledge among nurses in Turkey who regularly read literature on pressure ulcer prevention. Similar findings were reported by Gonzaga de Faria et al. [32] and Ferreira et al. [33]. They not only observed the use of informal knowledge sources but also identified a lack of protocol or guideline utilization in the clinical setting. They found that while theoretical knowledge was satisfactory, staff often struggled to apply it in practice.

The data obtained in our research indicates that most respondents lack specialized knowledge in pressure ulcer care. We found that nearly one-third of the respondents had never attended any seminars, and an equal proportion had not read any literature on pressure ulcers in the past year. While Sever and Bregar [34] noted that nursing students are already aware of the need for specialization due to new technologies, new knowledge, an increasing number of patients with chronic illnesses, longer life expectancies, a burdened healthcare system, and growing healthcare service demands, the survey results are somewhat surprising. Continuous knowledge enhancement and the development of evidence-based healthcare are essential for maintaining the quality and advancing the nursing profession. This responsibility applies to every healthcare professional [35, 36].

Based on the findings, we can conclude that healthcare professionals are well-versed in stages 1 and 2 of pressure ulcers but less so in stages 3 and 4. The issue may stem from the confusion between pressure ulcer stages and the assessment of a patient's risk for developing pressure ulcers, which are not equivalent. Also, Gul et al. [37], similar to Cox and Roche [38], discovered a knowledge deficit among nurses, particularly concerning wound classification. Fulbrook et al. [14] similarly found that among Australian nurses, their weakest area of knowledge was in wound descriptions. Ferreira et al. [33] identified knowledge deficiencies in various aspects of wound care, such as the accurate classification of pressure ulcers by stages, unfamiliarity with clinical guidelines and protocols in specific clinical settings, and improper choice of dressings, among other issues. We can infer that healthcare personnel partly use wound classification in their work and attempt to assess the stage of wounds, but struggle with recognizing stages 3 and 4 of pressure ulcers.

With the third research question, we assessed knowledge about pressure ulcer prevention. We were surprised to find that over half of the respondents incorrectly believed that ring-shaped cushions help prevent pressure ulcers and that massaging bony prominences is necessary for quality skin care. In Australia, Fulbrook et al. [14] also obtained a high percentage of incorrect answers related to the use of doughnut-shaped cushions. Lawrence et al. [39] were also surprised by the responses related to prevention. Incorrect answers from respondents were associated with doughnut-shaped cushions, heel protectors, massaging exposed areas, and the timeframe within which erythema is still reversible. Saleh et al. [40] and Gedamu et al. [41] reported unsatisfactory knowledge of pressure ulcer prevention and treatment. Beeckman et al. [42] reported that 70% of nurses mentioned regular skin observation as a common practice in the presence of erythema in patients at high risk of pressure ulcers. Respondents had a good understanding of when to perform anogenital care, which incontinence products to use, the appropriate intervals for repositioning patients, and similar aspects. We presume that in our research, healthcare professionals may not have been informed about the latest guidelines and recommendations.

The analysis of the fifth research question focused on the use of a modern approach in pressure ulcer care. A significant proportion of our respondents correctly answered that dressings should keep the wound bed moist and the peri-wound area dry, that assessing pain intensity is necessary, and that a nutritional assessment of the patient should be conducted. However, most respondents did not know that wound healing does not slow down in the proliferative phase of healing, that biofilm on a wound is not associated with reduced wound exudate, and that pressure ulcers can be cleaned with drinking water. Sharp et al. [43] found that nursing staff were knowledgeable about and used modern dressings for the care of stage 2 and 3 ulcers such as hydrocolloids, foams, and alginates. They also observed that outdated methods, such as iodine preparations, saline solutions, hydrogen peroxide, gauze, and others, were still in use. Gillespie et al. [44] aimed to investigate the practice of nurses in wound care in an Australian hospital. In their survey, 75.6% of respondents reported that the appearance of the wound was the most crucial factor in choosing a suitable dressing. Almost half of the respondents did not consider national standards for chronic wound care in their work. Therefore, the authors concluded that although hospital nurses were well-versed in wound healing processes, they did not use recommended clinical guidelines for wound care in their practice.

The research had some limitations. Some respondents wrote down primary education in the questionnaire, which was either an intentional or unintentional error. These questionnaires had to be excluded from the study before the analysis. The sample size was small, so the results cannot be generalized. The questionnaire, in our opinion and according to the respondents, was somewhat lengthy, and the concentration of respondents waned during completion. The questions were not logically sequenced, and they were intermingled, which could have contributed to the study's suboptimal results. It appears that the questionnaire might have been too demanding, and it should be revised and adapted to our specific context in the future. Further, research is called for, potentially involving a modified questionnaire, to ease meaningful comparisons with the questionnaire authors' results.

9. Conclusion

The results indicate that participants had varying levels of knowledge about pressure ulcers, their prevention, and care. While many participants proved good knowledge in some areas, there were gaps in their understanding in other areas. The findings highlight areas, where there is room for improvement in educating healthcare professionals or individuals about pressure ulcers and their management. These insights can be used to design more targeted training programs or materials. It is necessary to implement a comprehensive approach to elevate the knowledge, attitudes, and practices of healthcare staff with the goal of enhancing the quality of patient care. Emphasizing the importance of continuous knowledge and practice enhancement for nurses is imperative.

Author details

Melita Peršolja[1*] and Rosanda Drufovka[2]

1 Vipava Unit at Faculty of Health Sciences, University of Primorska, Vipava, Slovenia

2 Nova Gorica General Hospital, Šempeter pri Gorici, Slovenia

*Address all correspondence to: melita.persolja@fvz.upr.si

References

[1] Haesler E, editor. Prevention and Treatment of Pressure Ulcers: Quick Reference Guide. Perth, Australia: National Pressure Ulcer Advisory Panel, European Pressure Ulcer Advisory Panel and Pan Pacific Pressure Injury Alliance; 2014

[2] Alderden J, Rondinelli J, Pepper G, Cummins M, Whitney J. Risk factors for pressure injuries among critical care patients: A systematic review. International Journal of Nursing Studies. 2017;**71**:97-114. DOI: 10.1016/j.ijnurstu.2017.03.012

[3] Moore ZE, Cowman S. Repositioning for treating pressure ulcers. Cochrane Database of Systematic Reviews. 2015;**1**:1. DOI: 10.1002/14651858.CD006898

[4] Boyko TV, Longaker MT, Yang GP. Review of the current management of pressure ulcers. Advances in Wound Care. 2018;**7**(2):57-67. DOI: 10.1089/wound.2016.0697

[5] Perko D. Razjede zaradi pritiska. In: Perko VD, Borovničar A, editors. Kazalniki kakovosti v zdravstvu, Letno poročilo za leto 2019. Ljubljana: Nacionalni inštitut za javno zdravje, Ministrstvo za zdravje Republike Slovenije; 2019. pp. 20-21. Available from: https://www.gov.si/assets/ministrstva/MZ/DOKUMENTI/staro/1-PODROCJA-ZDRAVJE/1-Kakovost-varnost-in-dostopnost-zdravstvenega-varstva/1-Kakovost-zdravstvenega-varstva/Kazalniki-kakovosti-v-zdravstvu-2019.pdf

[6] Yavuz A, Çakmak M. Razjeda/poškodba zaradi pritiska. In: Hudin VD, editor. Sodobna oskrba kroničnih ran. Ljubljana: Srednja zdravstvena šola; 2020. pp. 45-63. Available from: http://szslj.splet.arnes.si/files/delightful-downloads/2020/11/SODOBNA-OSKRBA-KRONI%C4%8CNIH-RAN-PRIRO%C4%8CNIK.pdf [Accessed: December 09, 2022]

[7] Tomc D. Razjeda zaradi pritiska – preventiva in oskrba. In: Straus VKK, editor. Usmerjeni v stroko zdravstvene nege in oskrbe – usmerjeni v potrebe bolnikov: zbornik predavanj z recenzijo, Zreče 29.-30. marec 2019. Ljubljana: Zbornica zdravstvene in babiške nege Slovenije – Zveza strokovnih društev medicinskih sester, babic in zdravstvenih tehnikov Slovenije, Strokovna sekcija medicinskih sester in zdravstvenih tehnikov v socialnih zavodih; 2019. pp. 11-24

[8] Fatur M. Preprečevanje razjede zaradi pritiska pri osebah s paraplegijo (diplomska naloga). Ljubljana: Univerza v Ljubljani; 2020

[9] Šáteková L, Žiaková K, Zeleníková R. Predictive validity of the Braden scale, Norton scale and Waterlow scale in Slovak Republic. Central Europenal Jurnal Nursing and Midwifery. 2015;**6**(3):283-290. DOI: 10.1111/ijn.12499

[10] Edsberg LE, Black JM, Goldberg M, McNichol L, Moore L, Sieggreen M. Revised national pressure ulcer advisory panel pressure injury staging system: Revised pressure injury staging system. Journal of Wound, Ostomy, and Continence Nursing. 2016;**43**(6):585

[11] Simonič S. Majhni koraki-veliki prihranki: vloga medicinske sestreza preventivo razjede zaradi pritiskana oddelku intenzivne terapije. In: Doberšek VD, Kočevar R, Perko AN, Peternelj K, editors. Anesteziologija,

intenzivna terapija, transfuziologija: skupaj za pacienta: zbornik predavanj z recenzijo, Rogaška Slatina, 1.in 2. april.2016. Ljubljana: Zbornica zdravstvene in babiške Slovenije - Zveza strokovnih društev medicinskih sester, babic in zdravstvenih tehnikov Slovenije, Sekcija medicinskih sester in zdravstvenih tehnikov v anesteziologiji, intenzivni terapiji in transfuziologiji; 2016. pp. 35-39

[12] Moore ZE, Patton D. Risk assessment tools for the prevention of pressure ulcers. The Cochrane Database of Systematic Reviews. 2019;**1**(1):CD006471. DOI: 10.1002/14651858.CD006471.pub4

[13] Gaballah S, El-Deen DS. Pressure injury care program effects on nurses' performance and patients' pressure injury wound healing outcomes. American Journal of Nursing Research. 2021;**9**(3):76-84. DOI: 10.12691/ajnr-9-3-2

[14] Fulbrook P, Lawrence P, Miles S. Australian nurses' knowledge of pressure injury prevention and management: A cross-sectional survey. Journal of Wound, Ostomy, and Continence Nursing. 2019;**46**(2):106-112. DOI: 10.1097/WON.0000000000000508

[15] Soban LM, Kim L, Yuan AH, Miltner RS. Organisational strategies to implement hospital pressure ulcer prevention programmes: Findings from a national survey. Journal of Nursing Management. 2017;**25**(6):457-467. DOI: 10.1111/jonm.12416

[16] Fernandes C, Lima A, Santos M. Pressure injury prevention: Attitudes and knowledge of nursing students. Journal of Nursing & Healthcare. 2021;**11**(3):e2111320924. Available from: https://periodicos.ufpel.edu.br/ojs2/index.php/enfermagem/article/view/20924

[17] Pieper B, Zulkowski K. The Pieper-Zulkowski pressure ulcer knowledge test. Advances in Skin & Wound Care. 2014;**27**(9):413-420. DOI: 10.1097/01.ASW.0000453210.21330.00

[18] Official Gazette of the Republic of Slovenia. Uradni list RS. št.71/2014 (29.3.2014). 2014. Available from: https://www.uradni-list.si/glasilo-uradni-list-rs/vsebina/2014-01-2937/kodeks-etike-v-zdravstveni-negi-in-oskrbi-slovenije

[19] Miller DM, Neelon L, Kish-Smith K, Whitney L, Burant CJ. Pressure injury knowledge in critical care nurses. Journal of Wound Ostomy & Continence Nursing. 2017;**44**(5):455-457. DOI: 10.1097/WON.0000000000000350

[20] Eskes AM, Maaskant JM, Holloway S, van Dijk N, Alves P, Legemate DA, et al. Competencies of specialised wound care nurses: A European Delphi study. International Wound Journal. 2014;**11**(6):665-674. DOI: 10.1111/iwj.12027

[21] Barakat-Johnson M, Barnett C, Wand T, White K. Knowledge and attitudes of nurses toward pressure injury prevention. Journal of Wound, Ostomy and Continence Nursing. 2018;**45**(3):233-237. DOI: 10.1097/WON.0000000000000430

[22] Tirgari B, Mirshekari L, Forouzi MA. Pressure injury prevention: Knowledge and attitudes of Iranian intensive care nurses. Advances in Skin & Wound Care. 2018;**31**(4):1-8. DOI: 10.1097/01.ASW.0000530848.50085.ef

[23] Li Z, Zhou X, Cao J, Li Z, Wan X, Li J, et al. Nurses' knowledge and attitudes regarding major immobility complications among bedridden patients: A prospective multicentre study. Journal of Clinical Nursing. 2018;**27**(9-10):1969-1980. DOI: 10.1111/jocn.14339

[24] Parisod H, Holopainen A, Koivunen M, Puukka P, Haavisto E. Factors determining nurses' knowledge of evidence-based pressure ulcer prevention practices in Finland: A correlational cross-sectional study. Scandinavian Journal of Caring Sciences. 2022;**36**(1):150-161. DOI: 10.1111/scs.12972

[25] Ebi WE, Hirko GF, in Mijena, D. A. Nurses' knowledge to pressure ulcer prevention in public hospitals in Wollega: A cross-sectional study design. BMC Nursing. 2019;**18**(1):1-12. DOI: 10.1186/s12912-019-0346-y

[26] De Meyer D, Verhaeghe S, Van Hecke A, Beeckman D. Knowledge of nurses and nursing assistants about pressure ulcer prevention: A survey in 16 Belgian hospitals using the PUKAT 2.0 tool. Journal of Tissue Viability. 2019;**28**(2):59-69. DOI: 10.1016/j.jtv.2019.03.002

[27] Ilesanmi RE, Ofi BA, Adejumo PO. Nurses' knowledge of pressure ulcer prevention in Ogun state, Nigeria: Results of a pilot survey . Ostomy/Wound Management. 2012;**58**(2):24-32

[28] Nuru N, Zewdu F, Amsalu S, in Mehretie, Y. Knowledge and practice of nurses towards prevention of pressure ulcer and associated factors in Gondar University Hospital, Northwest Ethiopia. BMC Nursing. 2015;**14**(1):1-8. DOI: 10.1186/s12912-015-0076-8

[29] Al Shidi AS. Pressure ulcer management in Oman: Nurses' knowledge and views [doctoral thesis]. Glasgow: University of Glasgow; 2016. Available from: https://theses.gla.ac.uk/7635/

[30] Mccluskey P, Mccarthy G. Nurses' knowledge and competence in wound management. Wounds UK. 2012;**8**(2):37-47

[31] Sengul T, Karadag A. Determination of nurses' level of knowledge on the prevention of pressure ulcers: The case of Turkey. Journal of Tissue Viability. 2020;**29**(4):337-341. DOI: 10.1016/j.jtv.2020.06.005

[32] De Faria G, Begido G, Prado TN. Knowledge and practice of nurses on the care of wounds. Journal of Nursing UFPE/Revista de Enfermagem UFPE. 2016;**10**(12):4532-4538. DOI: 10.5205/reuol.9978-88449-6-ED1012201614

[33] Ferreira AM, Rigotti MA, da Silva Barcelos L, Simão CMF, Ferreira DN, Gonçalves RQ. Knowledge and practice of nurses about care for patients with wounds. Revista de Pesquisa Cuidado é Fundamental Online. 2014;**6**(3):1178-1190. DOI: 10.9789/2175-5361.2014v6n3p1178

[34] Sever M, Bregar B. Specializacije v zdravstveni negi: pogled študentov. Obzornik zdravstvene nege. 2015;**49**(1). DOI: 10.14528/snr.2015.49.1.49

[35] Kadivec S, Skela Savič B, Kramar Z, Zavrl Džananović D, Bregar B. Strategija razvoja zdravstvene nege in oskrbe v sistemu zdravstvenega varstva v republiki Sloveniji za obdobje od 2011 do 2020: povzetek. Slovenian Nursing Review. 2013;**47**(1):97-112

[36] Kramar Z. Kakovost in varnost v zdravstvu: priročnik. Ljubljana: Zbornica zdravstvene in babiške nege Slovenije - Zveza strokovnih društev medicinskih sester, babic in zdravstvenih tehnikov Slovenije. 2022. Available from: https://www.zbornica-zveza.si/wp-content/uploads/2022/03/Kakovost-in-varnost-v-zdravstvu_prirocnik.pdf [Accessed: February 04, 2023]

[37] Gul A, Andsoy II, Ozkaya B, Zeydan A. A descriptive, cross-sectional survey of Turkish nurses' knowledge

of pressure ulcer risk, prevention, and staging. Ostomy/Wound Management. 2017;**63**(6):40-46

[38] Cox J, Edsberg LE, Koloms K, VanGilder CA. Pressure injuries in critical care patients in US hospitals: Results of the international pressure ulcer prevalence survey. Journal of Wound, Ostomy, and Continence Nursing: Official Publication of The Wound, Ostomy and Continence Nurses Society. 2022;**49**(1):21-28

[39] Lawrence P, Fulbrook P, in Miles, S. A survey of Australian nurses' knowledge of pressure injury/pressure ulcer management. Journal of Wound, Ostomy and Continence Nursing. 2015;**42**(5):450-460. DOI: 10.1097/WON.0000000000000141

[40] Saleh MYN, Papanikolaou P, Nassar OS, Shahin A, Anthony D. Nurses' knowledge and practice of pressure ulcer prevention and treatment: An observational study. Journal of Tissue Viability. 2019;**28**(4):210-217. DOI: 10.1016/j.jtv.2019.10.005

[41] Gedamu H, Abate T, Ayalew E, Tegenaw A, Birhanu M, in Tafere, Y. Level of nurses' knowledge on pressure ulcer prevention: A systematic review and meta-analysis study in Ethiopia. Heliyon. 2021;**7**(7):e07648. DOI: 10.1016/j.heliyon.2021.e07648

[42] Manderlier B, Van Damme N, Verhaeghe S, Van Hecke A, Everink I, Halfens R, et al. Modifiable patient-related factors associated with pressure ulcers on the sacrum and heels: Secondary data analyses. Journal of Advanced Nursing. 2019;**75**(11):2773-2785. DOI: 10.1111/jan.14149

[43] Sharp C, Burr G, Broadbent M, Cummins M, Casey H, Merriman A. Pressure ulcer prevention and care: A survey of current practice. Journal of Quality in Clinical Practice. 2000;**20**(4):150-157. DOI: 10.1046/j.1440-1762.2000.00384.x

[44] Gillespie BM, Chaboyer W, Allen P, Morely N, Nieuwenhoven P. Wound care practices: A survey of acute care nurses. Journal of Clinical Nursing. 2014;**23**(17-18):2618-2627. DOI: 10.1111/jocn.12479

Chapter 14

Safeguarding Professional Intimate Care and Touch in Nursing Education: Humanistic Care in a Technological Era

Simangele Shakwane

Abstract

Facilitating intimate care and touch in the digital age advocates for quality humanistic care that is culturally, socially and religiously acceptable. The chapter attempts to create awareness of professional intimate care and touch on nursing education and practice to incorporate technology into humanistic care. The Participatory Action Research (PAR) process was used to allow for active participation in intimate care and touch activities to create new knowledge into humanistic intimate care practice. Symbolic interactionism's theoretical framework complemented the understanding of attitudes, motives, behaviors, and how individuals interpret experiences and events. Naïve sketches collected initial data to establish their diversity and understanding of intimate care. After that, facilitated diversity in intimate care and touch discussion sessions were conducted, humanistic intimate care and touch simulation sessions, drawing from intimate care and touch experiences, and post-interviews were conducted to narrate the drawing. These activities created a visual and multimodal experience for nursing students. Knowing one's socio-cultural beliefs and learning others' identities creates a sense of belonging and acceptance. When nursing students understand who they are (as individuals, collectively), it makes it easier to acknowledge the diverse patients requiring intimate care and touch. Thus, nursing students' preparedness in intimate care and touch is critical to allow them to practice in a safe space before being exposed to clinical placement.

Keywords: intimate care, nursing students, participatory action research, symbolic interactionism, nursing care, technology, humanistic care

1. Introduction

Nursing is an inherently human experience done for humans by humans. Nursing care basic activities require nurses to see and touch patients' bodies to promote healing and comfort. Caring in nursing involves human relationships between persons focused on knowing each other's uniqueness and sharing individual experiences to affirm each other's humanness in the world [1]. Through caring, a human person is valued, therefore, humanism in care is a necessity and global priority to improve quality of life [2]. Great emphasis is placed on nursing values to develop humanism and humanize the care provided. This means that nursing should be humanized to value and respect human life [3]. Therefore, caring rests on humanistic values that translate into attitudes and behaviors geared to protecting, enhancing or preserving the human dignity of patients [4]. Humanistic nursing care is further described as an interaction between nurses and patients/families as a response to the caring situation and is characterized by empathy, respect for human dignity, autonomy of patients and holistic care [5]. The authors [5] make a humanistic care distinctive shift from a task-oriented care model to a person-centered or relationship-centered model.

Nursing practice demonstrates technical skills performed following a standardized plan of care derived from the nursing process [1]. Every basic nursing procedure requires physical touch. The symbol of touch and being touched means different things to different people. It creates interpersonal relationships that can contribute to the student's failure or success. Intimacy is revealed as a site of connecting through which a sense of belonging is created [6]. A nurse and patient meet in a social space where human recognitions are established [7] to co-create a relationship between a nurse and patient, coordinated for the mutual purpose of knowing each other [1]. Intimate care is classified as closeness at a physical, psychological, and spiritual level. It is the care provided by the nurses that requires physical closeness or bodily contact and touch, thus invading the physical space and privacy of a patient [8]. Intimate care touch is task-oriented to areas of the patient's body that might produce feelings of discomfort, anxiety and fear or might be misinterpreted as having a sexual purpose [9]. Intimate care and touch are a significant element in the healthcare profession that defines the nursing profession as it requires a nurse to provide comprehensive physical, mental and emotional care. It transforms a very private, personal activity into a social process which impacts the providers and recipients of intimate care and touch [10].

Intimate care and touch may be threatened by the advancements in health technologies, where nurses rely on data technology produces, rather than incorporating it into quality nursing care. Technology is used in care, and interactions happen in diverse places, either private or social spaces. Technologies are conceptualized as embedded in relations with other tools, practices, groups, professionals, and patients [11]. Vast advancements in electronics, computing, and medicine have generated space for new dimensions of interactions between technology and the human body [12]. Technology at the clinical bedside has the power to become the point that nurses use to inform, direct, evaluate understand their nursing care [7]. Technological knowing is a way of understanding persons using technologies of health and human care and provides nurses with another way of knowing persons [1].

Yadal [12] indicates that as intimate technologies develop, it is important for healthcare practitioners to know how they will shape lived experiences and cultural issues and normative views to be addressed regarding the body. Even McCarthy [7] warns that technology may serve to further distance nurses from patients both proximally and emotionally, questioning the therapeutic nurse-patient relationship in healthcare environments. Thus, constant examination of how technology is created and used needs to be interpreted by the users and recipient of care [11]. Technologies used in nursing must increase proficient human caring, by providing opportunities to further the knowing of the person [1]. If technology is blindly accepted, it will serve to categorize and marginalize patients' illness experiences, especially if nurses practice without critically examining the overwhelming presence and impact of technology on knowledge development and nurses' interaction with patients.

This chapter illustrates the value of intimate care and touch in nursing education. It aims to safeguard the human element made visible through interaction and touch in caring for the body. It is important to conscientize the nursing fraternity to their pledge to service of humanity, which is realized through acknowledgement of human diversity, knowing a patient as a person, and respecting the touched body. There is no scientific dispute on the value of technology in advancing nursing science. However, moral and ethical decisions must be made when technology is used, and therapeutic nurse-patient relationships should be promoted. The future of the nursing profession lies in the nursing students' humanistic care competency and support.

2. Theoretical framework

Symbolic interactionism was used as a theoretical framework to direct the study. Symbolic interactionism is a theoretical perspective that addresses how society is generated and maintained through face-to-face, repeated, meaningful interactions among individuals [13]. The basic notion is that human action and interactions are understandable only through exchanging meaningful communication or symbols [14]. It takes a small-scale view of society by studying the interaction between individuals and through this approach, social order and changes in society are explained [14]. Therefore, individuals use language and significant symbols to communicate with others. The source of data is human interaction that focuses on individual perspectives through character, signs of facial expression, body language, gestures, and human behavior [15].

Several authors [13, 14, 16] describe the four tenets of symbolic interactionism: (i) individuals act based on the meanings objects have for them, (ii) interaction occurs within a particular social and cultural context in which physical and social objects and situations must be defined based on individuals meanings, (iii) meanings merge from interactions with other individuals and with society, and (iv) meanings are continuously created and recreated during interaction with others. Therefore, the communities are distinguished not only by a collectively shared symbolic knowledge but also by cultural activities in which they stage and perform such knowledge in rituals in which the particular social system is expressed, projected, and reproduced [17].

Symbolic interactionism is for understanding the relationship between individuals and society to empower nurse practitioners to provide holistic intimate care to diverse patients. The human body has various meanings attached to it; therefore, nursing students must understand these meanings to provide acceptable intimate care and touch to all patients. Symbolic interactionism was incorporated with the Model for facilitating the teaching of intimate care [8] that was implemented in this phase. The model posits four steps to the facilitation of intimate care which are summarized in **Table 1** and were used in Participatory Action Research that directed the study.

2.1 Research design

In this chapter, qualitative Participatory Action Research (PAR) was used to understand the intimate care and touch experiences of nursing students. A participatory approach is a qualitative methodology that values genuine and meaningful participation and direct engagement of local priorities and perspectives [5]. The PAR emphasizes the production of knowledge and empowerment, it seeks to transform social realities so that the lives of people are improved [18]. It affirms that experience

Intimate care facilitation steps	Descriptions
Step 1: Intimate care conflict	This step reflects the diversity of nursing students and patients when intimate care procedures are delegated. Lack of intimate care knowledge and experiences of caring for the body of the other person.
Step 2: Facilitation of Intimate care	In this step, nurse educators are empowered to facilitate intimate care. Reflecting on the current curriculum and creating intimate care realities for nursing students. Creating a safe space for the nursing students to experience touching a real human being using humanistic intimate care simulations using silicone masks.
Step 3: Intimate care support	Preparing nursing students for intimate care and touch, giving them tools to know when and how to touch. Strengthening intimate care support during clinical placement anticipating alleviating intimate care conflict.
Step 4: Therapeutic nurse-patient relationship	Intimate care knowledge and support, and debriefing sessions create a safe space for nursing students to experience intimate care realities. They will be able to establish a professional intimate care therapeutic relationship based on trust, respect, and dignity. Advocating for the provision of intimate care without fear of being stereotyped and the caring touch being misinterpreted.

Table 1.
Summary of the intimate care facilitation steps [8].

can be a basis for knowing and that experiential learning can lead to a legitimate form of learning that influences practice [19]. The PAR cyclic process and goals discussed in Ref. [20] were followed and discussed below.

2.1.1 Phase 1: collaboration

The researcher created relationships and ownership with the Nursing Education Institution (NEI) and nursing students who were part of the project. Entry into the research setting and initiating a mutual relationship is critical to establishing and nurturing the willingness to participate in the initiatives [21]. The researcher spent time in the NEI before the commencement of the project to establish trust and understand the intimate care practices in the NEI. Two nurse educators assisted with understanding the culture of the institution and the implemented curriculum. Meetings were held with the students during break times and after lectures to avoid disrupting teaching and learning. Informal discussions on the meaning of the body and cultural attributes were conducted. The process of the study was discussed with nursing students who were interested in participating in the study and were invited to complete a short survey with their names and contact details. All nursing students voluntarily signed informed consent before engaging in the research activities.

Twelve (n = 12) nursing students registered for a three-year Diploma in Nursing (Regulation 171) voluntarily participated in the activities of the project. They were in their second year of training. Ten (n = 10) females and two (male) nursing students with age range from 22 to 31 years. South Africa is a diverse country, with multiple cultural communities and in this objective, the participants were from five South African cultural groups which enhanced the diverse group and multiple voices on understanding intimate care and touch. **Table 2** displays the summary of the participants' characteristics.

Characteristics	Frequency (n)
Gender:	
Female	10 (83.3%)
Male	2 (16.7%)
Age:	
20-24	7 (58.3%)
25-29	3 (25%)
30-31	2 (16.7%)
Cultural backgrounds:	
Afrikaans	1 (8.3%)
Swati	4 (33.3%)
Tsonga	2 (16.7%)
Tshwana	2 (16.7%)
Zulu	3 (25%)

Table 2.
Summary of the participants' characteristics (n = 12).

2.1.2 Phase 2: incorporation of local knowledge

The knowledge of intimate care and touch was explored and analyzed to provide necessary support in the facilitation of intimate care and touch. The participation methods were built on the specific research site care, through understanding the context of the collaboration group. At the onset, four questions were asked to establish a diverse understanding of caring for the human body and they were based on step 1 of the Intimate Care Facilitation Model (see **Table 1**):

Q1: Discuss your beliefs on caring for the human body.
Q2: What is your understanding of intimate care and touch in nursing care?
Q3: Mention nursing procedures that you consider as intimate care.
Q4: Describe your experience when providing intimate care and touch.

The participants were given open-ended written questions to complete their answers. Narrative data analysis and coding for visual data were used to interpret the findings.

Narrative data is analyzed for the story they have to tell was conducted to understand the story of the touched body in nursing care. The large data patterns and meanings were organized into narrative segments and categories. Finally, the factors that shaped the participant's lives were identified. An analytic abstraction that highlights (a) the processes in an individual's life, (b) the different theories that relate to the participant's life experiences, and (c) the unique and general features of life. The author and an independent coder analyzed data individually and compared the findings. The presented findings were the final themes agreed upon by the two data analysts.

For drawing the participants used *"Sketchbook"* Application and Deco M Pen Tablet which they connected to their cellphones and were able to draw. Five Deco M Pen were used, and they were shared among the participants. After drawing, they could share the drawing with the researcher via Bluetooth and email. Visual data was analyzed using coding as described by Creswell [22] as follows:

1. Code the image by tagging areas of the image and assigning code labels.
2. Compile all the codes for the images on a separate sheet.
3. Review the codes to eliminate redundancy and overlap, reducing the codes to potential themes.
4. Grouping codes into themes that represent a common idea.
5. Assign the codes/themes to three themes: expected themes, surprising themes and unusual themes. This step helps to ensure the qualitative findings represent diverse perspectives.
6. Writing the narrative for each of them accompanied by the visual data.

In the visual data analysis, a member check was done when the researcher conducted short interviews to allow the participants to confirm that the themes attached to their drawings represented their experiences.

2.1.2.1 Theme 1: nursing education transforming lives

The visual data in this theme presents the participants' reactions to being accepted into a nursing training programme. It brought joy and hope to individuals who could not afford registration to higher education institutions. Receiving a call from a Nursing Education Institution regarding the positive outcome was a joyful occasion. **Figure 1** presents the expressions of being accepted in the nursing training programme.

The joy of being accepted in Nursing Education marks liberation and defiance of poverty for many nursing students. Access to higher education in South Africa

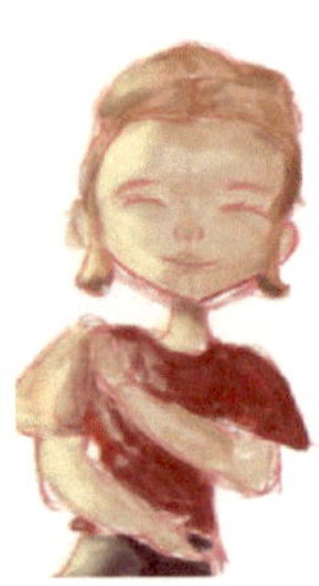	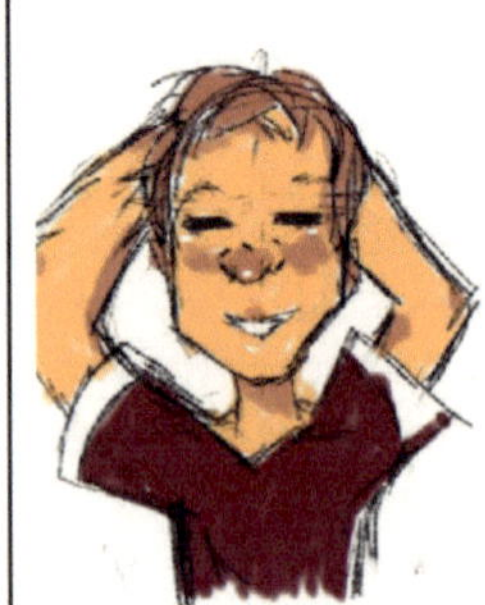	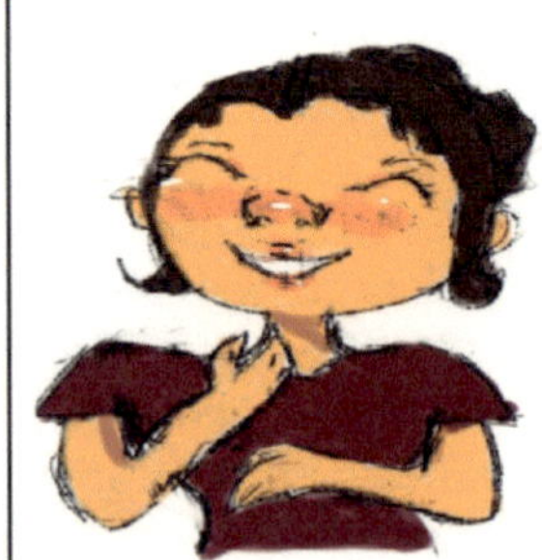
"My life changed; my family could have a better life" (FP3/25)	*"Wow, it was the best day of my life, [...]" (MP7/24)*	*"I can't describe the feeling. I could see my life changing after being at home for two years" (FP5/26)*

Figure 1.
Joyful expressions of being admitted to nursing education training.

is a long-standing challenge. Many young people complete basic education and cannot enroll for further education.

2.1.2.2 Theme 2: sacredness of the human body

The participants narrated their reflections on how African cultures influence the meaning of the body, including the power issues created by patriarchal gender roles. Two sub-themes were identified: *respect for the body and boundaries in accessing the body.*

2.1.2.2.1 Sub-theme 2.1: respect for the body

The body is multifaceted, which calls one to respect the physical and spiritual presence of the human person.

> *"[...], the human body must be respected by not being touched or doing anything on it. It must not be exposed unnecessarily" (MP7/24)*

> *"A human body is a very precious and sensitive gift from God [...] which need to be treated with respect, taking into consideration their feelings and asking for permission for any activity" (FP1-22)*

2.1.2.2.2 Sub-theme 2.2: cultural boundaries in accessing the body

Culture is the totality of the way of life evolved by people in their attempts to meet the challenge of living in their environment, which gives order and meaning to their social, political, and economic status that distinguishes them from others [23]. In African culture, each person has a role and children are not allowed to see and touch the body of the elders. Childhood is not limited to age but to the generational position in the family. The participants acknowledged the importance of knowing what is expected of a child from the body of an adult.

> *"A child is not supposed to see an adult body naked [...]" (FP3/25)*

> *"It is believed that it is not moral to see the naked body of an elderly person, especially their private parts" (FP7-31)*

> *"[...] for me as my young age I am not allowed to see and touch the body of an elderly person" (FP6-24)*

As African people, various moral and societal values are meant to regulate interpersonal relationships and the community. In African cultures, respect and honor for elders is important [24]. Gender boundaries also contribute to the care of the body. African cultures ascribe to patriarchal ideologies with defined gender roles. Cross-gender care is frowned upon and may limit quality care.

> *"A male is not supposed to see his mother or women naked, and females are not supposed to male or their father even when in need of their help. An elderly person of the same gender is requested to assist, at times a person is delegated to assist an elderly family member with physical needs" (FP7-31)*

> *"[...] only old women are allowed to care for the sick person because they are no longer sexually active, and they can handle the human body respectfully" (FP11-26)*

Interestingly, even though the participants were from various cultural communities, their understanding of the human body was of the communitarian outlook. Affirming the African notion of personhood that the reality of the communal world takes precedence over the reality of the individual. Even though there are many diverse African cultures, there are many commonalities in value systems, beliefs and systems which reflect the African communitarian worldview [25]. Kpanake [26] confirms that a person does not exist in isolation, therefore, each life and growing up in some specific social and cultural setting influences individual behavior, thoughts and the way of being in the world with others.

2.1.2.3 Theme 3: importance of intimate care in nursing

The nursing students understood that intimate care and touch are part of basic nursing care. It forms part of the daily routine of caring for the physical aspect of the human person.

2.1.2.3.1 Sub-theme 3.1: physical care requiring touch

> *"Intimate care is coming close to private parts or the whole human body, which makes one uncomfortable, especially during bathing, sometimes very uncomfortable [...]" (FP9-22)*

> *"Therapeutic touch you give to patients when caring for them, depending on the gender and age, even the body parts that are touched [...]. Well we do it to promote good health and comfort" (FP1-22)*

> *"[...] healing touch for care to another person, when you touch the patient, you need to do it gently and make the patient comfortable and safe" (FP8-30)*

The participants' definition of intimate care is coming near the body and touching the body for care. This understanding is congruent with [27] who define intimate physical touch as involving inspection of and possible physical contact with those parts of the body whose exposure can cause embarrassment to either the patient or the nurse. O'Lynn [9] expanded on this definition by emphasizing that intimate touch is task-oriented to areas of the patient's body such as genitalia, buttocks, perineum, inner thighs, lower abdomen and breasts that may produce in patients or caregivers, feelings of discomfort, anxiety and fear.

2.1.2.3.2 Sub-theme 3.2: touch-oriented basic nursing care

> *"I consider nursing procedures such as bed bath, vaginal examination and insertion of a urinary catheter. For me, any procedure that requires a patient to remove his or her clothes is intimate as it requires a high level of trust" (FP10-23)*

> *"[...] includes bathing the patient and touching sensitive areas of the body during physical examination [...]" (FP5-22)*

Unfortunately, intimate care procedures are often regarded as simple humble tasks and are thought to be less prestige than procedures requiring technical nursing skills [10]. Yet, physical and emotional encounters with the patient can be exhausting and create feelings of discomfort and fear when sensitive parts of the body are exposed and touched. Intimate care and touch fulfill the basic needs of a human person which are hygiene, elimination, and circulation to promote the dignity of the body.

2.1.2.4 Theme 4: learning nursing care

The visual data presents the participants' process of care learning journey starting from the lecture room (nursing theory), and skills laboratory where basic nursing care procedures were simulated and using high-tech equipment for simulated care. Thereafter, they had walkabouts in the hospital with their clinical facilitators to orientate them to the real hospital setting. **Figure 2** depicts the process of learning nursing care.

The simulations in the skills laboratory were basic nursing care procedures such as bed baths and physical examination of the manikins. This is in line with [28] who assert that many nursing students' experience of intimate care provision occurs during clinical placement, where they are in physical contact with the human body.

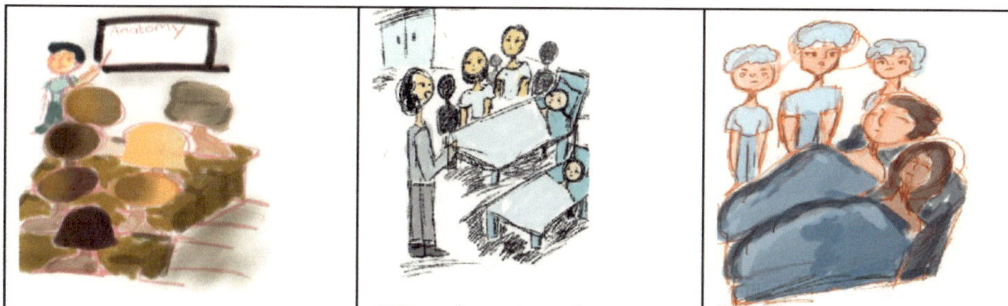

"We started in the lecture hall, where we learnt about anatomy & physiology [...]" (FP3-25)	*"After learning theory, we were in the skill lab doing bed bath, physical exams, etc. on the dolls" (MP7-24)*	*"After 5 weeks we went for orientation to the hospital with our clinical lecturers to see the wards" (FP11-26)*

Figure 2.
Facilitation of nursing care in nursing education institution.

2.1.2.5 Theme 5: not ready for the "other"

The participants drew on their experiences of intimate care and touch. From the visual data, one can see the emotions of the nursing students when caring for the body, feelings of embarrassment, fear and cultural taboo of cross-gender and age. **Figure 3** displays the visual data and verbatim extracts on intimate care experiences.

The two female participants' tears are prominent, with many tears in the toilets and students' residential rooms. These were tears of helplessness and knowing that they would go through the same process the next day. The male participant did not cry, but frustration and helplessness. These feelings are expected during intimate care and touch implementation as cultural boundaries are crossed and interacting with the naked body.

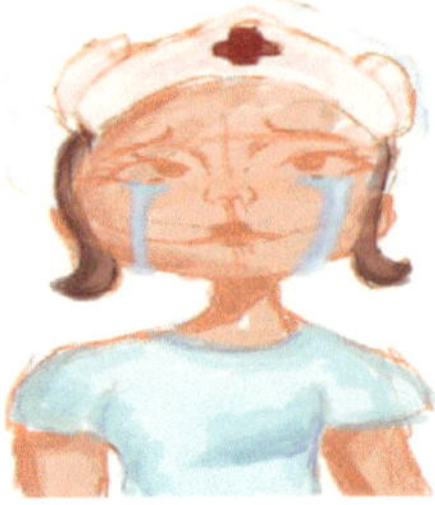	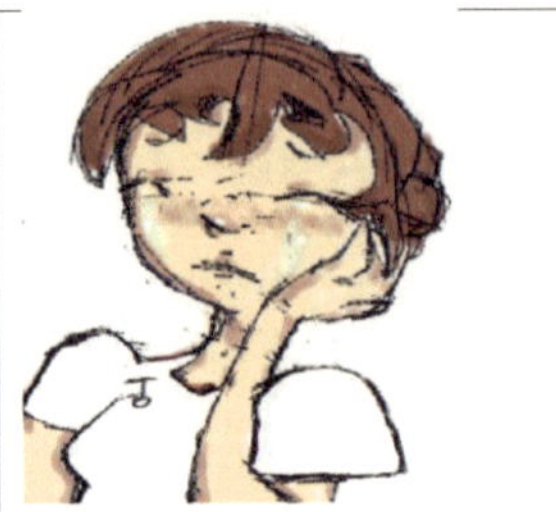	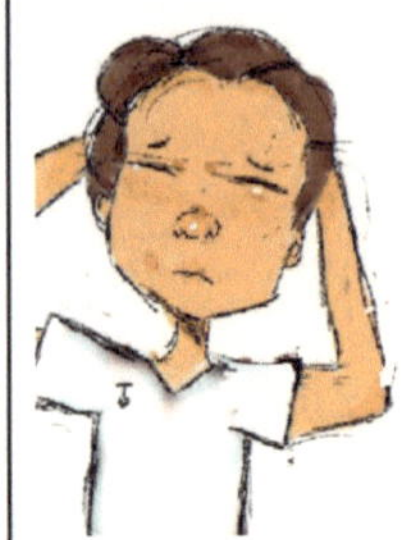
"[...], it was uncomfortable because I had to bath an elderly male patient who believed that a child must not see his naked bod [...]" (FP3-25)	*"It was like washing my father, the patient was unconscious, and I cried the whole time bathing. No one could rescue me, except coming to help with changing line [...]"(FP4-23)*	*"Having to see and touch the naked body of the patient, washing her whole body, I was scared and felt a sense of shame" (MP9-22)*

Figure 3.
Visual data of intimate care implementation experiences.

2.1.2.6 Theme 6: left in the dark: met with death

Nursing students have to care for patients who are critically ill, and they experience caring for dying and dying patients. Having to touch or prepare the cold body was not an easy task as it was not something that was a normal practice in African cultural practices. **Figure 4** shows the emotions surrounding caring for the lifeless body.

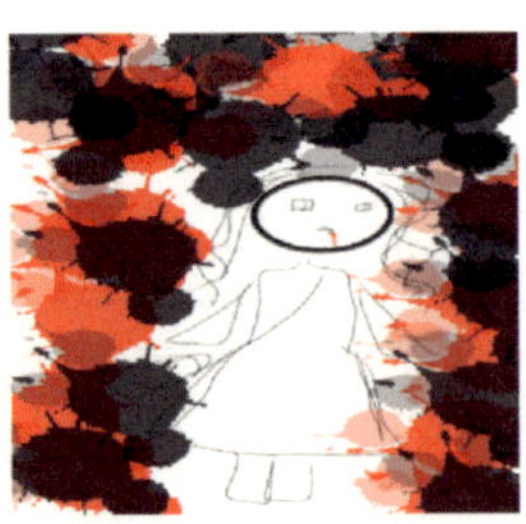	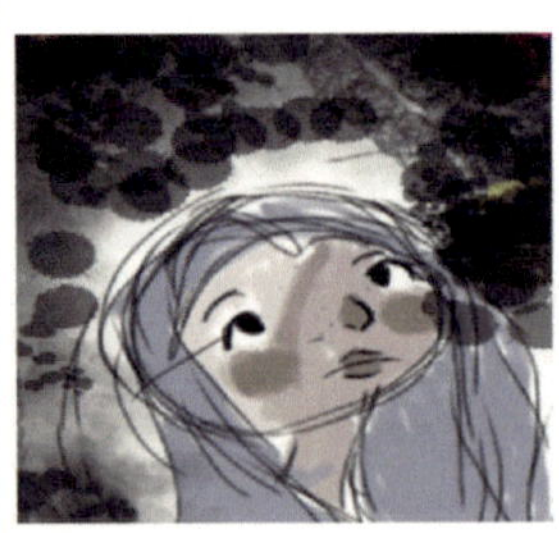	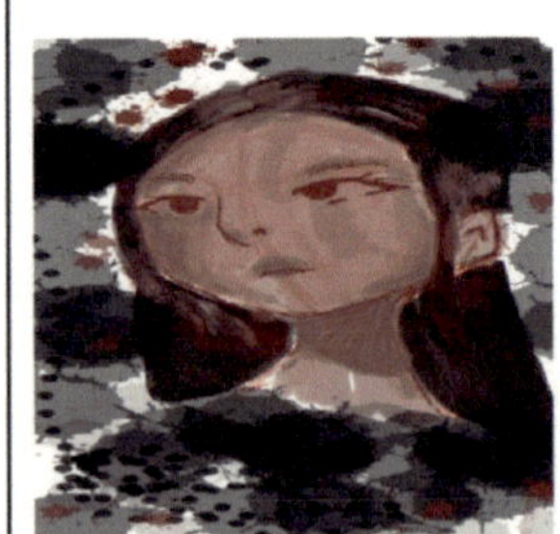
"I am a last born at home, have never seen a dead person. Having to clean and do the last office was worse than bathing a patient. I felt surrounded by darkness [...]" (FP5/22)	*"Working in the medical ward, seeing a dead body, I fainted as I had never seen a dead person, hoping someone will take over, well I had to recover fast as I had to do last office with the senior nurse" (FP10-23)*	*"It reminded me of the death of my mother, all the pain came back. I prayed that a nurse care for her dead body as I did for the patient [...]" (FP7-31)*

Figure 4.
Visual data of experiences for caring for a demised patient.

Death was an untapped territory, participants felt as if they were surrounded by darkness. Seeing a lifeless body for the first time was a shocking experience. In the drawings, the black, gray and red dots bring to life the pain of losing a patient, fear and trigger previous family member's losses.

2.1.3 Phase 3: emergent process

In this phase, intimate care activities were created and implemented. After understanding the local knowledge of the body and intimate care in phase 2. The major themes were used to create intimate care activities. Discussing matters of the body was not easy as the body is considered sacred and private in their cultural context. To break down the barrier, two nursing students were paired together and six groups were created. Deliberations on the diverse issues of age, gender, nakedness and touch were discussed. They were supported in finding *humor* and being appreciative of their cultural values.

After the discussions learning to negotiate physical space and touch content was presented. The main ethical principles were used to assist nursing students in preparing the patient for intimate care and touch. **Table 3** provides a guide for intimate care and touch planning.

Participants engaged in intimate care humanistic simulation in a skills laboratory where the cultural discourses on the human body were discussed.

Humanistic care simulations were conducted using silicone masks in the skills laboratory. Based on the findings in phase 2, the nursing students viewed the body as sacred. Seeing and touching the naked body of an elderly person was not an easy task to *fulfill*. Therefore, the activities focused on African elderly male and female patients. **Figure 5** offers visualization into intimate care humanistic simulation.

NB: the two procedures were conducted as the initial stage of establishing intimate care and touch for elderly patients. It offered nursing students an opportunity to apply the ethical principles in **Table 3**.

After the sessions, debriefing sessions were conducted in small groups of six. They had to discuss their experiences during intimate care and touch sessions. In each group, the masked patient revealed him/herself and shared the experience of being touched. Also, the nurse providing care had to share the experience of touching the

Ethical principles	Intimate care and touch discussion with the patient
1. Autonomy	• Tell me how you are going to touch me
2. Informed consent	• Ask permission to touch
3. Beneficence	• Benefits of intimate care and touch
4. Non-maleficence	• give me preferences before touching respect and dignity of the exposed body
5. Privacy, confidentiality	• Physical privacy (screening, avoiding unnecessary exposure of body)Emotional privacy (gender preferences)
6. Justice	• Equal treatment for all patients regardless of gender, age or cultural affiliations

Table 3.
Intimate care and touch interaction with the patient.

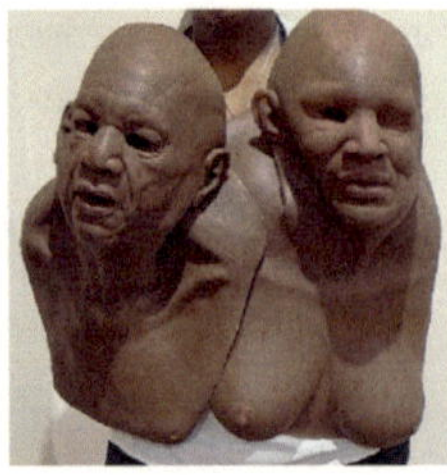	The two humanistic silicone masks (elderly male and female) were used to communicate intimate care with the elderly. Participants had to learn to talk to the elderly patients about the care they would provide, and the patient was able to respond. As cross-gender boundaries were emphasised, the nursing student had to enter into the experience of the "other" to understand the meaning of the touched body.
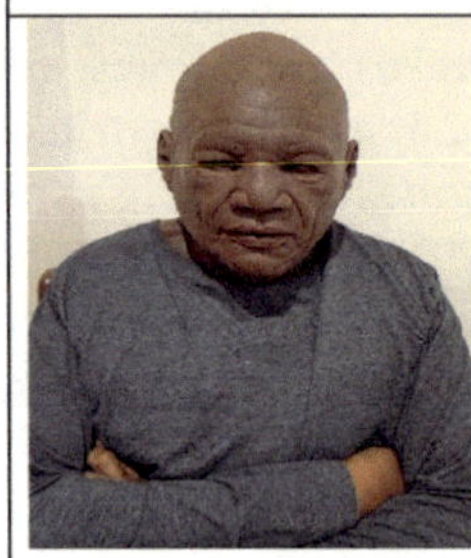 *Humanistic silicone: elderly man*	One female participant was transformed into an elderly male. The rest of the group did not know that the patient was one of their own. The simulated presence of an elder allowed nursing students to portray their cultural respect and discuss the challenges of touching the naked body of an elderly man (especially the female participants). Physical examination of the upper parts of the body was conducted using the principles indicated in Table 2.
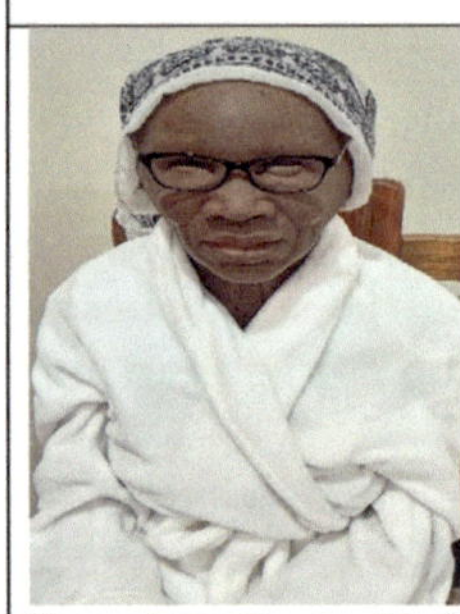 *Humanistic silicone: elderly woman*	A male nursing student was in the role of a female elderly woman. A breast examination procedure was conducted on the female elderly patient.

Figure 5.
Humanistic intimate care simulation for elderly patients.

"other". **Figure 6** provides the debriefing moments of post-intimate care and touch discussions and affirmation that they are not alone on the journey.

Humanistic aspects of caring might be neglected due to time limitations during clinical placement, shortage of competent nursing practitioners, heavy workload, and use of technology. Intimate care simulation using Mask-Ed™ allowed nursing students to authentically experience the shocking factor of caring for a naked elderly woman [28]. This indicates the importance of humanistic simulation in preparing nursing students for affective skills.

2.1.4 Phase 4: linking scientific understanding to social action

The research findings are presented to reflect the participants' understanding of intimate care and touch in their context. This section discusses the findings from

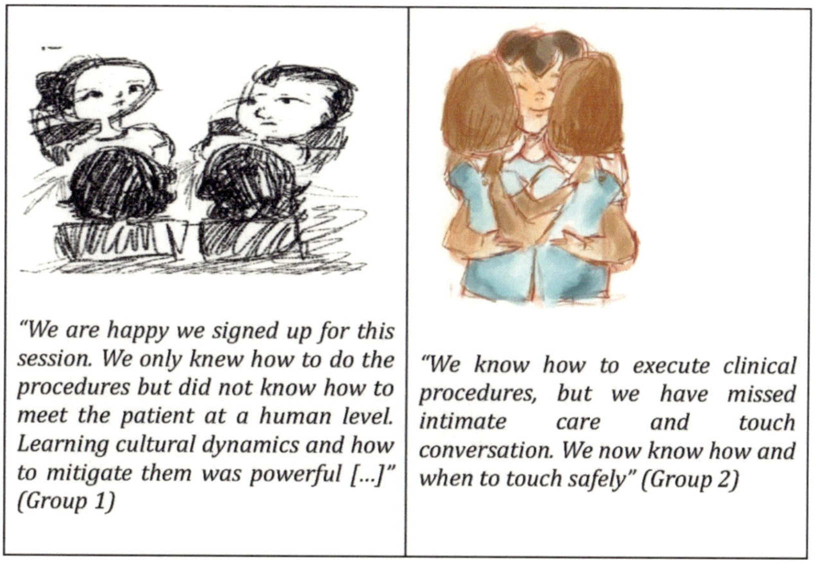
"We are happy we signed up for this session. We only knew how to do the procedures but did not know how to meet the patient at a human level. Learning cultural dynamics and how to mitigate them was powerful [...]" (Group 1)
"We know how to execute clinical procedures, but we have missed intimate care and touch conversation. We now know how and when to touch safely" (Group 2)

Figure 6.
Debriefing sessions post intimate care and touch sessions.

two phases of the activities (phase 2 – incorporation of local knowledge and phase 3 – emergent process).

2.1.4.1 Part 1: discussion of phase 2 – Incorporation of local knowledge

The participants viewed the body as a sacred entity that needs to be respected with its boundaries.

Nursing Education Transforming Lives: South Africa's democracy draws from its humble begins from apartheid where most black African students were excluded from higher education. After the democratic government election in 1994, the goal of access to higher education was set to achieve equity [29]. Therefore, Section 29 of the Constitution promises the right to quality education for all, expanding access and inclusion in higher education. Nursing education is regulated by the South African Nursing Council and Council of Higher Education. Acceptance to accredited NEI was the first entry to higher education for all the participants.

Learning Nursing Care: The nursing curriculum includes both theory and clinical learning. Clinical competency is the ability to effectively integrate cognitive, affective and psychomotor skills when delivering nursing care [30]. The simulation laboratories should function as a replicate of a real hospital for the nursing students to practice humanistic care. Many NEIs use technology-enhanced simulated learning such as videos to develop psychomotor clinical skills that are critical for patient care and challenging to teach students [31]. Unfortunately, the affective skills are not enhanced during this teaching strategy. As indicated earlier, intimate care requires a nurse to touch the body of the patient, if it is not facilitated in NEI, the student becomes exposed to the human body during clinical placement. A vast literature from humanistic care scholars such as [9, 28, 32, 33] has indicated that intimate care and touch are not facilitated in skills laboratories and nursing students learn it from trial and error and from other students. Since registered nurses are not knowledgeable about the supervision of intimate care, therefore, intimate care empowerment and support during clinical placement are lacking.

Respect for the human body: The body is a medium of culture, it is a social production of the self [34] which needs to be respected. Culture is a complex whole which includes knowledge, belief, art, custom and any other capabilities and habits acquired by an individual as a member of a society [24]. Body image refers to personal constructions and public projections of the human body involving perceptions, physical sensations and innated expected culture of the body [35]. Respect is often linked to the dignity of a person. The Constitution of the Republic of South Africa, Act 108 of 1996, in Section 9 outlines the fundamental human rights of human dignity, the achievement of equality and the advancement of human rights and freedom. Further Section 10 indicates that "everyone has inherent dignity and the dignity to have their dignity respected and protected". Dignity is about acknowledging the innate value in every individual, especially when they are feeling vulnerable and dependent on others for aspects of their care [36]. The authors [36] emphasize that treating someone with dignity is to treat them as being worthy, in a way that respects them as valued individuals within society.

Cultural boundaries in accessing the body: Gender and gender-defined roles are socially constructed with the opportunity to change and transform. Gender refers to the roles and responsibilities as well as opportunities that stem from the biological fact of being male or female [37]. Tamale [38] gives reasons for the boundaries in the nakedness of elderly women and mothers is symbolic in most African cultures and is considered the ultimate curse. The reason is that through pregnancy, childbirth and nurturing, women are givers of life, by stripping naked in front of men old enough to be her children or grandchildren, a mother is symbolically taking back the life that she has given, pronouncing social death. Unfortunately, in the nursing profession, young nursing students are exposed to the bodies of elderly people which may be a taboo for them as they cross the cultural norms. Therefore, the nursing curriculum should prepare students to be sensitive to patients' identity, culture, religion, age, gender and sexual orientation [39].

Importance of intimate care in nursing: Nursing students understood intimate care as physical care requiring touch and touch-oriented basic nursing care. In their intimate care facilitation model [8], intimate care involves physical or psychological closeness between a nurse and a patient. During this proximity, the nurse encounters a patient's body, and the patient must allow a nurse to touch their body. Therefore, during intimate care, the fragile body of the patient is seen and touched. It is in this view that technology should not be a barrier in humanistic care, not diminish the interaction between the nurse and the person in need of care [1].

Not ready for the "Other": During intimate care provision, the nurses touch the patients. Nurses use their hands to examine patients' bodies, bathe them and give physical comfort which may trigger feelings of fear and discomfort [40]. Intimate care procedures such as hygiene, elimination and pressure parts care may be considered simple, but have a psychological impact on those providing and receiving such care [10]. Readiness for intimate care is founded on clinical teaching and support.

Left in the dark – met with death: Death shocks everyone, whether young or old. In nursing life and death are often part of daily routine. Death after all healthcare professionals throughout their careers. There is no getting used to it. Nursing students do not feel ready to confront issues regarding death and dying, they are poorly prepared and vulnerable when providing care to dying patients [41]. In the study of [42] nursing students had terrible dreams of death, were shocked by the first death they encountered and were left insecure emotionally and physiologically. Therefore,

DOI: http://dx.doi.org/10.5772/intechopen.1004258

nursing students should be prepared for death and dying. Debriefing sessions should be conducted with nursing students to assist them in dealing with their experiences of encountering death.

2.1.4.2 Part 2: discussion of phase 2: emergent process

Teaching humanistic care is critical in creating a respectful environment for nursing students and patients. Technology will undoubtedly shape the future nursing profession but should not replace astute knowledge and humanistic nurse-patient interaction [43]. Humanistic care is characterized by empathy, respect for human dignity, patient autonomy, a friendly environment, and holistic care [44]. Humanization is intended to improve the healthcare delivered to the patients and contributes to understanding human beings in their own unique sense of dignity and identity [45]. In Mainey et al. [28] after participating in intimate care facilitating, there was a shift from fear of engaging in intimate touch to completing nursing tasks leading nursing students to experience patient-centered care. To provide intimate care and touch, the nursing student must be prepared to interact with a diverse patient. Importantly, the nurse and patient need to establish a therapeutic relationship based on respect, trust, and dignity [33]. The authors [33] further state the importance of including intimate care in the nursing curriculum as it will empower nursing students to provide intimate care to diverse patients competently, comfortably, and confidently.

3. Conclusions

This chapter presented the PAR grounded in symbolic interactionism theory. The meanings of the body were deliberated with their limitations. The nursing students' participation assisted in creating contextual intimate care activities linked to ethical principles of autonomy, informed consent, beneficence, non-maleficence, confidentiality, and justice. Even though NEIs in South Africa have moved to online teaching and learning following the COVID-19 trends, the patient's body still needs a human touch and interactions. Thus, technology should not replace the nurse. Therefore, the facilitation of intimate care and touch is at the centre of humanistic care. Through the findings, the nursing students indicate their competency in executing clinical procedures but fail to prepare themselves and the patients for intimate care and touch encounters. One cannot overemphasize the importance of establishing a nurse-patient relationship that is respectful and dignified during nursing care interactions. When nursing students are well prepared for diversities in patient care, and understand their cultural backgrounds, it is possible to provide intimate care in a collaborative manner, where there are no power struggles. It becomes important for the human body to be treated with respect and dignity for positive clinical outcomes. Unfortunately, intimate care and touch require time and dedication, and with the shortage of nurses, nursing students may continue struggling with humanistic care. Therefore, nurse educators and clinical preceptors should be vigilant and supportive in creating safe spaces for intimate care and touch activities.

Acknowledgements

I am grateful to UNISA for granting me time to focus on the intimate care project and NRF for the grant which made it easy to fulfill the objectives of the study (South African National Research Foundation Thuthuka Grant Reference: TTK210318590345). Thankful to all stakeholders who permitted to conduct the study in their institutions and all participants who dedicated their valuable time.

Conflict of interest

The author declares no conflict of interest.

Author details

Simangele Shakwane
University of South Africa, Pretoria North, South Africa

*Address all correspondence to: shakws@unisa.ac.za

References

[1] Locsin R. The co-existence of technology and caring in the theory of technological competency as caring in nursing. The Journal of Medical Investigation. 2017;**64**:160-164

[2] Taghinezhad F, Mohammadi E, Khademi M, Kazemnejad A. Humanistic care in nursing: Concept analysis using Rodgers' evolutionary approach. Iranian Journal of Nursing and Midwifery Research. 2022;**27**(2):83-91

[3] Khademi M, Mohammadi E, Vanaki Z. A grounded theory of humanistic nursing in acute care work environments. Nursing Ethics. 2017;**24**(8):908-921

[4] Lecocq D, Delmas P, Antonini M, Lefebvre H, Laloux M, Beghuin A, et al. Comparing feeling of competence regarding humanistic caring in Belgian nurses and nursing students: A comparative cross-sectional study conducted in a French Belgian teaching hospital. Nursing Open. 2020;**8**(1):104-114

[5] Zhu Y, Liu G, Shen Y, Wang J, Lu M, Wang J. Humanistic nursing care for patients in low-resourced clinical settings from students' perspectives: A participatory qualitative study. International Journal of Environmental Research and Public Health. 2022;**19**(19): 1-10

[6] Latimer J, López GD. Intimate entanglements: Affects, more-than-human intimacies and the politics of relations in science and technology. The Sociological Review. 2016;**67**:247-263

[7] O'Keefe-McCarthy S. Technologically-mediated nursing care: The impact on moral agency. Nursing Ethics. 2009;**16**(6):786-796

[8] Shakwane S, Mokoboto-Zwane S. Demystifying sexual connotations: A model for facilitating the teaching of intimate care to nursing students in South Africa. African Journal of Health Professions Education. 2020;**12**(3):103

[9] O'Lynn CO, Krautscheid L. "How Should I Touch you?": A Qualitative Study of Attitudes on Intimate Touch in Nursing Care. Faculty Publications-School of Nursing. American Journal of Nursing. 2011;**111**(3):1-8. Available from: https://digitalcommons.georgefox.edu/sn_fac

[10] Thompson GN, McClement SE, Peters S, Hack TF, Chochinov H, Funk L. More than just a task: Intimate care delivery in the nursing home. International Journal of Qualitative Studies on Health and Well-being. 2021;**16**(1):1-10

[11] Lehoux P, Saint-Arnaud J, Richard L. The use of technology at home: What patient manuals say and sell vs. what patients face and fear. Sociology of Health and Illness. 2004;**26**(5):617-644

[12] Yadav D, Balaam M, Lampinen A. Invisibility or visibility in intimate care at the workplace? Examining the use of breast pumps. In: Proceedings of the 2023 CHI Conference on Human Factors in Computing Systems (CHI '23), Hamburg, Germany. New York, NY, USA: ACM; 23-28 April 2023. p. 15. DOI: 10.1145/3544548.3581411

[13] Carter MJ, Fuller C. Symbolic Interactionism. Sociopedia.isa; 2015. pp. 1-16. DOI: 10.1177/205684601561

[14] Rehman T. Phenomenology, symbolic interactionism and research: From Hegel to Dreyfus. Science & Philosophy. 2019;**6**(2):197-209

[15] Husin SS, Ab Rahman AA, Mukhtar D. The symbolic interactionism theory: A systematic literature review of current research. International Journal of Modern Trends in Social Sciences. 2021;**4**(17):113-126

[16] Carter MJ, Fuller C. Symbols, meaning, and action: The past, present, and future of symbolic interactionism. Current Sociology. 2016;**64**(6):931-961

[17] Wulf C. Education as transcultural education: A global challenge. Educational Studies in Japan: International Yearbook. 2010;**5**:33-47

[18] Liamputtong P. Qualitative Research Methods. 4th ed. New Zealand: Oxford University Press; 2013

[19] Baum F, MacDougall C, Smith D. Participatory action research. Journal of Epidemiology and Community Health. 2006;**60**(10):854-857

[20] Greenwood DJ, Whyte WF, Harkavy I. Participatory action research as a process and as a goal. Human Relations. 1993;**46**(2):175-192

[21] Dearden A, Rizvi H. Participatory design and participatory development: A comparative review participatory IT design and participatory development: A comparative review [Internet]. Available from: http://shura.shu.ac.uk/29/

[22] Creswell JW, Creswell JD. Research Design: Qualitative, Quantitative, and Mixed Methods Approaches. 5th ed. Singapore: SAGE; 2018

[23] Idang GE. African culture and values. Phronimon. 2015;**16**(2):97-111

[24] Awoniyi S. African cultural values: The past, present and future. Journal of Sustainable Development in Africa. 2015;**17**(1):1-13

[25] Akpa-Inyang F, Chima SC. South African traditional values and beliefs regarding informed consent and limitations of the principle of respect for autonomy in African communities: A cross-cultural qualitative study. BMC Medical Ethics. 2021;**22**(1):1-17

[26] Kpanake L. Cultural concepts of the person and mental health in Africa. Transcultural Psychiatry. 2018;**55**(2):198-218

[27] Harding T, North N, Perkins R. Sexualizing men's touch: Male nurses and the use of intimate touch in clinical practice. Research and Theory for Nursing Practice. 2018;**22**(2):88-102

[28] Mainey L, Dwyer T, Reid-Searl K, Bassett J. High-level realism in simulation: A catalyst for providing intimate care. Clinical Simulation in Nursing. 2018;**17**:47-57

[29] Boughey C. From equity to efficiency: Access to higher education in South Africa. Arts & Humanities in Higher Education. 2003;**2**(1):65-71

[30] Hakimzadeh R, Ghodrati A, Karamdost N, Ghodrati H, Mirmosavie J. Assessing nursing students' clinical competency: Self-assessment. Quarterly Journal of Nursing Vision. 2012;**1**(1):17-25. Available from: WorldConferences.net

[31] Forbes H, Oprescu FI, Downer T, Phillips NM, McTier L, Lord B, et al. Use of videos to support teaching and learning of clinical skills in nursing education: A review. Nurse Education Today. 2016;**42**:53-56

[32] Shakwane S. Journey less travelled: Female nursing students' experiences in providing intimate care in two nursing education institutions in Gauteng

province, South Africa. Health SA Gesondheid. 2022;**27**:1-8

[33] Shakwane S, Mokoboto-Zwane S. Promoting intimate care facilitation in nursing education institutions in South Africa. International Journal of Africa Nursing Sciences. 2020;**13**:1-7

[34] Almeida T, Comber R, Balaam M. HCI and intimate care as an agenda for change in women's health. In: Conference on Human Factors in Computing Systems - Proceedings. USA: Association for Computing Machinery; 2016. pp. 2599-2611

[35] Oloruntoba T, Nigeria O. Understanding Human Sexuality Seminar Series Body Images, Beauty Culture and Language in the Nigeria, African Context. Nigeria: Africa Regional Sexuality Resource Centre; 2007

[36] Roberts GW, Machon A. Appreciative healthcare practice: A guide to compassionate, person-centred care. Nursing Management. 2016;**22**(9):15

[37] Prosen M. Nursing students' perception of gender-defined roles in nursing: A qualitative descriptive study. BMC Nursing. 2022;**21**(1):1-11

[38] Tamale S. Nudity, protest and the law in Uganda. Feminist Africa. 2019;**22**: 52-85

[39] Li P, Burgess Dowdell E, Speck PM. Recognition of trauma informed care responses in forensic nurses. Journal of the Academy of Forensic Nursing-JAFN. 2023;**1**(2):1-18

[40] Kelly MA, Nixon L, McClurg C, Scherpbier A, King N, Dornan T. Experience of touch in health care: A meta-ethnography across the health care professions. Qualitative Health Research. 2017;**28**(2):200-212

[41] Gorchs-Font N, Ramon-Aribau A, Yildirim M, Kroll T, Larkin PJ, Subirana-Casacuberta M. Nursing students' first experience of death: Identifying mechanisms for practice learning. A realist review. Nurse Education Today. 2020;**96**:1-16

[42] Park HS, Jee Y, Kim SH, YJI K. Nursing students' first clinical experiences of death. The Korean Journal of Hospice and Palliative Care. 2014;**17**(3):161-169

[43] Meissen H, Gong MN, Wong AKI, Zimmerman JJ, Nadkarni N, Kane-Gil SL, et al. The future of critical care: Optimizing technologies and a learning healthcare system to potentiate a more humanistic approach to critical care. Critical Care Explorations. 2022;**4**(3):1-9

[44] Zamaniniya Z, Khademi M, Toulabi T, Zarea K. The outcomes of humanistic nursing for critical care nurses: A qualitative study. Nursing and Midwifery Studies. 2021;**10**(2):114-120

[45] Mohamadi Asl S, Khademi M, Mohammadi E. The influential factors in humanistic critical care nursing. Nursing Ethics. 2022;**29**(3):608-620